THE YEAR IN
HYPERTENSION

THE YEAR IN HYPERTENSION

2000

H. L. ELLIOTT, J. M. C. CONNELL
and
G. T. McINNES

Department of Medicine and Therapeutics, University of Glasgow
Gardiner Institute, Western Infirmary, Glasgow

CLINICAL PUBLISHING SERVICES

OXFORD

Clinical Publishing Services Ltd

Oxford Centre for Innovation
Mill Street, Oxford OX2 0JX, UK

Tel: +44 1865 811116
Fax: +44 1865 251550
Web: www.clinicalpublishing.co.uk

Distributed by:

Radcliffe Medical Press
18 Marcham Road
Abingdon
Oxon OX14 1AA UK

Tel: +44 1235 528820
Fax: +44 1235 528830
e mail: orders@radcliffemed.com

A catalogue record for this book is available from the British Library
ISBN 0 9537339 0 4

The publisher makes no representation, express or implied, that the dosages in this book are correct. Readers must therefore always check the product information and clinical procedures with the most up-to-date published product information and data sheets provided by the manufacturers and the most recent codes of conduct and safety regulations. The authors and the publisher do not accept any liability for any errors in the text or for the misuse or misapplication of material in this work.

Typeset by Footnote Graphics, Warminster, Wiltshire
Printed by in Spain by
T G Hostench SA, Barcelona.

Contents

Part IV

Current issues in practice

Foreword

Michael A. Weber, MD

It is incongruous that despite all the ongoing developments in such basic sciences as vascular biology and genetics, the major focus of hypertension in 2000 appears to be blood pressure itself. Certainly for hypertensive patients with concomitant conditions like diabetes mellitus and renal insufficiency, lower is better as far as blood pressure is concerned. Supported by convincing clinical trial data, current treatment guidelines have reduced blood pressure targets for such patients to 130/85 mmHg or even 125/80 mmHg, rather than the traditional 140/90 mmHg. Of note is the fact that the systolic blood pressure has now eclipsed the diastolic as the primary guide to diagnosis and treatment, particularly in patients aged over 60. Pulse pressure, which is the difference between systolic and diastolic values, and may be a helpful index of arterial stiffness and disease in older patients, may turn out to be the single best predictor of cardiovascular events. Sadly, our performance as clinicians has not kept pace with this new understanding: worldwide, less than one-quarter of hypertensive people have blood pressures reduced below 140/90 mmHg, let alone the more aggressive targets that may be required. We have yet to learn why practitioners often fail to adjust treatment even when they recognize inadequate blood pressure responses and have effective and affordable remedies at hand.

Evidence for the role of the renin–angiotensin system in mediating the clinical endpoints of hypertension continues to mount. Much of the attention has focused on diabetic hypertensives whose high event rates make them appropriate candidates for clinical trials. Several of these studies now appear to confirm that the angiotensin-converting enzyme (ACE) inhibitors are especially beneficial in cardiovascular and renal protection, though effective blood pressure reduction is still required for optimal results. Even so, it is now evident that ACE inhibitors significantly decrease event rates in patients at high risk of vascular outcomes, regardless of whether these individuals are hypertensive. Not surprisingly, several major outcome trials with angiotensin receptor antagonists, which might be more selective blockers of the renin–angiotensin system than ACE inhibitors, are now under way in high-risk hypertensive patients. Such studies, though, are not helpful in monitoring progress in single patients, and so there is growing interest in surrogate measures of vascular changes. Simplified testing of endothelial function and, perhaps more practical, non-invasive measurements of arterial compliance, are two such approaches. More immediately, inexpensive methods that detect microalbuminuria, which is now recognized as a highly sensitive predictor of coronary events, are becoming part of routine clinical practice.

The Year in Hypertension 2000 provides a thoughtful and detailed account of these and other exciting developments in the field of hypertension.

Luis M. Ruilope, MD

Arterial hypertension is a highly prevalent disease that greatly contributes to the main cause of death in the Western world. I feel greatly honoured to have been invited to write this foreword to a book born at the Western Infirmary in Glasgow. Since the moment I decided to dedicate most of my time to the study of arterial hypertension, my knowledge has always been supplemented with information from this centre.

This book provides an overview of the current literature in hypertension, identifying the papers published in the past eighteen months that have potentially changed practice, or that lay the groundwork for future research. The work of compiling all this information has been done by an expert team, and the book covers most if not all the multidisciplinary aspects of arterial hypertension. What makes the reading of the book easy and practical is not only the expertise of the authors, but also the fact that because they work together in one of the leading centres in the field, there is a continuity throughout.

I am sure that any person interested in hypertension will profit from the reading of this book and will find ways to improve his/her daily clinical practice.

Part I

Clinical trials and guidelines

1

Recent trial results

Introduction

In epidemiological studies, there is a close relationship between blood pressure (systolic and diastolic) and the risk of stroke, coronary heart disease and other cardiovascular events [1]. The higher the blood pressure, the greater the risk. This relationship is consistent in different populations, in younger and older subjects, in men and women, and is independent of other cardiovascular risk factors. The relationship is continuous across the range of blood pressure, indicating that there is no lower threshold or safe level of blood pressure. The slope of the relationship between blood pressure and stroke is about 50% steeper than that between blood pressure and coronary heart disease. However, many more coronary events are experienced in Western populations, although strokes are the predominant events in individuals from South-East Asia.

Over the past four decades, numerous studies have examined the influence of drug treatment of hypertension on the risk of cardiovascular events [2]. The usual aim was to achieve a diastolic blood pressure less than 90 mmHg. The average reduction in diastolic blood pressure of 5–6 mmHg in these trials conferred a reduction of about 38% in stroke incidence, a 16% reduction in coronary heart disease events, a 21% reduction in all vascular events and a 12% reduction in all-cause mortality, all highly significant. Effects on fatal and non-fatal events were similar. The proportional reductions were the same in high- and low-risk individuals, in the young and the elderly, and in mild, moderate and severe hypertension.

The average time to events was 2–3 years. Epidemiological data suggest that a difference in usual blood pressure of the magnitude seen in the trials in the long term would result in a reduction in stroke incidence of 35–40% and of 20–25% for coronary heart disease events. Thus only a few years' treatment attains much or all of the long-term potential benefits. Since most of the trials used diuretics, with no known benefits beyond blood pressure reduction, it is unlikely that the results could be explained by anything other than change in blood pressure.

Benefits are likely to be greater with larger reductions in blood pressure. Epidemiological data indicate no lower threshold for risk, and observational findings suggest that patients with the lowest on-treatment blood pressure have the best prognosis [3].

The evidence base for the treatment of hypertension is among the strongest in medicine. The results of 18 unconfounded prospective trials in over 50 000 subjects attest to the benefits of antihypertensive drug therapy. However, several unanswered questions remain.

- What is the optimal target blood pressure during therapy?
- Does anti-platelet therapy confer benefits in treated hypertensives?
- Do newer agents have advantages over the older drugs used in the trials?
- Does the benefit of treatment extend to older patients with predominantly systolic hypertension?

Target blood pressure

The Hypertension Optimal Treatment (HOT) study

Effects of intensive blood pressure lowering and low-dose aspirin in patients with hypertension: principal results of the Hypertension Optimal Treatment (HOT) randomized trial.

L Hansson, A Zanchetti, S G Carruthers, B Dahlöf, D Elmfeldt, S Julius, *et al.* for the HOT Study Group. *Lancet* 1998; **351**: 1755–62.

BACKGROUND. The objective was to assess the optimum target diastolic blood pressure and the potential benefit of a low dose of acetylsalicylic acid in the treatment of hypertension.

INTERPRETATION. Intensive lowering of blood pressure in patients with hypertension was associated with a low rate of cardiovascular events. Acetylsalicylic acid significantly reduced major cardiovascular events, with the greatest benefit seen in all myocardial infarction. There was no effect on fatal bleeds, but non-fatal major bleeds were twice as common.

The Hypertension Optimal Treatment (HOT) Study. Patient characteristics: randomization, risk profiles, and early blood pressure results.

L Hansson, A Zanchetti. *Blood Press* 1994; **3**: 322–7.

BACKGROUND. Inclusion of patients in the HOT study was completed on 30 April, 1994. At that time 19 196 patients had been randomized.

INTERPRETATION. The average reduction in diastolic blood pressure after 3 months was 87 ± 7 mmHg in the ≤ 90 mmHg group, 85 ± 8 mmHg in the ≤ 85 mmHg group, and 83 ± 8 mmHg in the ≤ 80 mmHg group. After 6 months the corresponding values were 86 ± 7 mmHg in the ≤ 90 mmHg group, 84 ± 7 mmHg in the ≤ 85 mmHg group, and 82 ± 7 mmHg in the ≤ 80 mmHg group. These preliminary data indicated that it would be possible to fulfil the primary aims of the HOT study.

Comment

The principal objective of the HOT study was to determine the optimal target blood pressure for cardiovascular protection.

Nearly 19 000 patients aged 50–80 years (mean 61.5 years) with diastolic blood pressure 100–115 mmHg (mean 105 mmHg) were randomized to target diastolic blood pressure $\leq$ 90 mmHg, $\leq$ 85 mmHg or $\leq$ 80 mmHg. The design was a Prospective, Randomized, Open, Blinded Endpoint (PROBE) evaluation. Antihypertensive treatment was based on felodipine, and follow-up averaged 3.8 years. At study conclusion, 78% of patients were taking felodipine, 41% angiotensin-converting enzyme (ACE) inhibitor, 38% beta-blocker and 22% diuretic. Mean achieved diastolic blood pressures in the groups were 85.2 mmHg, 83.2 mmHg and 81.1 mmHg, respectively (Fig. 1.1); corresponding systolic blood pressure levels were 143.7 mmHg, 141.4 mmHg and 139.7 mmHg. The diastolic blood pressures associated with the lowest risk of cardiovascular events and cardiovascular mortality were 82.6 mmHg and 86.5 mmHg, respectively. For achieved systolic blood pressure, the lowest points of risk were at 138.5 mmHg and 138.8 mmHg (Fig. 1.2). Risk was not increased significantly at lower levels.

In the subset of 1501 patients with diabetes mellitus, there was a significant 51% reduction in major cardiovascular events in the target diastolic blood pressure $\leq$ 80 mmHg group compared with that in the target $\leq$ 90 mmHg group; reductions of approximately 50% in myocardial infarction and 30% in stroke were not signifi-

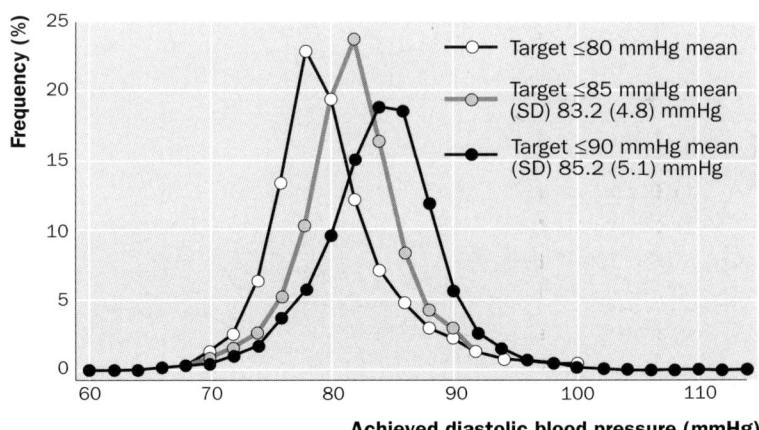

Fig. 1.1 Distribution of mean diastolic blood pressure from 6 months' follow-up to end of HOT study. SD = standard deviation.

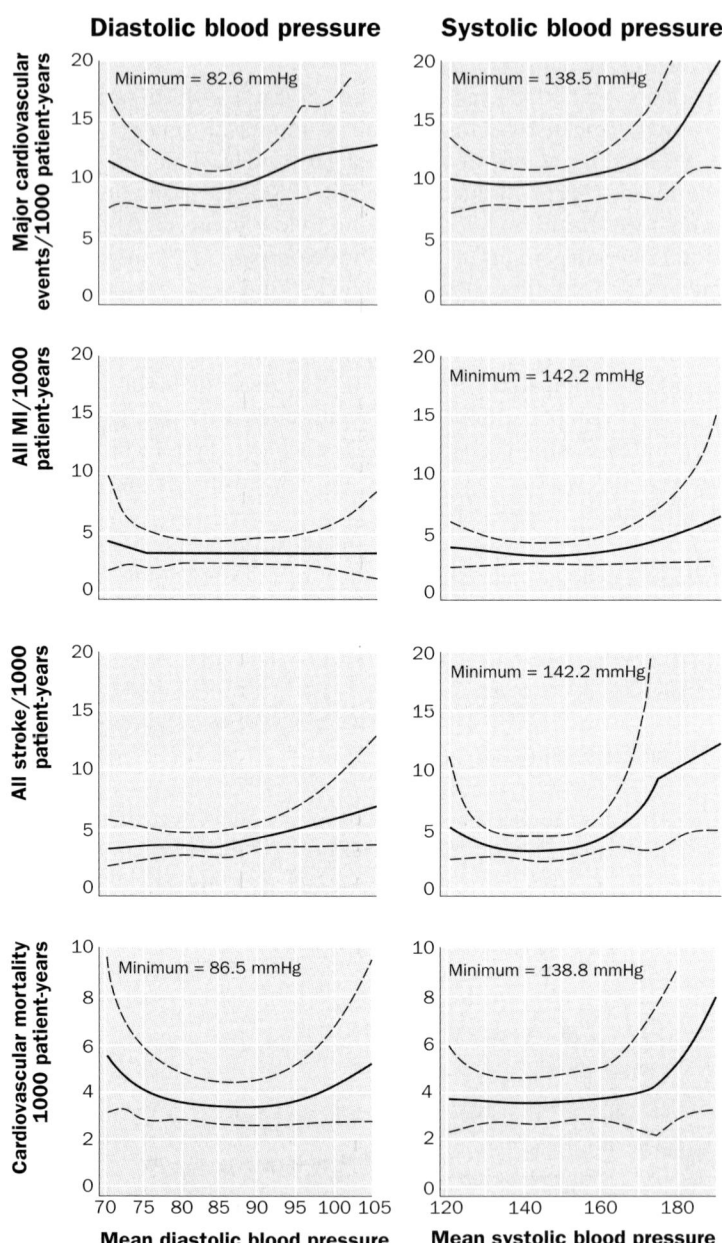

Fig. 1.2 Estimated incidence (95% confidence interval) of cardiovascular events in relation to achieved mean diastolic and systolic blood pressure in HOT study. Minimum = blood pressure at lowest point of curve; MI = myocardial infarction.

cant. However, the difference in achieved blood pressure was much less than planned. Cardiovascular mortality was reduced by two-thirds ($P=0.016$) and total mortality by three-quarters ($P=0.068$) by lowering diastolic blood pressure from 85.2 to 81.1 mmHg. In 3080 patients with ischaemic heart disease at baseline, major cardiovascular events and strokes were reduced with declining target blood pressure.

The small differences in blood pressure reduction between the three target groups made it difficult to detect differences in event rates. Furthermore, the number of events was fewer than that expected—only 724 rather than the 1100 anticipated. Thus the power of the study was less than that expected.

Nevertheless, the findings suggest that from 5 to 10 cardiovascular events can be prevented for every 1000 patients treated for 1 year by lowering blood pressure from the highest value present before randomization to the minimum blood pressure. Most of the benefit is achieved by lowering systolic blood pressure to about 140 mmHg and diastolic blood pressure to about 90 mmHg, with only a small further benefit to be gained by reducing blood pressure further.

The HOT study provided the first prospective evidence to support 'normalization' of blood pressure in patients with hypertension and diabetes even in the absence of nephropathy. In non-diabetic hypertensives, lowering blood pressure below minimum values was not harmful. There was no evidence of increased risk for any cardiovascular endpoints down to 70 mmHg diastolic and 120 mmHg systolic. Notably, this was true in the subgroup of patients with a history of ischaemic heart disease, a group which has been postulated to be at particular risk in conditions of low pressure [4]. A small, non-significant increase in all-cause mortality with declining blood pressure may be explained by the hypotensive effect of poor health rather than by treatment.

The cardiovascular event rate in the HOT study was surprisingly low—much lower than in actively treated patients in other studies [2] and in general control populations of similar age [3]. The low event rate may reflect the overall highly effective blood pressure control in the HOT study, the use of modern antihypertensive agents or the reluctance of investigators to enrol truly high-risk, particularly elderly, patients in clinical trials.

Blood pressure control

The HOT study demonstrated that diastolic blood pressure could be reduced to ≤ 90 mmHg in approximately 90% of patients and to ≤ 80 mmHg in nearly 60% of patients with mild to moderate hypertension treated with standard stepped-care drugs in general practice (Fig. 1.3). Compared with blood pressure at randomization, average diastolic blood pressure was reduced by 20.3 mmHg, 22.3 mmHg and 24.3 mmHg and systolic blood pressure by 26.2 mmHg, 28.0 mmHg and 29.9 mmHg in the target groups ≤ 90 mmHg, ≤ 85 mmHg and ≤ 80 mmHg, respectively. Only 12% (≤ 90 mmHg group), 7% (≤ 85 mmHg) and 6% (≤ 80 mmHg) had a diastolic blood pressure > 90 mmHg at the end of the study.

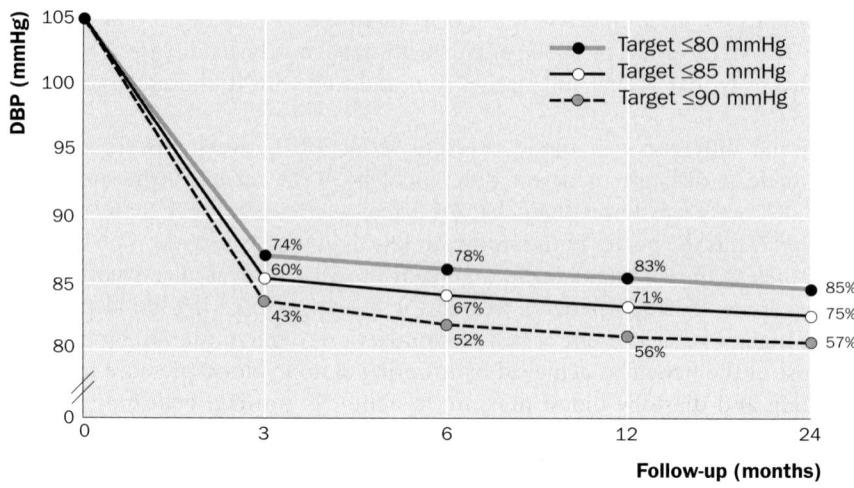

Fig. 1.3 Diastolic blood pressure (DBP) and percentage of patients on target during follow-up in HOT study.

Table 1.1 HOT study: drug treatment on completion

		Diastolic blood pressure target group		
		≤ 90 mmHg	≤ 85 mmHg	≤ 80 mmHg
Felodipine	(%)	77	78	79
ACE inhibitor	(%)	35	42	45
Beta-blocker	(%)	29	28	32
Diuretic	(%)	19	22	24

Even in these selected patients following a carefully predetermined protocol in a clinical trial, <50% were controlled adequately by monotherapy. About 10% of patients required three or more drugs. In the lowest target group, a large proportion of patients was taking ACE inhibitors, beta-blockers and diuretics (Table 1.1), and these drugs may have influenced the outcome of the trial.

The overall reduction in diastolic and systolic blood pressure was striking, although it must be remembered that this was in relation to baseline and not placebo control. The extent to which a placebo effect would have diminished the observed blood pressure reduction is unknown.

Tolerability of rigorous blood pressure control

The Hypertension Optimal Treatment (HOT) study: 24-month data on blood pressure and tolerability.
L Hansson, A Zanchetti for the HOT Study Group. *Blood Press* 1997; **6**: 313–7.

BACKGROUND. **This is a report on the blood pressure achieved, the tolerability and other available data after 24 months of follow-up of all patients in the HOT study.**

INTERPRETATION. On average, patients in the ≤ 90 mmHg diastolic blood pressure target group had reached 85 mmHg, in the ≤ 85 mmHg target group patients had reached 83 mmHg and in the 80 ≤ mmHg target group patients had reached 81 mmHg. The percentage of those achieving target blood pressure in each target group at 24 months of follow-up was 85% in the ≤ 90 mmHg target group, 75% in the ≤ 85 mmHg target group and 57% in the ≤ 80 mmHg target group. There had been relatively few side-effects. The 24-month data indicated that it should be possible to fulfil the primary aims of the HOT study.

Comment

There was a similar low incidence of side-effects in each of the three target blood pressure groups, suggesting that rigorous control of blood pressure can be achieved without an unacceptable burden of side-effects. With increasing dose titration steps, there was a gradual increase in the total number of side-effects, although the proportion of patients who reported side-effects decreased gradually throughout the trial from 16.9% at 3 months to 2.2% at the final visit. The main side-effects were ankle oedema and cough.

Randomized patients had a quality of life better than that of the population average at baseline, and during treatment quality of life improved in all groups |5|. The greatest improvement was in patients with the lowest target blood pressure and in those with the lowest achieved pressure, suggesting that even intensive treatment with antihypertensive drugs is not associated with impaired quality of life.

Concordance with therapy

Compliance with aspirin or placebo in the hypertension optimal treatment (HOT) study.
B Waeber, G Leonetti, R Kolloch, G T McInnes. *J Hypertens* 1999; **17**: 1041–5.

BACKGROUND. **Compliance with double-blind administration of aspirin or placebo added to antihypertensive treatment was evaluated for 1 year in a subset (n=530) of the HOT study population (n=18790) by placing the medication in a container closed with an electronic cap that recorded precisely the time of each opening.**

INTERPRETATION. Compliance rate was high (78%) and was not influenced by age, sex or country (Germany, Italy, Switzerland, UK). It was also similar irrespective of whether or not the patients had reached their target blood pressure. Therefore non-compliance cannot explain failure to achieve desired blood pressure control.

Comment

As assessed by an electronic monitoring device, about 80% of patients took the study medication as intended. Concordance was not affected by age or gender. There was no difference in concordance between those patients who achieved target blood pressure and those who did not (Fig. 1.4), strongly suggesting that patient non-compliance with therapy is unlikely to be the cause of treatment failure. Failure to achieve target blood pressure is more likely to be due to the reluctance of prescribers to intensify therapy (professional non-compliance).

Influence of anti-platelet therapy in treated hypertension

A major objective of the HOT study was to examine the influence of concomitant anti-platelet therapy on the rate of major cardiovascular events. Although acetyl-salicylic acid (aspirin) is established in secondary prevention, benefits in hypertension have not been examined because of concern about increased risk of cerebral haemorrhage.

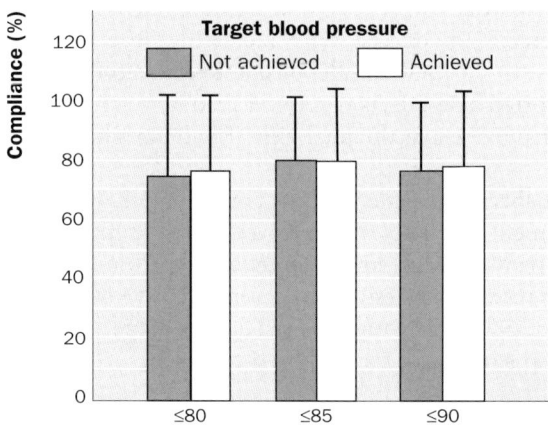

Fig. 1.4 Compliance in patients having achieved or not achieved target blood pressure during antihypertensive treatment in the HOT study. Compliance with aspirin or placebo, expressed as a percentage of days with one opening per day, inpatients having achieved their target diastolic blood pressure (group $\leq$ 80 mmHg, n=80; group $\leq$ 85 mmHg, n=126; group $\leq$ 90 mmHg, n=139) or not (group $\leq$ 80 mmHg, n=79; group $\leq$ 85 mmHg, n=54; group $\leq$ 90 mmHg, n=23) during antihypertensive treatment. Mean (vertical bars, standard deviation) results.

After allocation to blood pressure target groups, patients were randomized secondarily to additional aspirin 75 mg daily (n=9399) or placebo (n=9391). There were no differences in achieved blood pressure between patients randomized to aspirin or placebo.

The HOT study provided the first evidence for the benefit of low-dose aspirin in hypertensive patients. Aspirin was associated with a significant 15% reduction in major cardiovascular events, but rates of stroke and all-cause mortality were not altered. A particular benefit was seen for myocardial infarction (reduced 36%), but event rates were low, and many patients would need to be treated to prevent one heart attack. The relative benefit of aspirin was about the same in the groups of patients with diabetes mellitus and ischaemic heart disease as in the whole HOT population.

The prevention of 1.5 myocardial infarctions for 1000 patients treated for 1 year (2.5 per 1000 patient-years in patients with diabetes mellitus) was in addition to the benefit achieved by blood pressure reduction. This was achieved without any additional risk of stroke. Aspirin did not appear to influence the incidence of silent myocardial infarction, suggesting that the main benefit may be prevention of more severe myocardial infarction.

There was a twofold excess of non-fatal major bleeds in the aspirin group. Therefore, an overall advantage of aspirin is only likely in those with high cardiovascular risk. The absolute benefit in well-treated hypertension is less than in those with prior myocardial infarction, because of their much lower risk of myocardial infarction. An advantage of aspirin may not be seen in less well-treated patients.

Implications of the HOT study

Rigorous control of blood pressure is associated with reduced risk of cardiovascular events. Addition of low-dose aspirin further improves outcome in well-controlled hypertension, but at the expense of bleeding complications, limiting its advantage to those at high cardiovascular risk. Attainment of low blood pressure was achievable in a high proportion of patients without unacceptable side-effects and was associated with improved quality of life. Concordance with therapy was high in all groups. Therefore, failure to achieve target blood pressure cannot be attributed to side-effects or patient non-compliance.

Influence of newer antihypertensive agents

The Captopril Prevention Project (CAPPP)

Effect of angiotensin-converting enzyme inhibition compared with conventional therapy on cardiovascular morbidity and mortality in hypertension: the Captopril Prevention Project (CAPPP) randomized trial.
L Hansson, L H Lindholm, L Niskanen, J Lanke, T Hednel, A Niklasson, *et al.* for the Captopril Prevention Project (CAPPP) Study Group. *Lancet* 1999; **353**: 611–6.

BACKGROUND. **The Captopril Prevention Project (CAPPP) is a randomized intervention trial to compare the effects of ACE inhibition and conventional therapy on cardiovascular morbidity and mortality in patients with hypertension.**

INTERPRETATION. Captopril and conventional treatment did not differ in efficacy in preventing cardiovascular morbidity and mortality. The significant excess of stroke risk in captopril-treated patients was probably due to the lower levels of blood pressure attained in patients randomized to conventional therapy.

Comment

ACE inhibitors are used widely in the treatment of high blood pressure, and appear to offer benefits equal to or greater than those of conventional antihypertensive treatment for intermediate endpoints such as regression of left ventricular hypertrophy. The Captopril Prevention Project (CAPPP) was designed to compare the potential benefits on cardiovascular morbidity and mortality of a regimen based on the ACE inhibitor captopril with a conventional antihypertensive regimen of diuretics or beta-blockers.

CAPPP utilized a PROBE design. Of 10 985 eligible patients, 5492 were assigned randomly to captopril and 5493 to conventional treatment. Average age was 52.5 years (range 25–66 years) and baseline blood pressure was around 161/99 mmHg. Captopril was administered once or twice daily; beta-blockers and diuretics were given once daily. To achieve the goal diastolic blood pressure (≤ 90 mmHg), a diuretic could be added to captopril, beta-blocker and diuretic could be combined, and a calcium antagonist could be added to either group. Follow-up averaged 6.1 years.

The primary endpoint (fatal and non-fatal myocardial infarction and other cardiovascular deaths) did not differ between the treatment groups (Fig. 1.5). Cardiovascular mortality, defined as fatal stroke and myocardial infarction, sudden death and other cardiovascular deaths, was slightly lower in the captopril group,

	Relative risk* (95% CI)	P	Favours captopril	Favours conventional
Primary endpoint	1.05 (0.90–1.22)	0.52		
Fatal cardiovascular events	0.77 (0.57–1.04)	0.092		
Stroke, fatal and non-fatal	1.25 (1.01–1.55)	0.044		
Myocardial infarction, fatal and non-fatal	0.96 (0.77–1.19)	0.68		
All fatal events	0.93 (0.76–1.14)	0.49		
All cardiac events	0.94 (0.83–1.06)	0.30		
Diabetes mellitus	0.86 (0.74–0.99)	0.039		

Fig. 1.5 Relative risk during captopril versus conventional therapy in CAPPP. *Adjusted for age, sex, diabetes, systolic blood pressure and previous treatment. CI = confidence interval.

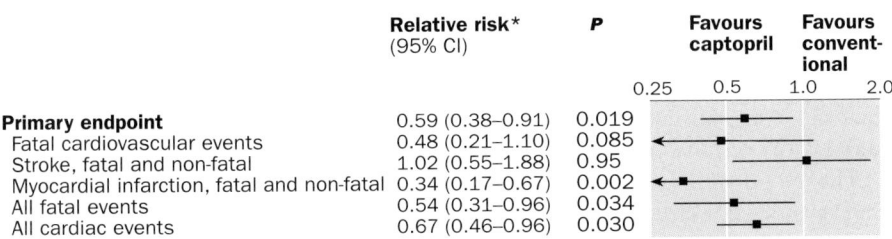

	Relative risk* (95% CI)	P	Favours captopril		Favours conventional	
			0.25	0.5	1.0	2.0
Primary endpoint	0.59 (0.38–0.91)	0.019				
Fatal cardiovascular events	0.48 (0.21–1.10)	0.085				
Stroke, fatal and non-fatal	1.02 (0.55–1.88)	0.95				
Myocardial infarction, fatal and non-fatal	0.34 (0.17–0.67)	0.002				
All fatal events	0.54 (0.31–0.96)	0.034				
All cardiac events	0.67 (0.46–0.96)	0.030				

Fig. 1.6 Relative risk during captopril versus conventional therapy in patients with diabetes at baseline (n=572) in CAPPP. *Adjusted for age, sex, systolic blood pressure and previous treatment. CI=confidence interval.

but fatal and non-fatal strokes were more common in that group. The rates of fatal and non-fatal myocardial infarction, all-cause mortality and all cardiac events were similar in the two groups. The incidence of new diabetes mellitus was significantly lower in captopril-treated patients. In subjects with diabetes mellitus at baseline (n=572), there were significant advantages for captopril with respect to the primary endpoint, all myocardial infarction, all cardiac events and all-cause mortality (Fig. 1.6).

The lower risk of stroke in the conventional treatment group might reflect differences in blood pressure between the groups. At baseline, both systolic and diastolic blood pressure were approximately 2 mmHg higher in the captopril group and remained higher throughout the study. Such a difference could account for a 15% difference in the risk of cerebrovascular events |**1**|. In diabetic patients, blood pressure was identical in the two groups and the incidence of stroke was the same. Long-term follow-up data from the Glasgow Blood Pressure Clinic suggest that the reduction in fatal stroke in patients treated with ACE inhibitors is at least as great as in patients who have never received ACE inhibitors |**6**|.

Significantly fewer patients in the captopril group developed diabetes. This is more likely to reflect the known detrimental effect of diuretic and beta-blocker therapy on carbohydrate metabolism than a beneficial effect of captopril. However, patients with diabetes at baseline did significantly better if randomized to captopril. Although an ACE inhibitor may be appropriate in a patient with diabetes, rigorous control of blood pressure is likely to be more important than the choice of drug.

Implications of CAPPP

The overall findings indicate that antihypertensive therapy based on an ACE inhibitor is no better than therapy based on diuretics and beta-blockers in prevention of cardiovascular events, and may be less effective in prevention of stroke, although ACE inhibitors may have an advantage in patients with diabetes mellitus. ACE inhibitors had been widely used in the management of hypertension for almost twenty years without outcome data. Was CAPPP worth the wait?

The use of captopril once daily in half the patients randomized to this form of therapy was illogical in view of the short duration of action of this drug. The excuse that this was routine practice among some practitioners is untenable and an example of excessive pragmatism.

The blood pressure differences between the groups cannot be explained by chance in such a large sample size, and are almost certainly related to the use of envelopes for randomization. The excess of stroke in captopril-treated patients is probably the consequence of the trial-long difference in blood pressure; statistical adjustment cannot compensate for such an effect.

The open nature of the trial makes the findings of excess diabetes in the conventionally treated group unsurprising. Clinicians expect such an effect and are likely to have looked for it. The incidence of diabetes was greater in patients allocated to captopril, strongly suggesting that investigators had a preference for use of ACE inhibitors in such patients, and providing further evidence for a failure of randomization.

The results in the diabetic subgroup are difficult to interpret in the absence of data on blood pressure and the actual drug regimens. It is unclear whether this subgroup was defined in advance and how many other subgroups were examined. Little emphasis should be placed on these findings. At present, for most hypertensive patients (including those with type II diabetes), drugs other than diuretics or beta-blockers should be selected infrequently.

The most damning comment on CAPPP comes from Sir Richard Peto |7| who considers the findings completely invalid because of the clear statistical evidence of failure of the randomization procedure. Sadly, it appears that CAPPP was not worth the wait.

Swedish Trial in Old Patients with Hypertension–2 (STOP-Hypertension–2) study

Randomized trial of old and new antihypertensive drugs in elderly patients: cardiovascular mortality and morbidity. The Swedish Trial in Old Patients with Hypertension–2 study.

L Hansson, L H Lindholm, T Ekbom, J Lanke, B Dahlöf, B Schersten, et al. Lancet 1999; **354**: 1751–6.

BACKGROUND. The STOP-Hypertension–2 study compared the effects of conventional and newer antihypertensive drugs on cardiovascular morbidity and mortality in elderly patients.

INTERPRETATION. Old and new antihypertensive drugs were similar in prevention of cardiovascular mortality or major events. Decrease in blood pressure was of major importance for the prevention of cardiovascular events.

Comment

The STOP-Hypertension–2 study was designed to compare cardiovascular morbidity and mortality during treatment with conventional drugs (diuretics, beta-blockers or both) with that during treatment with new drugs (ACE inhibitors and calcium antagonists) in older hypertensive patients. In total, 6628 subjects were enrolled. Blood pressure criteria were ≥ 180 mmHg systolic and/or ≥ 105 mmHg diastolic. Mean age was 76 years (range 70–84 years).

The study had a PROBE design. Patients were assigned randomly to treatment with conventional antihypertensive drugs (hydrochlorothiazide 25 mg plus amiloride 2.5 mg, atenolol 50 mg, metoprolol 100 mg or pindolol 5 mg daily), ACE inhibitors (enalapril 10 mg or lisinopril 10 mg daily) or calcium antagonists (felodipine 2.5 mg or isradipine 2.5 mg daily). The choice of drugs within the groups was not randomized. Target blood pressure was < 160/95 mmHg. Additional therapy to achieve target was hydrochlorothiazide plus amiloride in the beta-blocker group, beta-blocker in the diuretic or calcium antagonist group and hydrochlorothiazide 25–50 mg in the ACE inhibitor group.

Average blood pressure at randomization was 194/98 mmHg. After a mean of 5 years' treatment, blood pressure in all three groups was similar (159/81 mmHg). The decrease in blood pressure from baseline to last visit was 35/17 mmHg in the conventional drug group, 35/16 mmHg in the ACE inhibitor group and 35/18 mmHg in the calcium antagonist group. At the last visit, more than 60% of patients in each group were still taking randomized therapy and 46% of all patients were receiving more than one antihypertensive drug.

Prevention of cardiovascular deaths, the primary endpoint, was similar in all groups (Fig. 1.7). Risk of other cardiovascular events, including stroke, was also evenly distributed between the groups. There was little indication of any advantage of ACE inhibitor or calcium antagonist, even in the 719 patients who had diabetes at baseline.

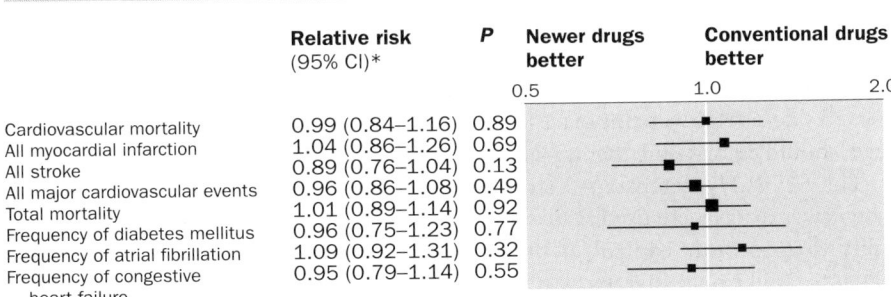

Fig. 1.7 Relative risk of cardiovascular mortality and morbidity for all newer drugs versus conventional drugs in STOP-Hypertension–2 study. *Adjusted for age, sex, diabetes, diastolic blood pressure and smoking. CI = confidence interval.

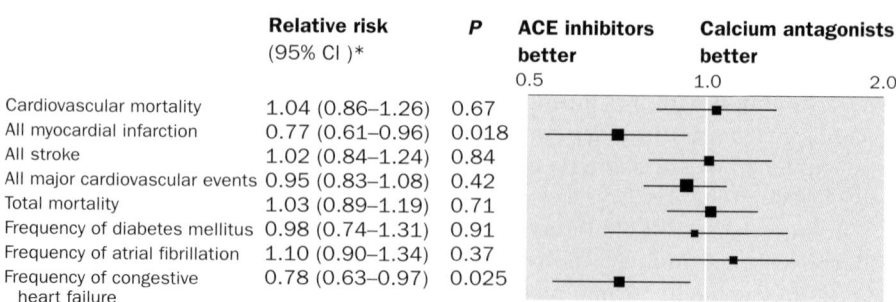

	Relative risk (95% CI)*	P	ACE inhibitors better	Calcium antagonists better
Cardiovascular mortality	1.04 (0.86–1.26)	0.67		
All myocardial infarction	0.77 (0.61–0.96)	0.018		
All stroke	1.02 (0.84–1.24)	0.84		
All major cardiovascular events	0.95 (0.83–1.08)	0.42		
Total mortality	1.03 (0.89–1.19)	0.71		
Frequency of diabetes mellitus	0.98 (0.74–1.31)	0.91		
Frequency of atrial fibrillation	1.10 (0.90–1.34)	0.37		
Frequency of congestive heart failure	0.78 (0.63–0.97)	0.025		

Fig. 1.8 Relative risk of cardiovascular mortality and morbidity for ACE inhibitors versus calcium antagonists in STOP-Hypertension–2 study. *Adjusted for age, sex, diabetes, diastolic blood pressure and smoking. CI = confidence interval.

There were significantly fewer fatal and non-fatal myocardial infarctions during treatment with ACE inhibitors compared with calcium antagonists (Fig. 1.8). Moreover, the frequency of heart failure in ACE inhibitor-treated patients was significantly lower than in those taking calcium antagonists. These results should be treated with caution, since 48 statistical comparisons were carried out, raising the possibility of spurious statistical significance. Calcium antagonists were associated with the lowest total mortality, cardiovascular mortality and stroke risks, although differences from ACE inhibitors and conventional therapy were small and not significant.

Implications of STOP-Hypertension–2

Older and newer antihypertensive drugs are equally useful in the management of elderly patients with hypertension. The hypothesis that some classes of drugs would have advantages was not substantiated. The choice of treatment must depend on concomitant disease, cost and adverse events. Adverse events were not less frequent with newer drugs. Among those randomized to conventional drugs, beta-blocker-related side-effects were more frequent. Therefore, thiazides, with their cost advantage, should be first-line therapy in elderly patients with hypertension.

The STOP-Hypertension–2 study has potential weaknesses and uncertainties. The newer drugs were used at low doses in a once-daily regimen, raising the possibility that 24-hour control of blood pressure might be less complete in these patients. Additional therapy was with older drugs, regardless of the randomized group, reducing the distinction between older and newer drugs. This is particularly relevant, since around 50% of patients required older drugs and at least one-third of patients discontinued randomized therapy during the course of the trial. Until details of the actual treatments administered are published, there must be uncertainty about the conclusions.

Benefit in older patients

The prevalence of hypertension and particularly systolic hypertension rises dramatically through adult life. By the later part of the sixth decade of life, isolated systolic hypertension accounts for 60–70% of hypertension.

Three trials have examined the treatment of isolated systolic hypertension. In the Systolic Hypertension in the Elderly Program (SHEP) |8|, 4736 patients aged ≥60 years with systolic blood pressure 160–219 mmHg and diastolic blood pressure <90 mmHg were treated with low-dose chlorthalidone-based therapy (with additional atenolol or reserpine) or placebo for an average 4.5 years, with a target systolic blood pressure ≤159 mmHg. Achieved blood pressure was 143/68 mmHg and 155/72 mmHg in the active and control groups, respectively. Active treatment reduced stroke by 36% and all cardiovascular events by 32%. Similar reductions in stroke (42%) and cardiovascular events (33%) were seen in the Systolic Hypertension in Europe (SYST-EUR) trial |9|, where elderly subjects were treated with nitrendipine-based therapy (supplemented by enalapril and hydrochlorothiazide as necessary). Target systolic blood pressure was <150 mmHg. After 2 years' follow-up, systolic blood pressure fell by 13 mmHg on placebo (n=2297) and 23 mmHg on active therapy (n=2398). In the Syst-China trial |10| alternate patients (n=1253) were assigned to nitrendipine (with the possible addition of captopril or hydrochlorothiazide or both) or placebo (n=1141). The aim was to reduce systolic blood pressure by at least 20 mmHg to below 150 mmHg. At entry, sitting blood pressure averaged 170/80 mmHg and age averaged 66.5 years. After 2 years, blood pressure fell by 20/5 mmHg and by 11/2 mmHg in the active and placebo groups, respectively. Active treatment was associated with 38% reduction in stroke and 37% reduction in all cardiovascular endpoints.

The vascular dementia substudy of the SYST-EUR trial

Prevention of dementia in randomised double-blind placebo-controlled Systolic Hypertension in Europe (SYST-EUR) trial.

F Forette, M-L Seux, J A Staessen, L Thijs, W H Birkenhager, M R Babarskiene, et al. Lancet 1998; **352**: 1347–51.

BACKGROUND. The vascular dementia project, set up in the framework of the double-blind placebo-controlled Systolic Hypertension in Europe (SYST-EUR) trial, investigated whether antihypertensive drug treatment could reduce the incidence of dementia.

INTERPRETATION. In elderly patients with isolated systolic hypertension, antihypertensive treatment was associated with a lower incidence of dementia. If 1000 hypertensive patients were treated with antihypertensive drugs for 5 years, 19 cases of dementia might be prevented.

Comment

This aimed to investigate whether antihypertensive treatment could prevent vascular dementia in older patients with isolated systolic hypertension. As well as satisfying the entry criteria for the main study (age at least 60 years, systolic blood pressure 160–219 mmHg and diastolic blood pressure <95 mmHg), eligible patients had to be free of dementia. Participants were screened for cognitive impairment at randomization and at annual follow-up, using the mini-mental state examination (MMSE) and further diagnostic tests as appropriate.

At randomization, patients allocated placebo (n=1180) and those allocated active treatment (n=1238) had similar characteristics. Active treatment reduced the rate of dementia by 50% from 7.7 to 3.8 cases per 1000 patient-years ($P=0.05$). However, among the 32 incident cases of dementia in the intention-to-treat analysis (21 in placebo and 11 in the active treatment group), 23 were Alzheimer's disease and only two were vascular dementia.

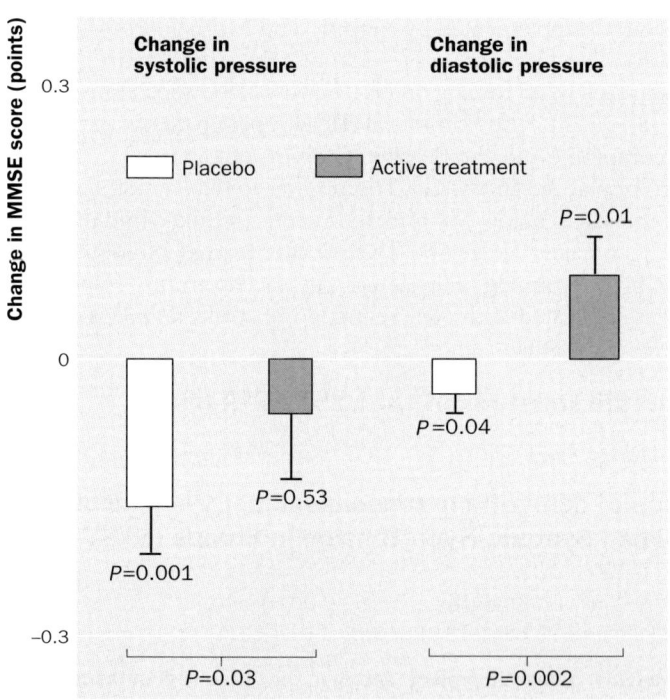

Fig. 1.9 Changes in mini-mental state examination (MMSE) score associated with mean decrease in systolic and diastolic blood pressure on placebo and active treatment in the SYST-EUR vascular dementia project. Values adjusted for age, sex, education level, previous cardiovascular complications, prior antihypertensive treatment, smoking and alcohol consumption.

The between-treatment difference in blood pressure was 8.3/3.8 mmHg ($P<0.001$). In the placebo group, the MMSE score decreased when systolic and diastolic blood pressure decreased, whereas in the active treatment group, the scores remained unchanged or increased slightly (Fig. 1.9); the between-group differences in these associations were significant for systolic ($P=0.03$) and diastolic ($P=0.002$) blood pressure.

Implications of the vascular dementia substudy of SYST-EUR

A reduction by 50% in the incidence of dementia by antihypertensive drug treatment would have important public health implications in view of the increasing longevity of the population. Treatment of 1000 hypertensive patients for 5 years could prevent 19 cases; the benefit could be even larger in unselected high-risk groups. This is in addition to the reduction in cardiovascular risk by reducing systolic blood pressure.

Only two vascular dementia events were detected, and a large number of participants was lost to follow-up. The analysis relied on 32 incident cases of dementia. Differences were of borderline statistical significance. The possible impact of active treatment ranged from no effect to a 76% reduction in rate of dementia. Thus the findings should be interpreted with caution.

A relevant proportion of patients was on combination treatment with enalapril and/or hydrochlorothiazide, and treatment was unknown for several participants. Hence, a specific beneficial effect of calcium channel blockers cannot be assumed.

Antihypertensive therapy in the very elderly

Antihypertensive drugs in very old people: a subgroup meta-analysis of randomised controlled trials.
F Gueyffier, C Bulpitt, J-P Brossel, E Schron, T Ekbom, R Fagard, *et al.*
Lancet 1999; **353**: 793–6.

BACKGROUND. Beneficial clinical effects of treatment with antihypertensive drugs have been shown in middle-aged patients and in those hypertensive patients over 60 years old, but whether treatment is beneficial in patients over 80 years old is not known.

INTERPRETATION. Results of a large-scale specific trial are needed for a definitive conclusion that antihypertensive treatment is beneficial in very elderly hypertensive patients. Meanwhile, an age threshold beyond which hypertension should not be treated cannot be justified.

Comment

Antihypertensive drug treatment might be less effective or even harmful in individuals above the age of 80 years. A meta-analysis has included all subgroup data from randomized controlled trials to give a non-biased estimate of the effect of treatment

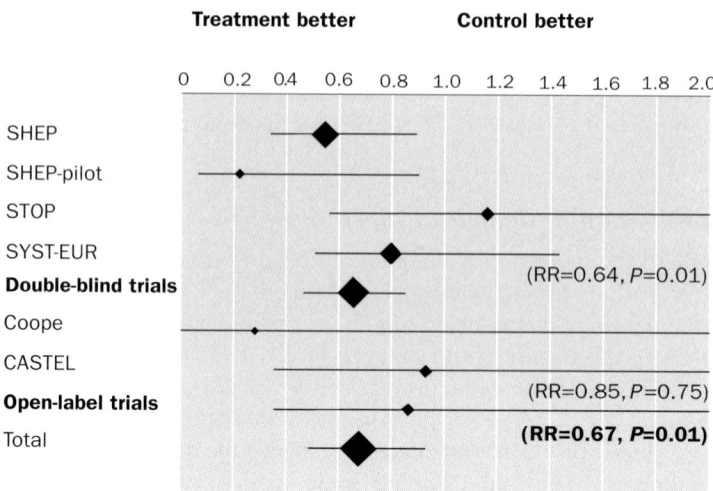

Fig. 1.10 Treatment effect on relative risk of stroke in very old people. Area of symbols proportional to information available; error bars = confidence intervals. RR = relative risk.

in hypertensive people of 80 years or older compared with that of placebo, no treatment or lower dosage.

In 1670 trial participants, the risk of fatal events was high, with a mortality rate of more than 20% after a mean follow-up of 3.5 years. For the primary outcome of stroke, treatment was associated with a 34% lower rate of fatal and non-fatal events (Fig. 1.10). The only two secondary outcomes that achieved a significant difference between treatment and control were major cardiovascular events and heart failure (Fig. 1.11). Results for major coronary events showed a non-significant trend towards treatment benefit. Treatment effect was not significant for fatal outcomes, but there was a non-significant trend for increased total mortality, with 2% relative excess of deaths from all causes.

The results for fatal outcomes raise some concern about possible harmful effects of treatment, especially for total mortality. Stroke events may be so disabling that patients will risk a treatment that causes some reduction in overall survival if it is associated with good quality of life.

Implications of this subgroup meta-analysis

A properly and specifically designed trial is needed to confirm these results. Meanwhile, these findings do not suggest that there is an age threshold above which hypertension should not be treated.

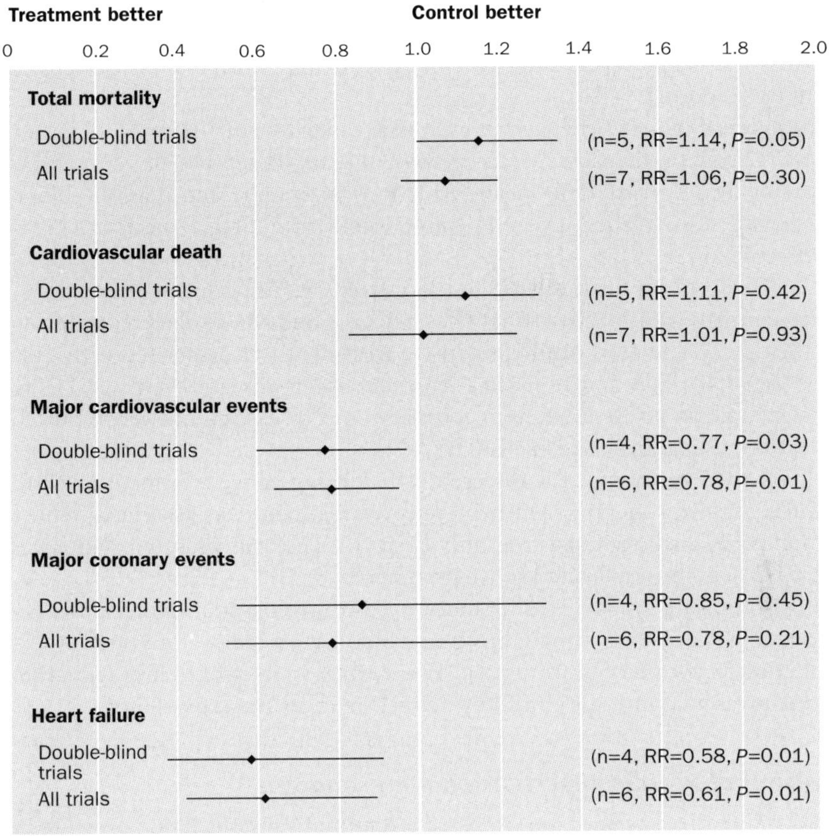

Treatment better   **Control better**

| 0 | 0.2 | 0.4 | 0.6 | 0.8 | 1.0 | 1.2 | 1.4 | 1.6 | 1.8 | 2.0 |

Total mortality

Double-blind trials   (n=5, RR=1.14, P=0.05)

All trials   (n=7, RR=1.06, P=0.30)

Cardiovascular death

Double-blind trials   (n=5, RR=1.11, P=0.42)

All trials   (n=7, RR=1.01, P=0.93)

Major cardiovascular events

Double-blind trials   (n=4, RR=0.77, P=0.03)

All trials   (n=6, RR=0.78, P=0.01)

Major coronary events

Double-blind trials   (n=4, RR=0.85, P=0.45)

All trials   (n=6, RR=0.78, P=0.21)

Heart failure

Double-blind trials   (n=4, RR=0.58, P=0.01)

All trials   (n=6, RR=0.61, P=0.01)

Fig. 1.11 Treatment effect on relative risk of secondary outcomes in very old patients. Error bars = confidence intervals; RR = relative risk.

Systolic hypertension

Elevated systolic blood pressure as a risk factor for cardiovascular and renal disease.

J He, P K Whelton. *J Hypertens* 1999; **17** (Suppl 2): S7–S13.

BACKGROUND. The aim was to review published literature on the relationship between systolic blood pressure and risk of cardiovascular and renal disease.

INTERPRETATION. Observational epidemiological studies and randomized controlled trials have demonstrated that systolic blood pressure is an independent and strong predictor of risk of cardiovascular and renal disease.

Comment

A recent meta-analysis has reviewed 10 randomized trials in which the efficacy of reduction in systolic blood pressure on clinical outcomes during antihypertensive treatment was reported.

The number of patients enrolled in each trial ranged from 143 to 4736, with a total of 18 542 trial participants. Mean age was 70 years (range 44–76 years). Average follow-up was 4 years. The mean reductions in systolic and diastolic blood pressure during active treatment were 14.4 mmHg and 6.5 mmHg, respectively, compared with controls.

Overall, 412 coronary heart disease and 385 stroke events occurred during active treatment, compared with 520 coronary heart disease and 596 stroke events during control therapy (Table 1.2). Antihypertensive treatment was associated with 21% reduction in total (fatal and non-fatal) coronary heart disease events and 37% reduction in fatal stroke. Reductions in coronary heart disease events were reported in nine of 10 trials and in stroke in all 10 trials.

There were 467 cardiovascular disease deaths during active treatment and 617 deaths during control therapy. Antihypertensive treatment was associated with a 25% reduction in cardiovascular mortality (5 of 10 trials). All-cause mortality was reduced by 13% in those allocated active treatment.

Pooling of the data available from randomized controlled trials indicate that an average reduction of 14–15 mmHg in systolic blood pressure over 4 years confers 21% reduction in coronary heart disease, 37% reduction in stroke, 25% reduction in total cardiovascular mortality and 13% reduction in all-cause mortality.

Implications of systolic hypertension meta-analysis

These data emphasize the need for increased attention to systolic blood pressure in the effort to reduce the hypertension-related risk of coronary heart disease and stroke.

Table 1.2 Meta-analysis of trials of systolic hypertension*

	Events		% risk reduction	
	Active	**Control**	**(95% CI)**	**P-value**
Total coronary heart disease	412	520	21 (10, 31)	< 0.001
Fatal coronary heart disease	250	341	27 (13, 38)	< 0.001
Total stroke	385	596	37 (28, 45)	< 0.001
Fatal stroke	101	158	36 (18, 50)	< 0.001
Cardiovascular deaths	467	617	25 (15, 34)	< 0.001
All-cause mortality	906	1028	13 (4, 21)	0.005

*Results from 10 randomized trials with 9278 active treatment and 9264 control participants.
CI = confidence interval.

Isolated systolic hypertension

Overview of the outcome trials in older patients with isolated systolic hypertension.

J A Staessen, J G Wang, L Thijs, R Fargard. *J Hum Hypertens* 1999; **13**: 859–63.

BACKGROUND. **The aim was to review each of the three published placebo-controlled outcome trials of antihypertensive drug therapy of isolated systolic hypertension in the elderly and to present the pooled estimates of benefit of antihypertensive drug treatment in isolated systolic hypertension in the elderly.**

INTERPRETATION. The pooled results of the outcome trials in older patients with isolated systolic hypertension indicated that antihypertensive drug treatment should be prescribed if, on repeated measurement, systolic blood pressure is 160 mmHg or higher.

Comment

The results of the three outcome trials in older patients with isolated systolic hypertension were pooled. Overall, active treatment reduced all-cause mortality by 17% and cardiovascular mortality by 25% compared with placebo (Fig. 1.12). For fatal

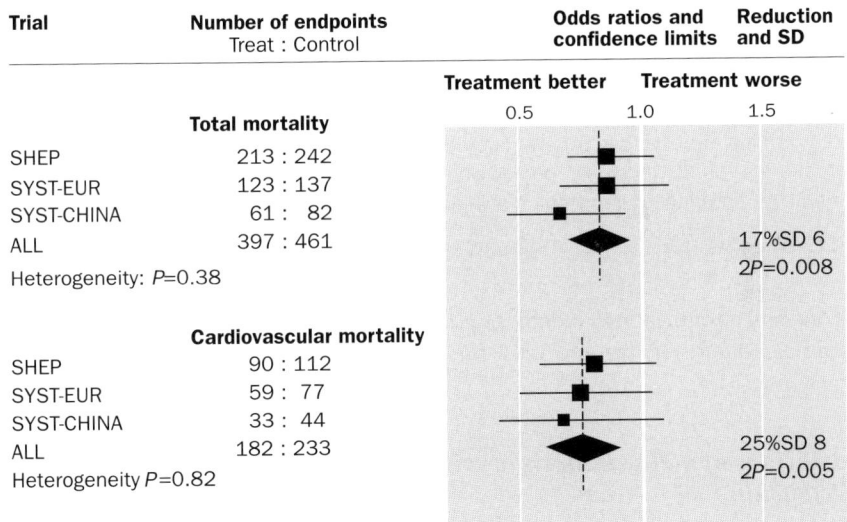

Fig. 1.12 Treatment effect on total and cardiovascular mortality in older patients with isolated systolic hypertension. *Solid squares* = simple odds ratios for individual trials. *Solid triangles* = pooled odds ratios with 95% confidence interval. Areas of symbols proportional to information available. SD = standard deviation.

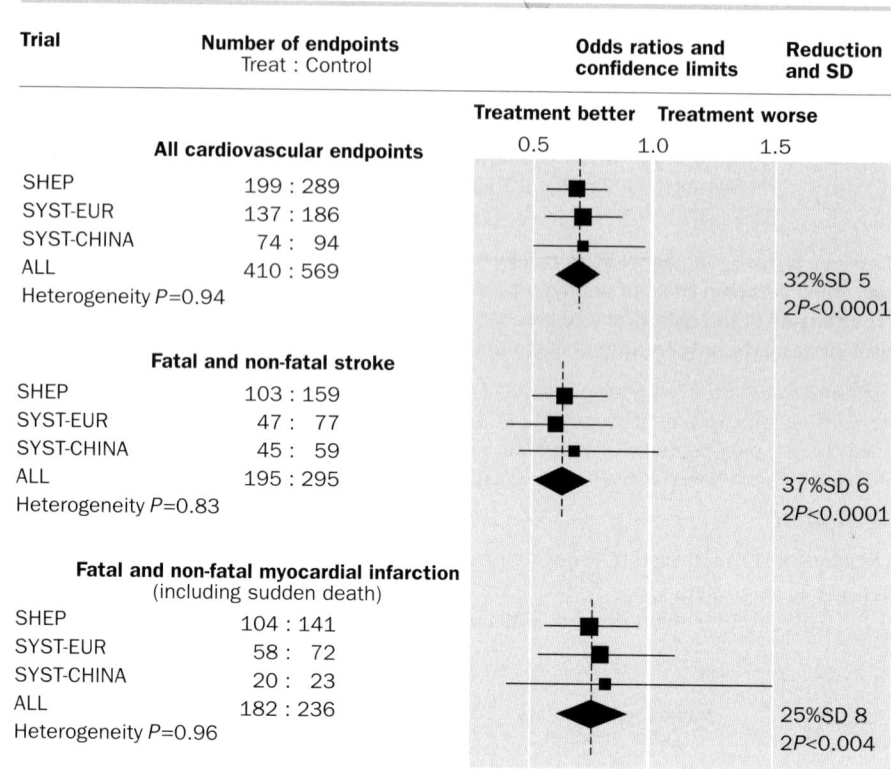

Fig. 1.13 Treatment effect on fatal and non-fatal cardiovascular endpoints in older patients with isolated systolic hypertension. *Solid squares* = simple odds ratios for individual trials. *Solid triangles* = pooled odds ratios with 95% confidence interval. Areas of symbols proportional to information available. SD = standard deviation.

and non-fatal complications combined, reductions were 32% for all cardiovascular endpoints, 37% for stroke and 25% for myocardial infarction including sudden death (Fig. 1.13).

Implications of meta-analysis of trials of isolated systolic hypertension

The pooled results provide strong evidence in support of antihypertensive drug treatment if, on repeated measures, systolic blood pressure is 160 mmHg or higher. The low entry and achieved diastolic blood pressures in these trials negate the hypothesis that rigorous lowering of diastolic blood pressure would compromise the coronary circulation and provoke rather than prevent coronary complications.

Conclusions

The results of recent trials have provided answers to several questions concerning the management of hypertension. The value of rigorous control of blood pressure, particularly in high-risk patients, has been established. The benefits and risks of concurrent anti-platelet therapy in the form of low-dose aspirin have been clarified; aspirin is cheap but not cheerful. At last, we have evidence of the potential advantage of newer drugs, although results have been inconclusive. The findings in support of treatment of older individuals with mainly systolic hypertension are more compelling. Although much has been achieved, continued efforts are needed to refine further the drug treatment of hypertension.

References

1. MacMahon S, Peto R, Cutler J, Collins R, Sorlie P, Neaton J, *et al.* Blood pressure stroke and coronary heart disease. Part 1, Prolonged differences in blood pressure: prospective observational studies corrected for the regression dilution bias. *Lancet* 1990; **335**: 765–74.

2. Collins R, MacMahon S. Blood pressure, antihypertensive drug treatment and the risks of stroke and of coronary heart disease. *Br Med Bull* 1994; **50**: 272–98.

3. Isles CG, Walker LM, Beevers DG, Brown I, Cameron HL, Clarke J, *et al.* Mortality in patients of the Glasgow Blood Pressure Clinic. *J Hypertens* 1986; **4**: 141–56.

4. Cruickshank JM, Thorp JM, Zacharias FJ. Benefits and potential harm of lowering high blood pressure. *Lancet* 1987; **i**: 581–4.

5. Wiklund I, Halling K, Rydén-Bergsten T, Fletcher A. Does lowering of blood pressure improve mood? Quality-of-life results from the Hypertension Optimal Treatment (HOT) Study. *Blood Press* 1997; **6**: 357–64.

6. McInnes GT, Hole D, Lever AF, Meredith PA, Murray LS, Reid JL. ACE inhibitors and mortality at the Glasgow Blood Pressure Clinic. *J Hum Hypertens* 1999; **13**: 897–8.

7. Peto R. Failure of randomisation by 'sealed' envelope. *Lancet* 1999; **354**: 73.

8. SHEP Co-operative Research Group. Prevention of stroke by antihypertensive drug treatment in older persons with isolated systolic hypertension: final results of the Systolic Hypertension in the Elderly Program (SHEP). *JAMA* 1991; **265**: 3255–64.

9. Staessen JA, Fagard R, Thijs L, Celis H, Arabidze GG, Birkenhager WH, *et al.* Randomised double-blind comparison of placebo and active treatment for older patients with isolated systolic hypertension. *Lancet* 1997; **350**: 757–64.

10. Liu L, Wang JG, Gong L, Liu G, Staessen JA. Comparison of active treatment and placebo for older patients with isolated systolic hypertension. *J Hypertens* 1998; **16**: 1823–9.

2

Current guidelines

Introduction

The conclusive evidence for the benefits of treating hypertension has encouraged the treatment of patients at risk. Unfortunately, the standards of care are extremely variable, ranging from total neglect to over-intensive use of drugs in individuals who stand to gain little if anything from treatment. These considerations have stimulated the publication of guidelines to assist practitioners in the management of hypertension.

Various national and international guidelines have endeavoured to distil the plethora of available information into practical recommendations. The guidelines range from lengthy and extremely detailed reports to relatively succinct advice. Each guideline is a consensus, a compromise among different views, and therefore subject to change which is not always evidence-based.

The guidelines essentially address three questions: when to treat; how to treat; and the target blood pressure. Despite a general consensus, health care practices in different countries can dictate various interpretations of the evidence. Earlier guidelines differed in their views of the optimal threshold for treatment, the choice of first-line drugs and the goals of treatment. Recent guidelines have come closer together in these respects. The new wave of guidelines reviewed in this chapter are united in their recognition of the need to include other risk factors for cardiovascular disease in determining the threshold for intervention, the role of other cardio-protective drugs and the optimal target blood pressure.

The sixth report of the Joint National Committee on Prevention, Detection, Evaluation, and Treatment of High Blood Pressure (JNC VI) [1]

This comprehensive and lengthy document embraces many aspects of the epidemiology and management of hypertension. It follows the pattern of earlier reports and expands on advice, sometimes on the basis of new evidence. JNC VI places more emphasis on absolute risk and benefit, and uses risk stratification as part of the treatment strategy.

Table 2.1 Trends in awareness, treatment and control of high blood pressure in adults in the United States, 1978–1994

	Adults 18–74 years		
	1976–80	**1988–91**	**1991–94**
Awareness (%)	51	73	68
Treatment (%)	31	55	53
Control (%)	10	29	27

Threshold blood pressure 140/90 mmHg. Source: NHANES II, III.

Hypertension awareness, treatment and control rates have increased during the last three decades. However, the rates of increase have lessened since the publication of the JNC V report in 1993 |2| (National Heart and Nutrition Examination Surveys: NHANES II, III: Table 2.1). Age-adjusted mortality rates for stroke and coronary heart disease (CHD) declined during this time, but thereafter were levelling. The incidence of end-stage renal disease and the prevalence of heart failure were increasing.

In considering the evidence to formulate clinical policy, absolute rather than relative changes were used, because the absolute benefit derived from treating hypertension depends on the absolute risk, i.e. those with the greatest risk achieve the greatest benefit (Fig. 2.1). Despite limitations, evidence from randomized clinical trials was given emphasis.

Blood pressure measurement and clinical evaluation

Although classification of adult blood pressure (BP) is somewhat arbitrary, it is useful for clinicians who must make treatment decisions based on a constellation of factors including the actual level of BP (Table 2.2). When systolic BP (SBP) and diastolic BP (DBP) fall into separate categories, the higher category should be selected to classify the individual BP.

Table 2.2 JNC VI guidelines classification of blood pressure for adults aged 18 years and older

	Systolic (mmHg)		Diastolic (mmHg)
Optimal	< 120	and	< 80
Normal	< 130	and	< 85
High–normal	130–139	or	85–89
Hypertension (≥ 2 readings at ≥ 2 visits after screening)			
Stage 1	140–159	or	90–99
Stage 2	160–179	or	100–109
Stage 3	≥ 180	or	≥ 110

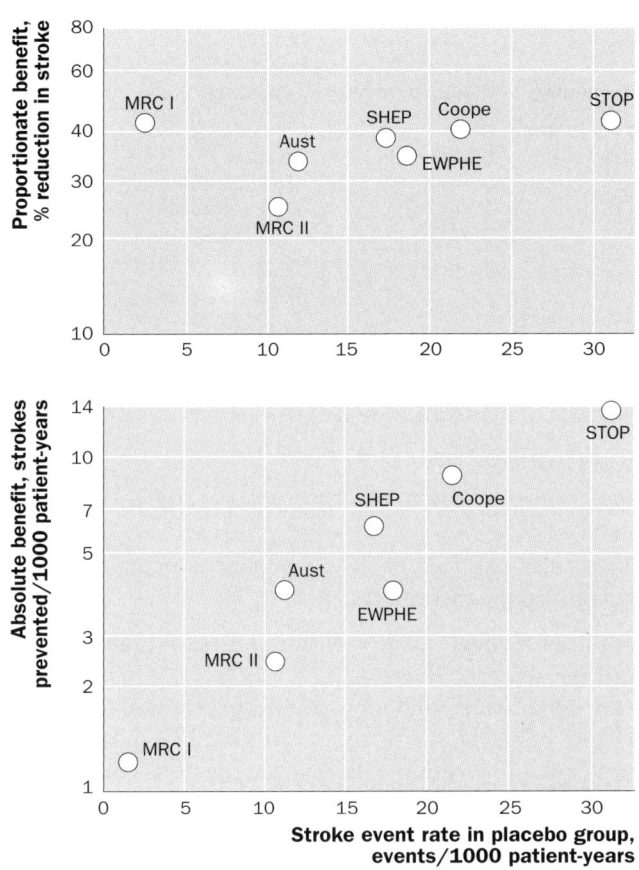

Fig. 2.1 Comparison of proportionate (relative) and absolute benefit from reduction in the incidence of stroke.
MRC I = Medical Research Council trial I; MRC II = MRC trial II; Aust = Australian study; SHEP = Systolic Hypertension in the Elderly Program; EWPHE = European Working Party on High Blood Pressure in the Elderly trial; Coope = Coope and Warrender |3|; STOP = Swedish Trial in Old Patients with Hypertension–2.

Recommendations for detection, confirmation and evaluation of high BP remain consistent with those in the JNC V report |2|. Two or more readings should be carried out on each occasion, and periodic re-measurement is essential (Table 2.3).

Measurement of BP outside the clinician's office—self-measurement or ambulatory blood pressure monitoring (ABPM)—may have a role in some patients. However, these procedures should not be used indiscriminately in the routine evaluation of patients with suspected hypertension. Since BP tends to be higher when measured in the clinic than when measured outside, new definitions of

Table 2.3 JNC VI guidelines recommendations for follow-up based on initial BP measurement in adults

Systolic (mmHg)	Diastolic (mmHg)	Follow-up
< 130	< 85	2 years
130–139	85–89	1 year
140–159	90–99	≤ 2 months
160–179	100–109	≤ 1 month
≥ 180	≥ 110	≤ 1 week

hypertension are proposed: ≥ 135/85 mmHg for self-measured and mean daytime BP (ABPM) and ≥ 120/75 mmHg for mean night-time BP (ABPM).

Evaluation of patients with documented hypertension has three objectives:

- to identify known causes of hypertension;
- to assess the presence or absence and extent of target organ damage (TOD) and cardiovascular disease; and
- to identify other cardiovascular risk factors (RFs) and concomitant disorders that may define prognosis and guide treatment.

Data for evaluation are acquired through medical history, physical examination, laboratory tests and other diagnostic procedures.

Laboratory tests recommended before initiation of therapy are tests to determine the presence of TOD and other RFs—urinalysis, complete blood cell count, blood chemistry (potassium, sodium, creatinine, fasting glucose, total cholesterol, high density lipoprotein cholesterol) and 12-lead electrocardiogram (ECG). Optional tests include microalbuminuria, blood calcium and uric acid, and echocardiography.

Risk stratification

This depends not only on the level of BP but also on the presence or absence of TOD (Table 2.4a) and other RFs (Table 2.4b). Three stages of BP and three levels of risk form a matrix against which physicians can determine therapy (Table 2.5). In

Table 2.4a Components of cardiovascular risk stratification in patients with hypertension–1

Major risk factors

- Smoking
- Dyslipidaemia
- Diabetes mellitus
- Age > 60 years
- Male/post-menopausal female
- Family history

Source: JNC VI, 1997.

Table 2.4b Components of cardiovascular risk stratification in patients with hypertension–2

Target organ damage

- Left ventricular hypertrophy
- Clinical ischaemic heart disease
- Heart failure
- Stroke/TIA
- Nephropathy
- Peripheral vascular disease
- Retinopathy

TIA = transient ischaemic attack. Source: JNC VI, 1997.

Table 2.5 Risk stratification and treatment

BP (mmHg)	Risk group A No RF/TOD	Risk group B ≥ 1 RF*/No TOD	1991–94 TOD ± RF+
130–139/85–89	Lifestyle	Lifestyle	Drugs++
140–159/90–99	Lifestyle (1 yr)	Lifestyle (6/12)	Drugs
≥ 160/≥ 100	Drugs	Drugs	Drugs

*Not DM   ++HF, RI, DM   +Including DM
RF = risk factor; TOD = target organ damage; DM = diabetes mellitus; HF = heart failure;
RI = renal insufficiency. Source: JNC VI, 1997.

patients with stage 1 hypertension, drug therapy should be instituted if lifestyle modification does not achieve goal BP. In risk group B, clinicians should consider antihypertensive drugs as initial therapy if multiple RFs are present.

Treatment of high blood pressure

The goal of treatment is to achieve and maintain an SBP < 140 mmHg and a DBP < 90 mmHg, and lower if tolerated. Goals based on out-of-office measurements should be lower than those based on office readings.

The first step in hypertension management is lifestyle modification (Table 2.6). This can also reduce other cardiovascular RFs at little cost and minimal risk. Even when lifestyle modifications alone are not adequate to control hypertension, they may reduce the number and dosage of antihypertensive medications needed for management. Implementation of lifestyle modification should not delay the start of an effective antihypertensive drug regimen in those at higher risk.

A diuretic or beta-blocker should be used as initial therapy unless there are compelling or specific indications for another drug. For most drugs, a low dose should be used, slowly titrating upwards according to response. Formulations that provide 24-hour control are recommended, although no advice is given on how such agents

Table 2.6 Lifestyle modifications for hypertension prevention and management

- Lose weight if overweight
- Limit alcohol intake
- Increase aerobic exercise
- Reduce sodium intake ($\leq$ 100 mmol/day)
- Maintain potassium intake (90 mmol/day)
- Maintain calcium and magnesium intake
- Stop smoking and reduce saturated fats

Source: JNC VI, 1997.

should be selected. Examples of compelling and specific indications for and contraindications to individual drugs are shown in Table 2.7. An algorithm for the treatment of hypertension is given in Fig. 2.2. The use of immediate-release nifedipine is not recommended, because of the risk of precipitating ischaemic events.

Table 2.7a Considerations for individualizing antihypertensive drug therapy–1

Compelling indications for drugs

- DM (type 1) with proteinuria   ACE inhibitor (ARB)
- Heart failure   ACE inhibitor (ARB)
  Diuretic
- ISH in elderly   Diuretic
  Long-acting DHP
- MI   Beta-blocker
  —systolic dysfunction   ACE inhibitor (ARB)

DM = diabetes mellitus; ACE = angiotensin-converting enzyme; ARB = angiotensin receptor blocker; ISH = isolated systolic hypertension; DHP = dihydropyridine; MI = myocardial infarction.
Source: JNC VI, 1997.

Table 2.7b Considerations for individualizing antihypertensive drug therapy–2

Specific indications for drugs

- Angina   Beta-blocker
  Calcium antagonist
- DM (types 1 and 2)   ACE inhibitor (ARB)
  with proteinuria   Calcium antagonist
- DM (type 2)   Diuretic
- Dislipidaemia   Alpha-blocker
- Renal insufficiency   ACE inhibitor (ARB)

DM = diabetes mellitus; ACE = angiotensin-converting enzyme; ARB = angiotensin receptor blocker.
Source: JNC VI, 1997.

Table 2.7c Considerations for individualizing antihypertensive drug therapy–3

Contraindications for drugs

● Bronchospasm	Beta-blocker
● Depression	Reserpine
● Gout	Diuretic
● Heart block (2° or 3°)	Beta-blocker
	Rate-limiting calcium antagonist
	ACE inhibitor (ARB)

ACE = angiotensin-converting enzyme; ARB = angiotensin receptor blocker. Source: JNC VI, 1997.

If the response to the initial drug advice is inadequate after reaching the full dose, two options for subsequent therapy should be considered—combination or substitution (Fig. 2.2). Treatment decisions should be made after at least 4 weeks of a particular therapy. The control of BP, avoiding side-effects, may take several months. A diuretic should be selected as first- or second-step therapy, because addition will enhance the effect of other agents.

Before proceeding to each successive treatment step, clinicians should consider possible reasons for lack of responsiveness (Table 2.8). Stepwise decrease of dosage and number of antihypertensive drugs should be considered after hypertension has been controlled effectively for at least 1 year, with careful follow-up arrangements.

Resistant hypertension is defined as SBP $\geq$ 140 mmHg ($\geq$ 160 mmHg in older patients with isolated systolic hypertension) or DBP $\geq$ 90 mmHg despite adequate adherence to triple therapy including a diuretic, with all drugs at near-maximal dose. Management strategies can improve concordance (adherence) with therapy (Table 2.9). Strategies for management of hypertensive emergencies and urgencies are described.

Special population and situations

Coexisting cardiovascular disease

In patients with *coronary artery disease*, a goal BP even lower than the usual target is desirable if angina persists. Beta-blockers and calcium antagonists may be

Table 2.8 Reasons for lack of responsiveness to therapy

- Pseudotolerance, e.g. white-coat hypertension
- Non-adherence to therapy
- Volume overload, e.g. excess salt intake or inadequate diuretic therapy
- Drug interactions, e.g. non-steroidal anti-inflammatory drugs
- Associated conditions, e.g. smoking, chronic pain
- Secondary hypertension

Source: JNC VI, 1997.

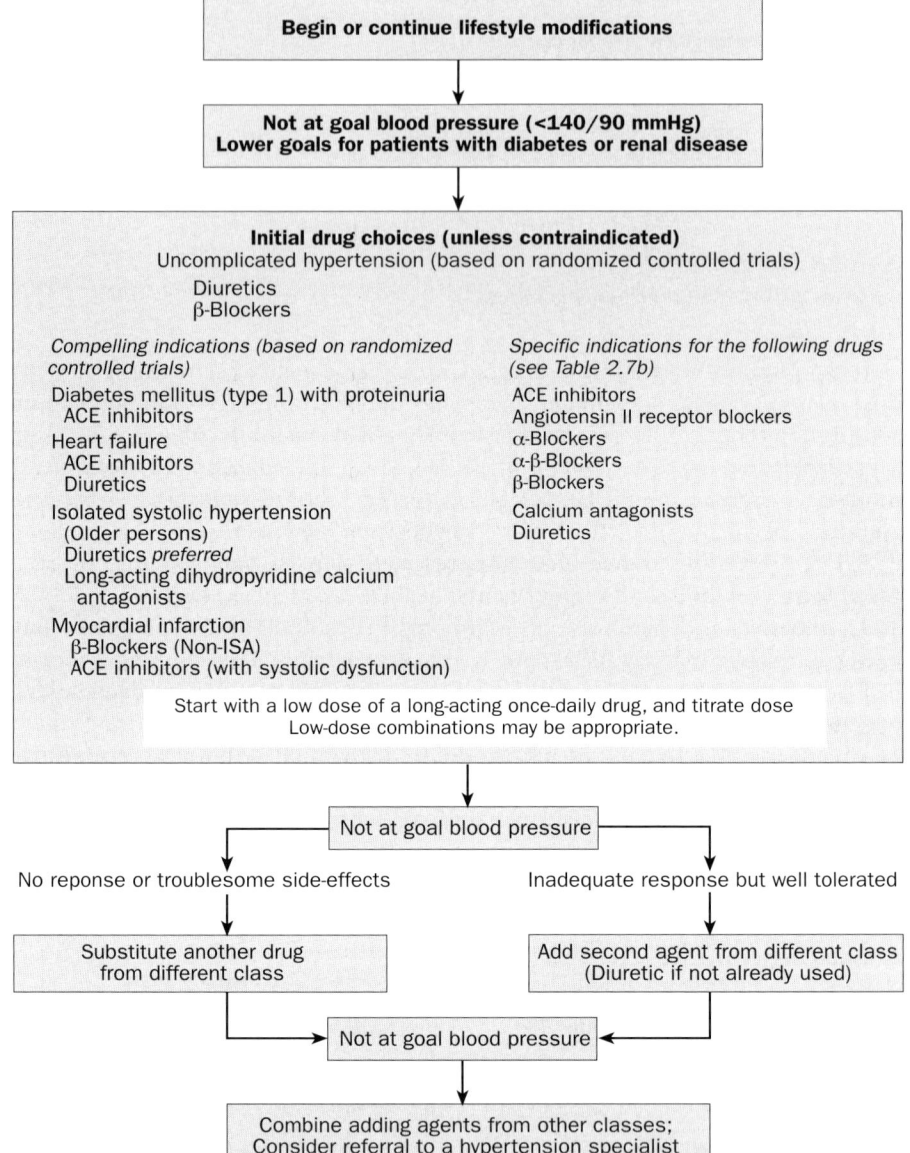

Fig. 2.2 Algorithm for the treatment of hypertension. ISA = intrinsic sympathomimetic activity.

Table 2.9 General guidelines to improve patient adherence to antihypertensive therapy

- Consider non-adherence
- Establish goals with patient
- Educate patients/families
- Maintain contact
- Avoid expensive management
- Respond to patient needs/concerns
- Avoid adverse drug effects
- Consider nurse care management

Source: JNC VI, 1997.

specifically useful, but short-acting calcium antagonists should not be used. After *myocardial infarction*, beta-blockers without intrinsic sympathomimetic activity should be given, and ACE inhibitors are also useful if there is left ventricular systolic dysfunction. If beta-blockers are ineffective or contraindicated, verapamil or diltiazem may be used. Identification of patients with *left ventricular hypertrophy* should be based on the ECG, with echocardiography reserved for patients with untreated stage 1 hypertension, no cardiovascular RFs, no evidence of clinical cardiovascular disease and no TOD. Lifestyle modification and all antihypertensive drugs (except direct vasodilators such as hydralazine and minoxidil) reduce left ventricular mass. Patients with *cardiac failure* should receive an ACE inhibitor; addition of carvedilol has been shown to be beneficial. When an ACE inhibitor is contraindicated or not tolerated, the combination of hydralazine and isosorbide dinitrate is also effective, and an angiotensin receptor blocker (ARB) should be considered. Amlodipine and felodipine appear relatively safe in treating patients with chronic heart failure when used in addition to an ACE inhibitor, a diuretic and digoxin; other calcium antagonists are not recommended.

Renal insufficiency

Reversible causes of renal failure should always be sought. Thus patients with proteinuria > 1 g/day should be treated to a goal BP of 125/75 mmHg; if proteinuria is less, the target BP is 130/85 mmHg. The most important action to slow progressive renal failure is to lower BP to goal. All classes of antihypertensive drugs are effective and, in most cases, multiple drugs are necessary. ACE inhibitors appear to have additional renal protective effects and should be included in the regimen (in most cases along with a diuretic) unless contraindicated. In patients with serum creatinine ≥ 265.2 μmol/l (3 mg/dl), ACE inhibitors should be used with caution. If serum creatinine rises by ≥ 88.4 μmol/l (1 mg/dl) and persists on re-checking, the diagnosis of renal artery stenosis should be considered and any ACE inhibitor (or ARB) discontinued. Thiazide diuretics are not effective at serum creatinine ≥ 221 μmol/l (2.5 mg/dl) and loop diuretics (often at high doses) are needed. Potassium-sparing diuretics should be avoided.

Diabetes mellitus

The goal of antihypertensive therapy is a BP < 130/85 mmHg. Drugs from all of the main classes can be used, and combinations are usually necessary. ACE inhibitors (or ARBs if these are not tolerated) are preferred as the first step in diabetic nephropathy.

Comment

JNC VI provides comprehensive advice on the prevention, evaluation and treatment of hypertension. It emphasizes risk factor stratification and multiple risk factor intervention. The new targets for therapy are rigorous. JNC VI represents a major effort that should help clinicians to appreciate the importance of treating hypertension. However, it has uncertain relevance to health care systems outside the United States.

1999 World Health Organization–International Society of Hypertension Guidelines for the Management of Hypertension |4|

The second half of the twentieth century saw a progressive decline in cardiovascular mortality in North America, Western Europe, Japan and Australasia. At the same time, the control of hypertension in these regions improved considerably, although most hypertensive subjects have imperfect control (or no treatment at all). Moreover, given the ageing population structure of most developed countries, the total numbers of strokes and CHD events are increasing or remaining static. Even more worrying is the rapid development of the 'second wave' epidemic of cardiovascular disease (CVD) that is flowing through developing countries and the former socialist republics.

Scope and purpose

These guidelines concentrate on the practical clinical management of mild hypertension. The primary aim is to offer balanced information to guide clinicians who

Table 2.10 Cardiovascular disease risk factors–1: the relative contribution of blood pressure and selected other factors

BP (mmHg)	Age (yrs)	DM	TIA	Risk
140/90	40	No	No	1
170/105	40	No	No	×2–3
145/90	65	Yes	Yes	×20

BP = blood pressure; DM = diabetes mellitus; TIA = transient ischaemic attack.

Otherwise healthy male. Source: WHO–ISH Guidelines 1999.

Table 2.11 Cardiovascular disease risk factors–2: factors other than blood pressure

- Age
- Male sex
- Prior event
- Renal disease
- IGT
- Cigarettes
- Lipids

- Obesity
- Fibrinogen
- Alcohol
- Physical activity
- Socio-economic status
- Ethnicity
- Geographical region

IGT = impaired glucose tolerance. Source: WHO–ISH Guidelines 1999.

manage patients from a wide range of ethnic and cultural backgrounds with very different health systems and varying availabilities of resources.

Contribution of blood pressure and other risk factors to cardiovascular risk

Differences in risk of CVD are determined not only by the level of BP, but also by the presence or levels of other RFs (Table 2.10). Thus differences in the absolute level of cardiovascular risk between patients with hypertension will often be determined to a greater extent by other RFs than by the level of BP. Examples of other cardiovascular RFs are shown in Table 2.11.

Clinical evaluation

The aims of the clinical and laboratory evaluation of hypertensive patients are summarized in Table 2.12. A comprehensive clinical history and full physical examination are essential. Because BP is characterized by large spontaneous variations, the diagnosis of hypertension should be based on multiple BP measurements taken on several occasions.

Home and ABPM provide useful additional clinical information and have a limited place in the management of hypertensive patients (Table 2.13). The information from these methods must be regarded as supplementary to conventional measurements, and not a substitute. Average 24-hour BP values of around 125/80 mmHg

Table 2.12 Aims of clinical evaluation of the hypertensive patient

- Sustained blood pressure level
- Target organ damage
- Other cardiovascular risk factors
- Conditions that may influence treatment
- Secondary hypertension

Source: WHO–ISH Guidelines 1999.

Table 2.13 Circumstances in which ambulatory blood pressure monitoring should be considered

- Variability in blood pressure
- Low cardiovascular risk
- Symptoms suggesting hypotension
- Resistant hypertension

Source: WHO–ISH Guidelines 1999.

correspond to a clinic BP of 140/90 mmHg. Home devices that measure BP in the fingers or the arm below the elbow should be avoided.

In a few patients, office BP is persistently elevated, whereas daytime BP outside the office environment is not ('white-coat' or better 'isolated office' hypertension). Physicians should aim at its identification (by use of home BP or ABPM) whenever clinical suspicion is raised. The decision to treat or not should be based on the overall risk profile and the presence or absence of TOD. Close follow-up is essential for subjects with isolated office hypertension when the physician chooses not to treat.

Routine investigations should include urinalysis for blood, protein and glucose, microscopic examination of urine, blood potassium, creatinine, fasting glucose and total cholesterol, and ECG. Optional investigations are guided by the findings from history, examination and routine investigations. Echocardiography should be performed whenever the clinical assessment reveals the presence of TOD or suggests the possibility of left ventricular hypertrophy or other cardiac disease. Vascular ultrasonography should be performed whenever the presence of arterial disease is suspected in the aorta or the carotid or peripheral arteries. Renal ultrasonography should be performed if renal disease is suspected. Whether such expensive high-technology investigations are appropriate in all health care systems is not discussed.

Definition and classification of hypertension

To reduce confusion and provide more consistent advice to clinicians, the WHO–ISH guidelines adopt in principle the definition and classification provided by JNC VI |**1**|. However, the term 'grade' rather than 'stage' has been chosen to avoid implying progression. The guidelines emphasize that the decision to lower BP in particular patients is not based on the level of BP alone but on assessment of the total cardiovascular risk.

Stratification of patients by absolute level of cardiovascular risk

These guidelines provide a simple method by which to estimate the combined effect of several RFs and conditions on the future absolute risk of cardiovascular events. The estimates in Table 2.14 are based on the RFs, TOD and associated clinical conditions (ACC) listed in Table 2.15. Among individuals in the low-risk group, the risk of a major cardiovascular event in the next 10 years is typically < 15%; in the medium-risk group 15–20%; and in the high-risk group 20–30%. Patients with

Table 2.14 Stratifying risk to quantify prognosis

Other risk factors and disease history	Blood pressure (mmHg)		
	Grade 1 (mild hypertension) SBP 140–159 or DBP 90–99	Grade 2 (moderate hypertension) SBP 160–179 or DBP 100–109	Grade 3 (severe hypertension) SBP ≥ 180 or DBP ≥ 110
I. no other risk factors	Low risk	Medium risk	High risk
II. 1–2 risk factors	Medium risk	Medium risk	Very high risk
III. 3 or more risk factors or TOD or diabetes	High risk	High risk	Very high risk
IV. ACC	Very high risk	Very high risk	Very high risk

TOD = target organ damage; ACC = associated clinical conditions, including clinical cardiovascular disease or renal disease. The typical 10-year risk of stroke or myocardial infarction is shown, where 'low risk' corresponds to below 15%, 'medium risk' to 15–20%, 'high risk' to 20–30%, and 'very high risk' to 30% or higher.

Table 2.15a Factors influencing prognosis. A: risk factors

- Men > 55 years
- Women > 65 years
- Cigarette smoking
- Total cholesterol > 6.5 mmol/l
- Diabetes mellitus
- FH of premature CVD

FH = family history; CVD = cardiovascular disease.

Source: WHO–ISH Guidelines 1999.

Table 2.15b Factors influencing prognosis. B: target organ damage

- LVH (ECG/echo/CXR)
- Proteinuria/slight elevation ser cr
- Atherosclerotic plaque (US/X-ray)
- Retinopathy (grade II)

LVH = left ventricular hypertrophy; ECG = electrocardiogram; CXR = chest X-ray; ser cr = serum creatinine; US = ultrasound.

Source: WHO–ISH Guidelines 1999.

Table 2.15c Factors influencing prognosis. C: associated clinical conditions

- Cerebrovascular disease
- Heart disease
- Renal disease
- Vascular disease
- Advanced retinopathy

Source: WHO–ISH Guidelines 1999.

grade 3 hypertension and one or more RFs and all patients with CVD or renal disease carry the very highest risk of cardiovascular events (around 30% over 10 years) and qualify for the most intensive and rapidly instituted therapeutic regimens.

Goals of treatment

Effective treatment requires management of all reversible RFs and ACCs as well as of raised BP. BP targets are < 130/85 mmHg in young, middle-aged and diabetic subjects; and < 140/90 mmHg in the elderly. When home or ABP measurements are used, targets should be lower: 10–15 mmHg for SBP and 5–10 mmHg for DBP.

Management strategy

Lifestyle measures

Lifestyle measures should be instituted wherever appropriate in all patients including those who require drug therapy:

- to lower BP;
- to reduce the need for antihypertensive drugs and maximize their efficacy; and
- to address other RFs present.

Lifestyle measures that are widely agreed to lower BP and that should be considered in all patients are weight reduction, reduction of excessive alcohol consumption, reduction of high salt intake and increase in physical activity. Particular emphasis should be placed on cessation of smoking and on healthy eating patterns that contribute to the treatment of associated RFs and CVD.

Drug treatment

- Begin with the lowest dose to minimize adverse effects. If there is a good response and treatment is well tolerated but BP control remains inadequate, it is reasonable to increase the dose.
- Use appropriate drug combinations (Table 2.16). Using both drugs at low doses minimizes side-effects. Fixed low-dose combinations may be advantageous. Most patients are likely to require more than one drug.

Table 2.16 Effective drug combinations

- Diuretic + beta-blocker
- Diuretic + ACE inhibitor (or ARB)
- Calcium antagonist (dihydropyridine) + beta-blocker
- Calcium antagonist + ACE inhibitor
- Alpha-blocker + beta-blocker

ACE = angiotensin-converting enzyme; ARB = angiotensin receptor blocker. Source: WHO–ISH Guidelines 1999.

- Change to a different drug class if there is little response or poor tolerability to the first drug choice.
- Use long-acting drugs providing 24-hour efficacy on a once-daily basis to improve compliance with therapy and to minimize BP variability.

For patients in the high- and very high-risk groups, drug treatment should be instituted within a few days, as soon as repeated measurements have confirmed the patient's BP. For patients in the medium-risk groups, lifestyle measures with re-inforcement should be continued for 3–6 months before initiating drug treatment if goal BP is not achieved. For patients in the low-risk group, drug treatment should be initiated after 6 months to 1 year of assiduous lifestyle modification; in the border-line subgroup (DBP 90–94 mmHg and SBP 140–149 mmHg), lifestyle measures alone may be continued in the long-term. In contrast, in patients with high normal BP (130–139/85–95 mmHg) who also have diabetes mellitus and/or renal insufficiency, early antihypertensive drug therapy should be considered to reduce the risk of loss of renal function. A practical framework for the management of patients with grade 1 or 2 hypertension is shown in Fig. 2.3.

All available drugs are suitable for the initiation and maintenance of anti-hypertensive therapy, but the choice of drugs will be influenced by many factors (Table 2.17). The absolute effect of treatment on cardiovascular risk depends on absolute risk and BP reduction (Table 2.18).

Hypertension is termed refractory when a therapeutic plan that has included attention to lifestyle measures and the prescription of combination therapy at adequate doses has failed to lower BP to below 140/90 mmHg. Common causes of refractory hypertension are listed in Table 2.19.

Since the aim of treatment is the reduction of total cardiovascular risk, it is at least as important to treat the other RFs and ACCs in the individual hypertensive patient. It is reasonable to recommend, where BP has been rigorously controlled, the use of low-dose aspirin in hypertensive patients who are at high risk of CHD and who are not particularly at risk of bleeding from the gastrointestinal tract or from other sites. The use of cholesterol-lowering therapy can be recommended for hypertensive patients who have elevated serum cholesterol and who, for other reasons, are at high risk of CHD.

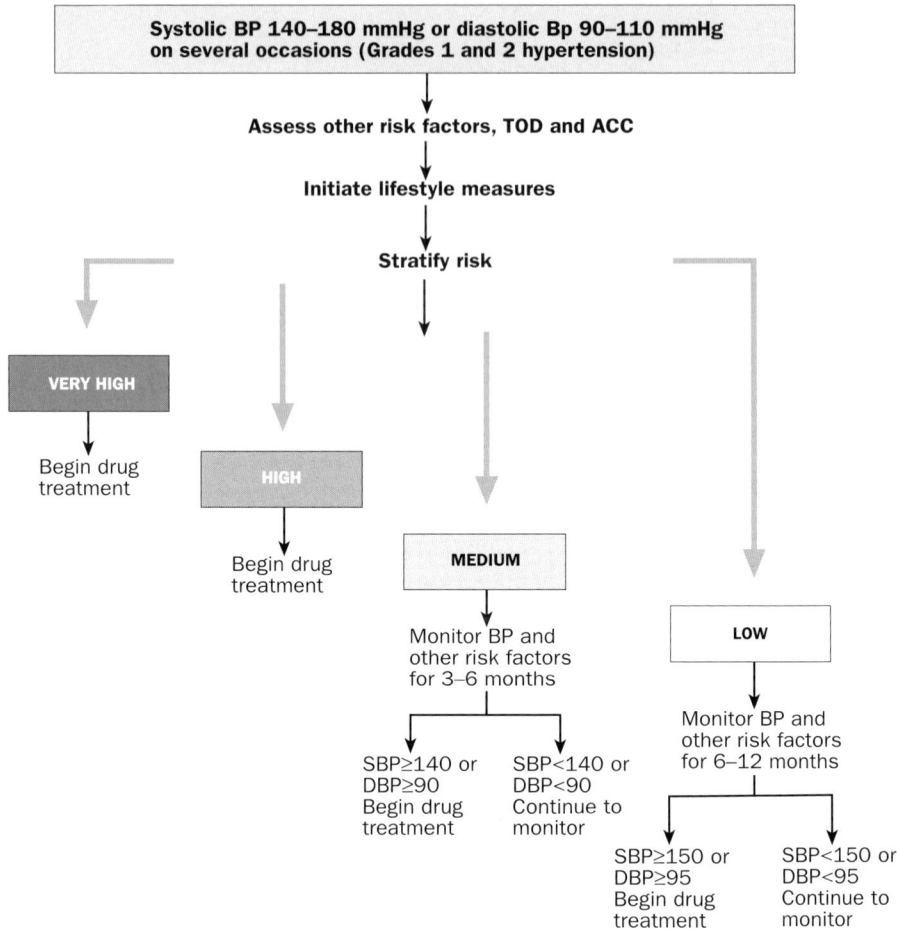

Fig. 2.3 A practical framework for the management of patients with grade 1 and grade 2 hypertension. TOD = target organ damage; ACC = associated clinical conditions; (S/D) BP = (systolic/diastolic) blood pressures.

Follow-up

The frequency of visits will depend on the overall risk category as well as the level of BP (Fig. 2.4). After prolonged BP control it may be possible to attempt careful progressive reduction in the dose and number of drugs used under careful supervision.

Implementation

These guidelines will be accompanied by a briefer companion set of 'Practice Guidelines' intended for translation into many languages and distribution to

Table 2.17 Guidelines for selecting drug treatment of hypertension

Class of drug	Compelling indications	Possible indications	Compelling contraindications	Possible contraindications
Diuretics	Heart failure Elderly patients Systolic hypertension	Diabetes	Gout	Dyslipidaemias Sexually active males
Beta-blockers	Angina After myocardial infarction	Heart failure Pregnancy	Asthma and COPD Heart block (a)	Dyslipidaemias Athletes and physically active patients Peripheral vascular disease
ACE inhibitors	Heart failure Left ventricular dysfunction After myocardial infarction Diabetic nephropathy		Pregnancy Hyperkalaemia Bilateral renal artery stenosis	
Calcium antagonists	Angina Elderly patients Systolic hypertension	Peripheral vascular disease	Heart block (b)	Congestive heart failure (c)
Alpha-blockers	Prostatic hypertrophy	Glucose intolerance Dyslipidaemias		Orthostatic hypotension
Angiotensin II antagonists	ACE inhibitor cough	Heart failure	Pregnancy Bilateral renal artery stenosis Hyperkalaemia	

(a) Grade 2 or 3 atrioventricular block; (b) Grade 2 or 3 atrioventricular block with verapamil or diltiazem; (c) verapamil or diltiazem COPD = chronic obstructive pulmonary disease. Adapted from WHO–ISH Guidelines 1999.

Table 2.18 Absolute effects of treatment on cardiovascular risk

Patient group	Absolute risk (CVD events/ 10 years)	Absolute treatment effect (CVD events prevented/ 1000 pt-years)	
		10/5 mmHg	20/10 mmHg
Low risk	< 15%	< 5	< 9
Medium risk	15–20%	5–7	8–11
High risk	20–30%	7–10	11–17
Very high risk	> 30%	> 10	> 17

CVD = cardiovascular disease; pt-years = patient treatment years. Source: WHO–ISH Guidelines 1999.

Table 2.19 Causes of refractory hypertension

- Secondary hypertension
- Poor concordance
- Drug interaction, e.g. NSAID
- Lifestyle, e.g. weight/alcohol
- Volume overload, e.g. inadequate diuretic
- Spurious, e.g. white-coat hypertension

NSAID = non-steroidal anti-inflammatory drug. Source: WHO–ISH Guidelines 1999

medical practitioners in many countries. The WHO–ISH guidelines can act as a model and a stimulus for the development of national recommendations adopted to suit the local culture and economic and social realities. It is hoped that such modified recommendations could be embedded in an implementation plan that reaches local medical practitioners and local communities alike.

Comment

The WHO–ISH guidelines provide recommendations that are based on the collective expert interpretation of the available evidence from epidemiological studies and clinical trials. The primary aim is to offer balanced information to guide clinicians rather than rigid rules that would constrain their judgement about the management of individual patients who will differ in their personal, medical, social, economic, ethnic and cultural characteristics.

These are both strengths and weaknesses. The guidelines are more a consensus statement than evidence-based recommendations, and there is a lack of clear practical advice. The WHO–ISH guidelines are written for a global audience of communities that vary widely in the nature of their health systems and the availability of resources. This challenge may have been beyond the capabilities of the authors.

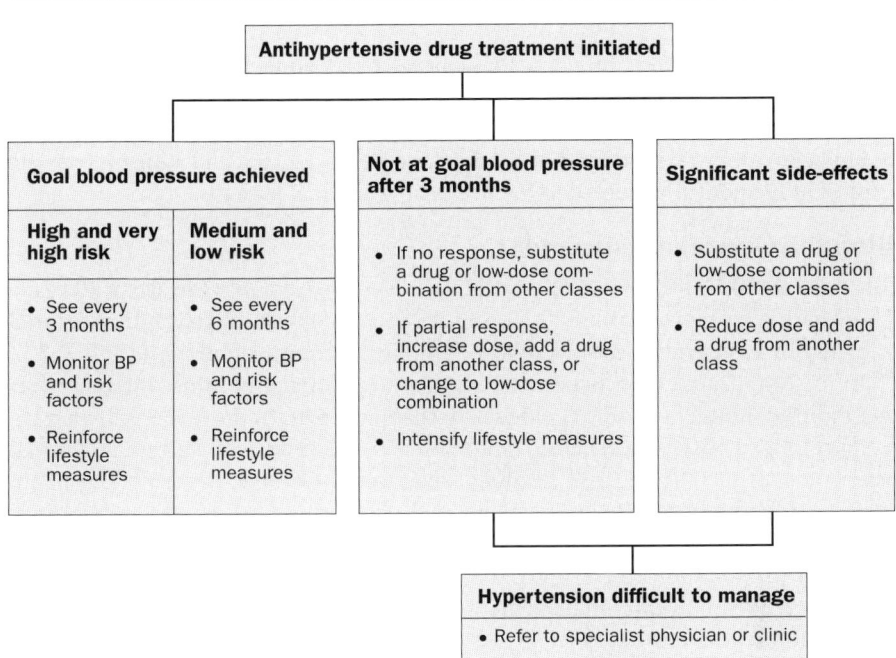

Fig. 2.4 Stabilization, maintenance and follow-up of patients with hypertension after initiation of drug therapy.

Guidelines for management of hypertension: report of the third working party of the British Hypertension Society [5, 6]

These guidelines update previous reports in 1989 [7] and 1993 [8]. Since the 1993 guidelines, much more evidence has emerged, notably on optimal BP targets during antihypertensive therapy, management of hypertension in diabetic patients and treatment of isolated systolic hypertension in the elderly. These important additions to an already formidable body of evidence provide the basis for the new recommendations. The guidelines embrace the concept that effective management of hypertension requires the identification of those at highest cardiovascular risk and the adoption of multifactorial intervention, targeting not only BP levels, but also associated cardiovascular RFs.

The guidelines recommend formal estimation of 10-year CHD risk using a computer program or risk chart. CHD risk is a good predictor of CVD risk (the proper focus of hypertension management), which can be approximated by multiplying the estimated 10-year CHD risk level by 4/3 (i.e. 30% CHD risk approximates to 40% CVD risk).

These guidelines are intended for general practitioners, practice nurses and generalists in hospital practice, and aim to present as clearly as possible the best currently available evidence on hypertension management. The guidelines should be applied with due regard to local circumstances and policies, and with appropriate clinical judgement with regard to the needs of individual patients.

Blood pressure measurement

All adults should have BP measured routinely every 5 years until the age of 80 years. Those with high–normal values (135–139/85–89 mmHg) should have BP measured annually. Measurement should follow standard recommendations (Table 2.20).

In uncomplicated mild hypertension, measurements at monthly intervals over 4–6 months should be used to guide the decision to treat. In more severe hypertension prolonged observation before treatment is not necessary or warranted. Formal assessment of CHD/CVD risk needs to take account of age, sex, smoking habit, diabetes, total high-density lipoprotein (HDL) cholesterol ratio and family history in addition to BP.

ABPM may be indicated in the circumstances shown in Table 2.21. Normal BP values by ABPM may alter management when there are no TOD or cardiovascular complications, the estimated CHD risk is < 15%, and elevated clinic BP (average ≥ 160/100 mmHg) is the only indication of high risk. The average daytime BP

Table 2.20 Blood pressure measurement

- Well-validated and maintained device
- Patient seated, arm at level of heart
- Bladder size appropriate
- Cuff deflated 2 mm/sec
- Measure ± 2 mmHg
- Phase V diastolic
- Two measurements per visit
- Repeated visits

Source: BHS Guidelines 1999.

Table 2.21 Circumstances where ambulatory blood pressure monitoring may be indicated

- Unusual variability in blood pressure
- Resistant hypertension
- Symptoms suggestive of hypotension
- White-coat hypertension

Resistant hypertension is defined as blood pressure > 150/90 mmHg on a regimen of three or more anti-hypertensive drugs. Source: BHS Guidelines 1999.

should be used for treatment decisions. Since ABP measurements are systematically lower than clinic measurements, treatment thresholds and targets must be adjusted downwards by about 12/7 mmHg when making decisions based on ABPM: i.e. an ABPM average daytime BP of 148/83 mmHg is approximately equivalent to a clinic BP of 160/90 mmHg, and may require treatment in some patients. Furthermore, a normal value from ABPM should be confirmed by a second ABPM record, because of within-patient variability and limited reproducibility. Also, patients left untreated on the basis of ABPM need reassessment of BP (perhaps repeated ABPM) and cardiovascular risk at least once a year. The same considerations apply to self-measurement of BP at home.

Non-pharmacological measures

Measures that lower blood pressure:

- weight reduction by calorie restriction
- reduced salt intake
- moderation of alcohol consumption
- physical exercise
- increased fruit and vegetable consumption
- reduced total and saturated fat intake

Measures to reduce cardiovascular risk:

- stop cigarette smoking
- increase polyunsaturated and monounsaturated fats
- increase oily fish consumption
- reduce total and saturated fat

Evaluation of hypertensive patients

All hypertensive patients should have a thorough history and physical examination (Table 2.22) but need only a limited number of routine investigations (Table 2.23). An echocardiogram is valuable to confirm or refute the presence of left ventricular hypertrophy when the ECG shows 'high' left ventricular voltage without T-wave abnormalities, as is often the case in young people. When the clinical evaluation or

Table 2.22 Aims of clinical evaluation of the hypertensive patient

- Causes of hypertension
- Contributory factors
- Complications of hypertension
- Cardiovascular risk factors
- Contraindications to specific drugs

Source: BHS Guidelines 1999.

Table 2.23 Routine investigations in the hypertensive patient

- Urine strip test
- U and E
- BS
- TC:HDL-C
- ECG

U and E = serum urea and electrolytes; BS = blood sugar; TC:HDL-C = serum total cholesterol: HDL cholesterol; ECG = electrocardiogram. Source: BHS Guidelines 1999.

Table 2.24 Indications for referral for specialist advice or treatment

- Urgent treatment
- Suspicion of secondary hypertension
- Therapeutic problem
- ABPM
- Pregnancy

ABPM = ambulatory blood pressure monitoring. Source: BHS Guidelines 1999.

the results of these simple investigations suggest a need for further investigation, it is usually best to refer for specialist advice. Indications for referral for specialist advice or treatment are summarized in Table 2.24.

Thresholds for antihypertensive therapy

Drug therapy should be started in all patients with sustained SBP ≥ 160 mmHg despite non-pharmacological measures (Fig. 2.5). Drug treatment is also indicated in patients with a sustained SBP of 140–159 mmHg or DBP of 90–99 mmHg if TOD or diabetes is present, or if the 10-year CHD risk is ≥ 15% (Fig. 2.6). The preferred method for estimation of risk is a computer program; but, where this is not practicable, a 'coronary risk chart' is recommended (Fig. 2.7). Thresholds for intervention and times to intervention are summarized in Fig. 2.6 and Table 2.25.

When a decision is reached not to treat a patient with mild hypertension, it is essential to continue observation and monitoring of BP and CHD risk at least once per year. These patients should be encouraged to continue with non-pharmacological measures to lower BP and cardiovascular risk.

Treatment goals

Recommendations for target BP during treatment are shown in Table 2.26. Systolic and diastolic targets should both be attained. The audit standard reflects the minimum recommended level of BP control.

BHS Guidelines

Threshold blood pressure

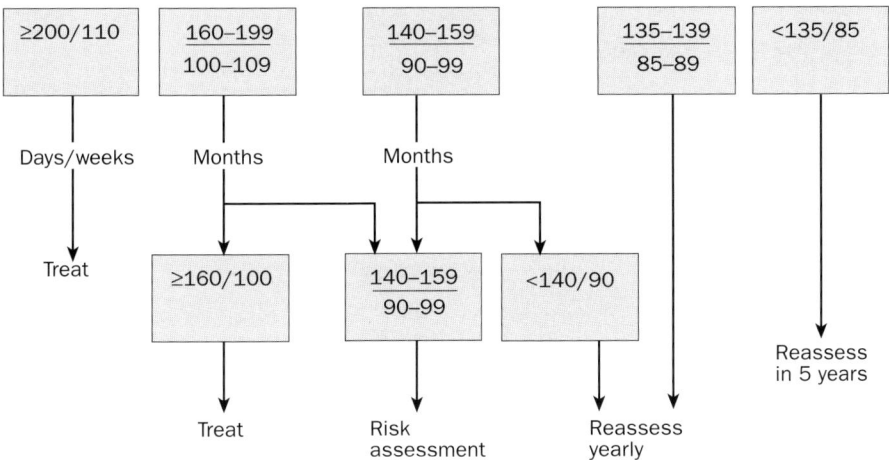

Fig. 2.5 Thresholds for antihypertensive drug therapy.

BHS Guidelines

Risk assessment

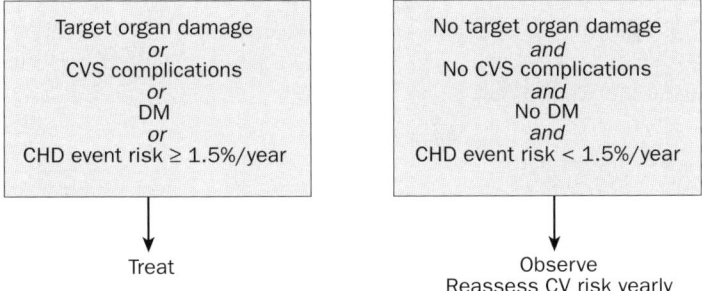

Fig. 2.6 Risk assessment in hypertensive patients. CVS = cardiovascular system; DM = diabetes mellitus; CHD = coronary heart disease; CV risk = cardiovascular risk.

No diabetes

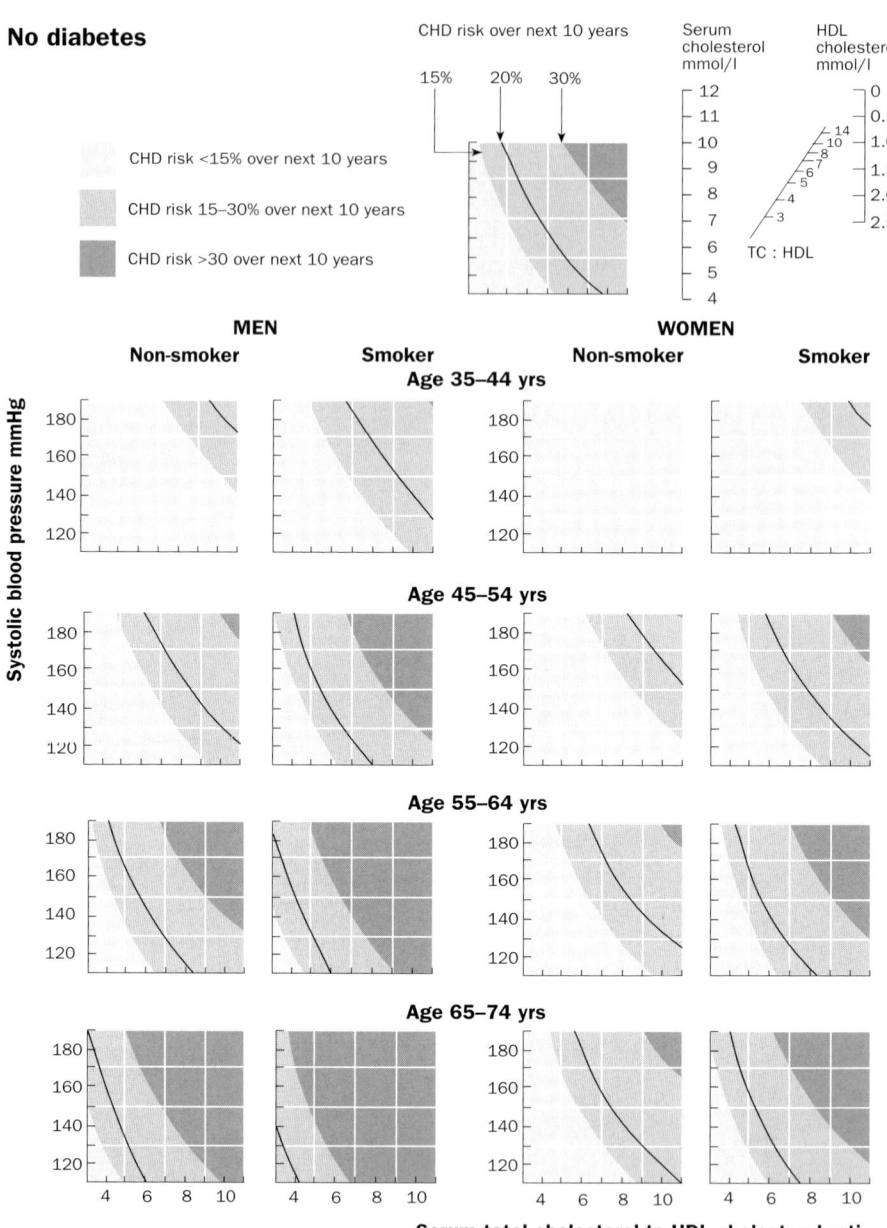

Fig. 2.7a Joint British Societies Coronary Risk Prediction Chart: without diabetes. CHD = coronary heart disease; HDL = high-density lipoprotein; TC = total serum cholesterol.

Diabetes

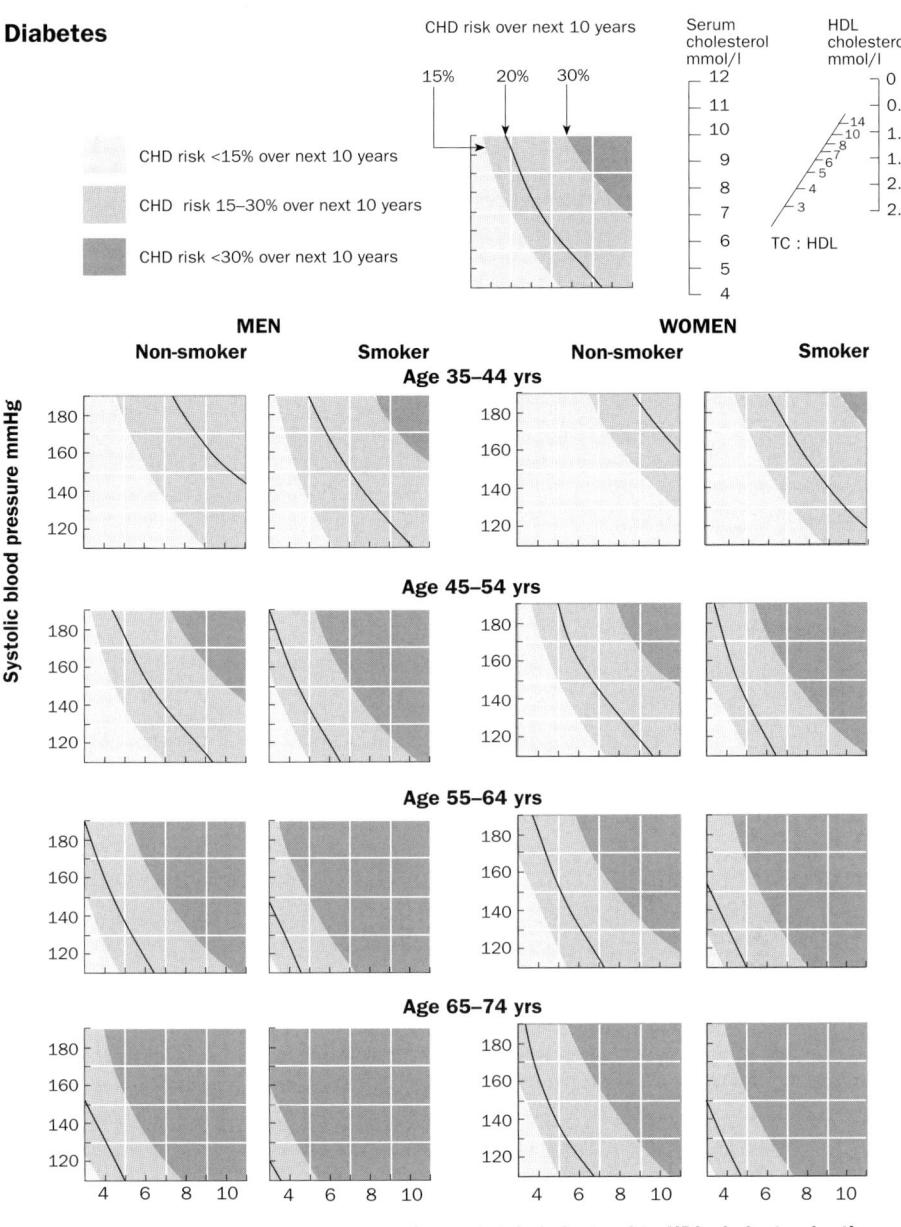

Fig. 2.7b Joint British Societies Coronary Risk Prediction Chart: with diabetes.
CHD = coronary heart disease; HDL = high-density lipoprotein; TC = total serum
cholesterol.

How to use the coronary risk prediction chart for primary prevention (Fig. 2.7)

These charts are for estimating coronary heart disease (CHD) risk (non-fatal myocardial infarction and coronary death) for individuals who have not developed symptomatic CHD or other major atherosclerotic disease.

The use of these charts is not appropriate for patients who have existing disease which already puts them at high risk. Such diseases are:

- CHD or other major atherosclerotic disease
- Familial hypercholesterolaemia or other inherited dyslipidaemia
- Established hypertension (SBP >160 mmHg and/or DBP >100 mmHg) or associated target organ damage (TOD)
- Diabetes mellitus with associated TOD
- Renal dysfunction

- To estimate an individual's absolute 10-year risk of developing CHD, find the table for their gender, diabetes (yes/no), smoking status (smoker/non-smoker) and age. Within this square define the level of risk according to SBP and the ratio of total cholesterol to HDL cholesterol. If there is no HDL cholesterol result, then assume this is 1.0 mmol/l and then the lipid scale can be used for total cholesterol alone.

- High-risk individuals are defined as those whose 10-year CHD risk exceeds 15% (equivalent to a cardiovascular risk of 20% over the same period). As a minimum, those at highest risk (30%) should be targeted and treated now, and as resources allow, others with a risk of >15% should be progressively targeted.

- Smoking status should reflect lifetime exposure to tobacco and not simply tobacco use at the time of risk assessment).

- The initial BP and the first random (non-fasting) total cholesterol and HDL cholesterol can be used to estimate an individual's risk. However, the decision on using drug therapies should be based on repeat risk factor measurements over a period of time. The chart should not be used to estimate risk after treatment of hyperlipidaemia or BP has been initiated.

- CHD risk is higher than indicated in the charts for:
  - Those with a family history of premature CHD (men <55 years and women <65 years), which increases the risk by a factor of approximately 1.5
  - Those with raised triglyceride levels
  - Those who are not diabetic but have impaired glucose tolerance
  - Women with premature menopause
  - Persons approaching the next age category. As risk increases exponentially with age the risk will be closer to the higher decennium for the last 4 years of each decade

- In ethnic minorities the risk chart should be used with caution, as it has not been validated for these populations.

- The estimates of CHD risk from the chart are based on groups of people, and in managing an *individual* the physician also has to use clinical judgement in deciding how intensively to intervene on lifestyle and whether or not to use drug therapies.

- An individual can be shown on the chart the direction in which the risk of CHD can be reduced by changing smoking status, BP, or cholesterol.

Table 2.25 Time to intervention in hypertension

- Immediate—malignant phase/emergencies
- 1–2 weeks—BP ≥ 200/110
- 3–4 weeks—BP ≥ 160/100 + complications/TOD/DM
- 4–12 weeks—BP ≥ 160/100
- 12 weeks—BP ≥ 140/90 + complications/TOD/DM
- 6 months—BP ≥ 140/90 + 10-year CHD risk ≥ 15%

BP = blood pressure; TOD = target organ damage; DM = diabetes mellitus; CHD = coronary heart disease. Source: BHS Guidelines 1999.

Table 2.26a Treatment targets for antihypertensive drug therapy–1: office blood pressure

	No diabetes	Diabetes
Optimal	< 140/85	< 140/80
Audit standard	< 150/90	< 140/85

Source: BHS Guidelines 1999.

Table 2.26b Treatment targets for antihypertensive drug therapy–2: ambulatory blood pressure monitoring

	No diabetes	Diabetes
Optimal	< 130/80	< 130/75
Audit standard	< 140/85	< 140/80

Source: BHS Guidelines 1999.

Choice of antihypertensive drug treatment

A low dose of thiazide is the first-line treatment unless there is a contraindication or a compelling indication for another drug. A long-acting dihydropyridine calcium antagonist is a suitable alternative for isolated systolic hypertension in the elderly when a low-dose thiazide is not tolerated or is contraindicated. The choice of drug will depend on relative indications and contraindications in individual patients (Table 2.27).

The drug or formulation used should ideally be effective when taken as a single daily dose. An interval of 4 weeks should be allowed to observe the full response, unless it is necessary to lower BP more urgently. The dose of thiazide diuretic should not be titrated upwards, whereas other drugs should be titrated according to the manufacturers' instructions. When the first drug is well tolerated but the

Table 2.27 Compelling and possible indications, contraindications and cautions for the major classes of antihypertensive drugs

Class of drug	Indications		Contraindications	
	Compelling	**Possible**	**Possible**	**Compelling**
α-blockers	Prostatism	Dyslipidaemia	Postural hypotension	Urinary continence
ACE inhibitors	Heart failure Left ventricular dysfunction Type I diabetic	Chronic renal disease Type II diabetic nephropathy	Renal impairment Peripheral vascular disease	Pregnancy Renovascular disease
Angiotensin II receptor antagonists	Cough induced by ACE inhibitor	Heart failure Intolerance of other antihypertensive drugs	Peripheral vascular disease	Pregnancy Renovascular disease
β-blockers	Myocardial infarction Angina	Heart failure	Heart failure Dyslipidaemia Peripheral vascular disease	Asthma or chronic obstructive pulmonary disease Heart block
Calcium antagonists (dihydropyridine)	Isolated systolic hypertension in elderly patients	Angina Elderly patients	—	—
Calcium antagonists (rate-limiting)	Angina	Myocardial infarction	Combination with β-blockade	Heart block Heart failure
Thiazides	Elderly patients	—	Dyslipidaemia	Heart failure

ACE = angiotensin-converting enzyme. Source: BHS Guidelines 1999.

response is insufficient, the options are to substitute another drug or add a second drug. Substitution is appropriate when hypertension is mild and uncomplicated, and the response to the initial drug is small. In more severe or complicated hypertension, it is safer to add drugs stepwise until BP control is attained. Treatment can be stepped down later if the BP falls substantially below the optimal level.

Drugs from the major classes have additive antihypertensive effects, but certain drugs should not be co-presented. These include beta-blockers with diltiazem or verapamil ACE inhibitors with ARBs and potassium-sparing diuretics with ACE inhibitors.

Other measures to reduce cardiovascular risk

Patients with established CVD or at high risk should be considered for aspirin and statin therapy.

- For *primary prevention*, aspirin 75 mg is recommended for hypertensive patients aged ≥50 years who have satisfactory control of BP (<150/90 mmHg) and TOD, diabetes or a 10-year CHD risk ≥ 15%; statin therapy is indicated when serum total cholesterol is ≥5% mmol/l and the 10-year CHD risk is ≥30% in patients aged ≤70 years.

- For *secondary prevention*, aspirin should be prescribed unless contraindicated; statin therapy is indicated when the serum total cholesterol is ≥5.0 mmol/l in patients aged ≤75 years.

Follow-up

The frequency of follow-up for treated patients after adequate BP control is attained is variable. A review every three months is sufficient when treatment and BP are stable, and the interval should not exceed 6 months.

Special patient groups

Elderly

Once started, antihypertensive therapy should be continued after patients reach the age of 80 years. Patients with newly diagnosed hypertension after the age of 80 years should be considered for treatment provided they are generally fit and have reasonable life expectancy, particularly if there are hypertensive complications or TOD. Similarly, doctors should consider the anticipated benefits and resource implications when reaching treatment decisions about patients aged >60 years with borderline isolated systolic hypertension (140–159/<90 mmHg).

Diabetes

In type I and type II diabetes, the threshold for starting antihypertensive therapy is ≥140/90 mmHg and the target BP is <140/80 mmHg. In type I diabetes with nephropathy, the target BP is <130/80 mmHg, or lower (<125/75 mmHg) when proteinuria is ≥1 g/24 hours; an ACE inhibitor titrated to the maximum dose recommended and tolerated is the preferred first-line therapy. In both forms of diabetes, rigorous control of BP invariably necessitates the use of combinations of antihypertensive drugs. As well as ACE inhibitors, low-dose diuretics, calcium antagonists, beta-blockers and alpha-blockers are all suitable.

Renal disease

In patients with chronic renal impairment, good BP control is essential to retard this process. Thresholds and targets are the same as for hypertensive patients with type I diabetes complicated by nephropathy. Multiple drugs, including a diuretic, are usually required. Since thiazide diuretics may be ineffective in patients with renal impairment, loop doses, frequently in high doses, are often required. Patients with renal failure have a very high risk of cardiovascular complications, and may need aspirin or statin in addition to antihypertensive management to reduce the burden of risk.

Oral contraceptives

BP should be measured before starting oral contraceptives and 6-monthly there-after. In hypertensive women, other non-hormonal forms of contraception should be sought, particularly if other RFs for CVD coexist. If other methods of contraception are unacceptable, changing to a progestogen-only pill is recommended. If BP does not fall to < 160/100 mmHg, antihypertensive medication should be instituted.

Hormone replacement therapy

Hormone replacement therapy is not contraindicated for women with hypertension provided BP can be controlled by antihypertensive medication. It is prudent to monitor BP 2–3 times in the first 6 months and then 6-monthly. Hormone replacement therapy should be discontinued temporarily in women with resistant hypertension to assess its contribution to BP.

Implementation

All practices and primary care groups should develop protocols for hypertension management, including methods for identifying and recalling patients who drop out of follow-up. Written confirmation should be available for patients. The practice policy should detail those aspects of management that are in the province of the practice nurse and the doctor, and the indications and procedures for passing management decisions from nurse to doctor and vice versa. It is recommended that implementation of the practice policy should be audited periodically.

Comment

The new British Hypertension Society guidelines are a natural progression from earlier reports. However, the new recommendations introduce the concept of formal risk assessment incorporating all cardiovascular risk factors, advocate much more rigorous treatment targets, formalize advice on other cardioprotective strategies, and promote greater efforts in implementations. The guidelines are supported by information material for patients and doctors prepared by and available from the Society.

In contrast to the JNC VI and WHO–ISH guidelines, the brevity of the British Hypertension Society guidelines will make them especially useful for clinicians. Perhaps the most controversial issue is the recommendation to initiate treatment on the basis of level of risk rather than level of BP in patients with the mildest hypertension. This algorithm represents an important new direction that will require evaluation, since it alters fundamentally the way in which doctors are encouraged to think about treatment of hypertension.

Joint British recommendations on prevention of coronary heart disease in clinical practice |9|

The British Cardiac Society, the British Hyperlipidaemia Association and the British Hypertension Society cooperated in preparing national recommendations, which have been endorsed by the British Diabetic Association. Previously, each society had worked independently, publishing independent guidelines. This professional isolation is mirrored in clinical practice, where major determinants of cardio-vascular risk can be overlooked.

It is hoped that collaboration among professional societies will result in a more unified and hence more effective approach to the prevention of CHD. To achieve this, it is necessary to include all cardiovascular RFs, rather than focusing on treat-ing a single RF. The authors concede that the recommendations are based on evidence rather than strictly 'evidence-based'.

Priorities and objectives

Individuals who present to doctors vary enormously in their risk of CHD. Priority should depend on risk, and the following is proposed:

- patients with established CHD or other major atherosclerotic disease; and
- individuals with hypertension, or other RFs, or combinations of RFs that put them at high risk of CHD.

The specific objectives are:

- in patients with established CHD or other major atherosclerotic disease, to pre-vent the risk of further major cardiac events and to reduce overall mortality; and
- in high-risk individuals in the general population, to reduce the risk of CHD or other major atherosclerotic disease.

Coronary heart disease risk

Patients with established CHD identify themselves to medical services, are at high risk and gain considerable benefit from treatment. Therefore, in these cases it is not necessary to calculate absolute coronary risk before deciding on intervention.

In the general 'healthy' population, individuals may be at high or low but unknown risk. Since benefit depends on risk, it is necessary to calculate absolute risk before taking treatment decisions.

A staged approach is recommended (Table 2.28). Those at highest risk should be targeted first, and, as a minimum, healthy individuals with $\geq 30\%$ CHD risk over 10 years should be identified and treated. This is consistent with advice from the Standing Medical Advisory Committee (SMAC) and the Scottish Intercollegiate Guidelines Network (SIGN). Patients with DBP ≥ 100 mmHg, familial hyperlipi-daemia and diabetes mellitus with TOD should be included in the priority group. As a next step, it is appropriate to expand RF intervention down to individuals with a 15% CHD risk over 10 years, provided those at higher levels of risk have already received effective preventive care.

To calculate risk, the computer program or coronary risk chart (Fig. 2.7) sub-sequently adopted by the British Hypertension Society is recommended. The RFs used to calculate CHD risk are listed in Table 2.29.

Table 2.28 Priorities for coronary heart disease (CHD) prevention

- Stage 1   Established vascular disease
- Stage 2   CHD risk ≥ 30%*
            plus
            SBP ≥ 160 mmHg
            DBP ≥ 100 mmHg
            Familial hypercholesterolaemia
            DM + TOD
- Stage 3   CHD ≥ 15%

* As recommended by the Standing Medical Advisory Committee (1998) and the Scottish Intercollegiate Guidelines Network (1999).
SBP = systolic blood pressure; DBP = diastolic blood pressure; DM = diabetes mellitus; TOD = target organ damage. Source: Joint British Recommendations 1998.

Secondary prevention

The interventions recommended are listed in Table 2.30. Lifestyle changes (Table 2.31) are the starting point, but only one component of management. Treatment of hypertension follows the British Hypertension Society guidelines (Table 2.32). Recommendations concerning serum lipids (≤ age 75 years), patients with diabetes mellitus, and the use of cardioprotective drugs are summarized in Tables 2.33–2.35.

Table 2.29 Risk factors used to calculate coronary heart disease (CHD) risk

- Smoking (current or recent)
- Blood pressure (repeated measures)
- Total cholesterol (repeated measures)
- HDL cholesterol (repeated measures)
- Diabetes
- FH of premature CHD
- ECG evidence of LVH

HDL = high-density lipoprotein; FH = family history; ECG = electrocardiogram; LVH = left ventricular hypertrophy. Source: Joint British Recommendations 1998.

Table 2.30 Management of risk factors in secondary prevention of coronary heart disease

- Lifestyle
- Blood pressure
- Serum lipids
- Glucose
- Cardioprotective drugs

Source: Joint British Recommendations 1998.

Table 2.31 Lifestyle modifications to prevent coronary heart disease

- Stop smoking
- Avoid obesity
- Reduce saturated fat intake
- Increase intake of poly(mono)unsaturated fat
- Increase fruit/vegetables/fish
- Moderate alcohol
- Increase physical activity

Source: Joint British Recommendations 1998.

Table 2.32 Treatment of blood pressure for secondary prevention of coronary heart disease

- Beta-blocker-based therapy
- Rate-limiting calcium antagonist
  —intolerant of beta-blocker
  —no LV dysfunction
- ACE inhibitor
  —LV dysfunction or failure
- Rigorous control
  —target SBP < 140 mmHg < 130 (DM)
         DBP < 85 mmHg < 80 (DM)
  —combination therapy often required

LV = left ventricular; ACE = angiotensin-converting enzyme; SBP = systolic blood pressure; DBP = diastolic blood pressure; DM = diabetes mellitus. Source: Joint British Recommendations 1998.

Table 2.33 Treatment of serum lipids for secondary prevention of coronary heart disease

- Dietary advice
- Statin if TC ≥ 5.0 mmol/l after diet
  or TC ≥ 6.0 mmol/l without diet
  (post-MI or unstable angina)
- Target TC < 5.0 mmol/l
  AND ≥ 33% reduction

TC = serum total cholesterol; MI = myocardial infarction. Source: Joint British Recommendations 1998.

Table 2.34 Management of diabetes mellitus for secondary prevention of coronary heart disease

- Lifestyle
- Blood pressure
- Serum lipids
- Glycaemic control

Source: Joint British Recommendations 1998.

Table 2.35 Cardioprotective drugs for secondary prevention of coronary heart disease

- Aspirin*
- Beta-blockers*
- Rate-limiting calcium antagonists+
- ACE inhibitors+
- Cholesterol-lowering drugs+
- Anticoagulants+

* Unless contraindicated. +Selected patients. ACE = angiotensin-converting enzyme. Source: Joint British Recommendations 1998.

Primary prevention

For patients without clinical atherosclerotic disease, the absolute risk of developing CHD or other atherosclerotic disease during the next 10 years should strongly influence the intensity of lifestyle and therapeutic intervention. The decision not to introduce a particular therapy for a particular individual should be reviewed regularly since risk increases with age, and may in the course of time become sufficient to justify intervention.

It is recommended that intervention is initiated at the absolute risk levels indicated in Table 2.28. For individuals with an absolute CHD risk < 15% over the next 10 years, drug therapy is not usually recommended.

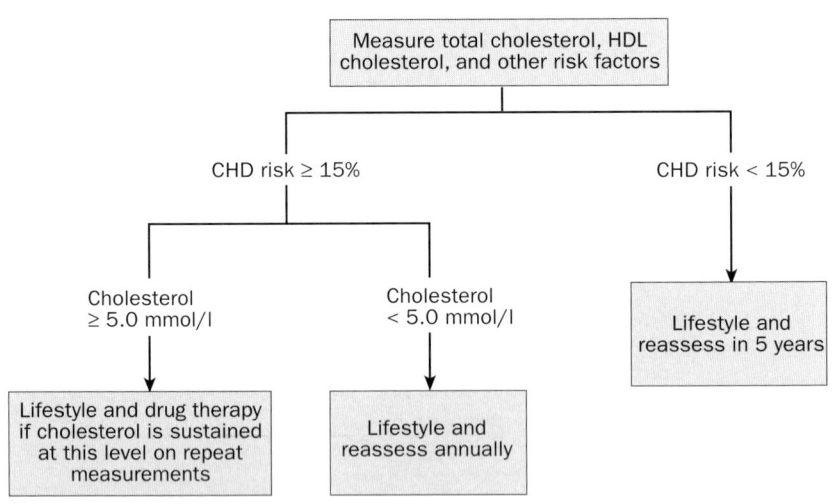

Fig. 2.8 Absolute coronary heart disease (CHD) risk and management of blood lipids in primary prevention of CHD and other atherosclerotic disease. HDL = high-density lipoprotein.

Lifestyle measures (Table 2.31) should be given priority, and will be the only approach offered to those with a CHD risk insufficient to justify pharmacotherapy. BP should be managed according to British Hypertension Society guidelines. The strategy for management of blood lipids in patients aged ≤69 years is shown in Fig. 2.8. In patients with type I and type II diabetes mellitus, efforts should be made to achieve not only tight glycaemic control, but also rigorous control of BP. The strategy for management of hypertension in diabetes is given in Table 2.36. Low-dose aspirin is recommended in selected high-risk patients using the criteria adopted in the British Hypertension Society guidelines. The management of patients with chronic renal failure is summarized in Table 2.37.

Table 2.36 Strategy for management of hypertension in a diabetic patient

- **Threshold**
  Type I   SBP ≥ 160   DBP ≥ 80 mmHg
  Type II SBP ≥ 160   DBP ≥ 90 mmHg
           SBP ≥ 140 mmHg (TOD)
- **Treatment**
  Type I   ACE inhibitor (ARB)
           + others
  Type II ACE inhibitor (ARB)
           or beta-blocker
           + thiazide/DHP calcium antagonist
- **Target**
  Type I/II SBP < 130   DBP < 80 mmHg
             SBP < 125   DBP <75 (proteinuria)

SBP = systolic blood pressure; DBP = diastolic blood pressure; TOD = target organ damage; ACE = angiotensin-converting enzyme; DHP = dihydropyridine; ARB = angiotensin receptor blocker. Source: Joint British Recommendations 1998.

Table 2.37 Strategy for management of hypertension in a patient with chronic renal failure

- **Blood pressure**
  —threshold SBP ≥ 140   DBP ≥ 90 mmHg
  —treatment ACE inhibitor (ARB)
              loop diuretic
              others
  —target   SBP ≥ 130   DBP ≥ 80 mmHg
- **Serum lipids**
  —statin
  —high risk

SBP = systolic blood pressure; DBP = diastolic blood pressure; ACE = angiotensin-converting enzyme; ARB = angiotensin receptor blocker. Source: Joint British Recommendations 1998.

Other recommendations

Screening of first-degree blood relatives (principally siblings and offspring aged ≥ 18 years) of patients with premature CHD or other atherosclerotic disease (men < 55 years and women < 65 years) is encouraged, and is essential in the context of familial hyperlipidaemia.

Auditing of the impact of common clinical protocols for hospital and general practice in the management of patients with CHD and other atherosclerotic diseases, and for the identification and management of high-risk individuals, is strongly recommended.

Comment

The Joint British Recommendations on Prevention of Coronary Heart Disease emphasize the need for practitioners to prioritize patients on the basis of risk, and advocate a staged approach to management. Patients with established CHD or other atherosclerotic diseases have the highest priority; therapeutic attention should be paid to individuals with hypertension and other risk predictors. The highest-priority patients should be treated appropriately and effectively. There is a need to calculate cardiovascular risk accurately in those without overt CVD.

Implementation requires an integrated care plan involving doctors and nurses in the primary and secondary care settings, and the patient. All RFs should be addressed by appropriate lifestyle measures and drug therapy. Regular audit of care protocols is essential.

Recommendations of the Second Joint Task Force of European and other Societies on Coronary Prevention |10|

These are similar in concept and objectives to the Joint British Recommendations (Fig. 2.9). The main differences relate to the threshold of absolute CHD risk at which drug treatment is recommended and the target BP. The Joint Task Force suggests an absolute CHD risk of ≥ 20% over 10 years or ≥ 20% if projected to the age of 60 years. A different risk chart is also recommended (Fig. 2.10). Optimal target BP is defined as < 140/90 mmHg in both primary and secondary prevention. Treatment algorithms for BP and blood lipids are shown in Figs. 2.11 and 2.12.

Comment

The differences from the British guidelines reflect national prejudices. The most controversial recommendation is the option to project an individual's predicted CHD risk to the age of 60 years. The accuracy of this approach is untested. An inevitable consequence will be a large number of individuals at currently low risk committed to long-term drug therapy. The advantages and disadvantages of this policy require careful scrutiny.

Lifestyle and therapeutic goals for patients with CHD, or other atherosclerotic disease, and for healthy high-risk individuals

| Patients with CHD or other atherosclerotic disease | Healthy high-risk individuals Absolute CHD risk ≥ 20% over 10 years, or will exceed 20% if projected to age 60 |

Lifestyle
Stop smoking, make healthy food choices, be physically active and achieve ideal weight

Other risk factors
Blood pressure <140/90 mmHg, total cholesterol <5.0 mmol/l (190 mg/dl)
LDL cholesterol <3.0 mmol/(115 mg/dl)
When these risk factor goals are not achieved by lifestyle changes, blood pressure and cholesterol-lowering drug therapies should be used.

Other prophylatic drug therapies

| Aspirin (at least 75 mg) for all coronary patients, those with cerebral atherosclerosis and peripheral atherosclerotic disease.
β-blockers in patients following myocardial infarction.
ACE inhibitors in those with symptoms or signs of heart failure at the time of myocardial infarction, or with chronic LV systolic dysfunction (ejection fraction <40%).
Anticoagulants in selected coronary patients. | Aspirin (75mg) in treated hypertensive patients, and in men at particularly high CHD risk. |

Screen close relatives

| Screen close relatives of patients with premature (men <55 yrs, women <65 yrs) CHD | Screen close relatives if familial hypercholesterolaemia or other inherited dyslipidaemia is suspected. |

Fig. 2.9 Framework for prevention of coronary heart disease (CHD) in clinical practice. LDL = low-density lipoprotein; ACE = angiotensin-converting enzyme; LV = left ventricular.

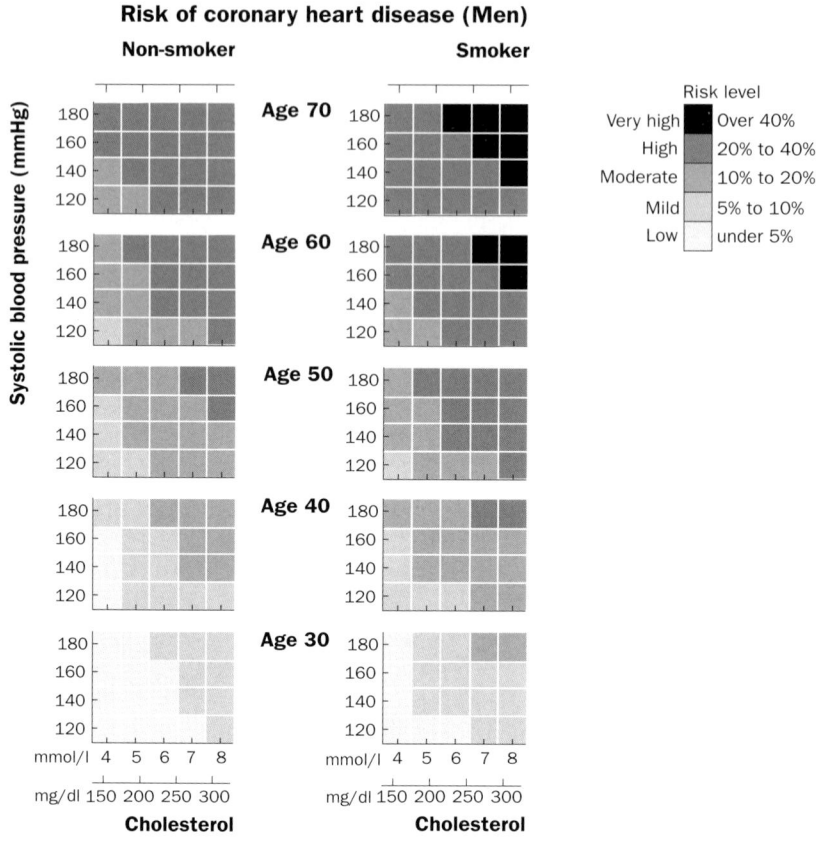

Fig. 2.10a Coronary risk chart: men.

How to use the coronary risk chart for primary prevention (Fig. 2.10)

- **To estimate a person's absolute 10-year risk of a CHD event**, find the table for their gender, smoking status, and age. Within the table, find the cell nearest to their systolic blood pressure (mmHg) and total cholesterol (mmol/l or mg/dl).
- **The effect of lifetime exposure to risk factors** can be seen by following the table upwards. This can be used when advising younger people.
- **High-risk individuals are defined as those whose 10-year CHD risk exceeds 20% or will exceed 20% if projected to age 60.**

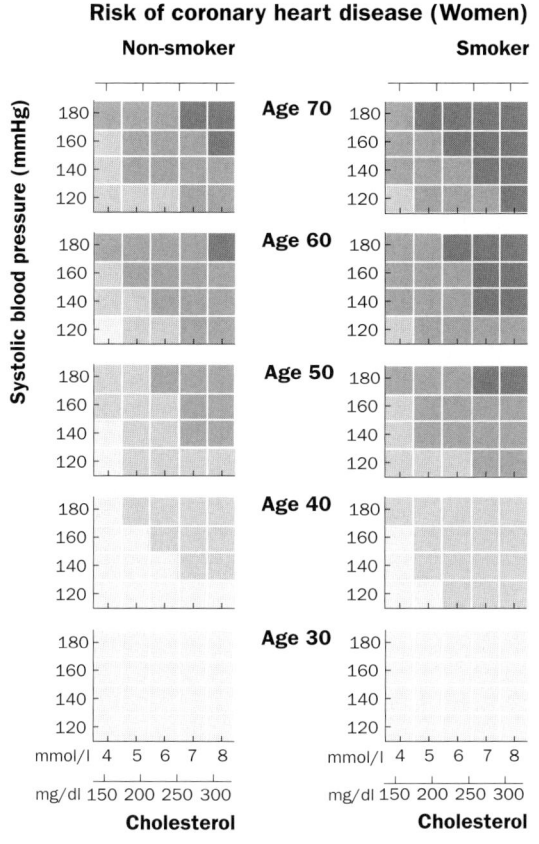

Fig. 2.10b Coronary risk chart: women.

- **CHD risk is higher than indicated** in the chart for those with:
  - Familial hyperlipidaemia (diabetes risk is approximately doubled in men and more than doubled in women);
  - Those with a family history of premature cardiovascular disease;
  - Those with low HDL cholesterol. These tables assume HDL cholesterol to be 1.0 mmol/l (39 mg/dl) in men and 1.1 (43) in women;
  - Those with raised triglyceride levels >2.0 mmol/l (>180 mg/dl);
  - As the person approaches the next age category.
- **To find a person's relative risk**, compare his/her risk category with that for other people of the same age. The absolute risk shown here may not apply to all populations, especially those with a low CHD incidence. Relative risk is likely to apply to most populations.
- **The effect of changing** cholesterol, smoking status, or BP can be read from the chart.

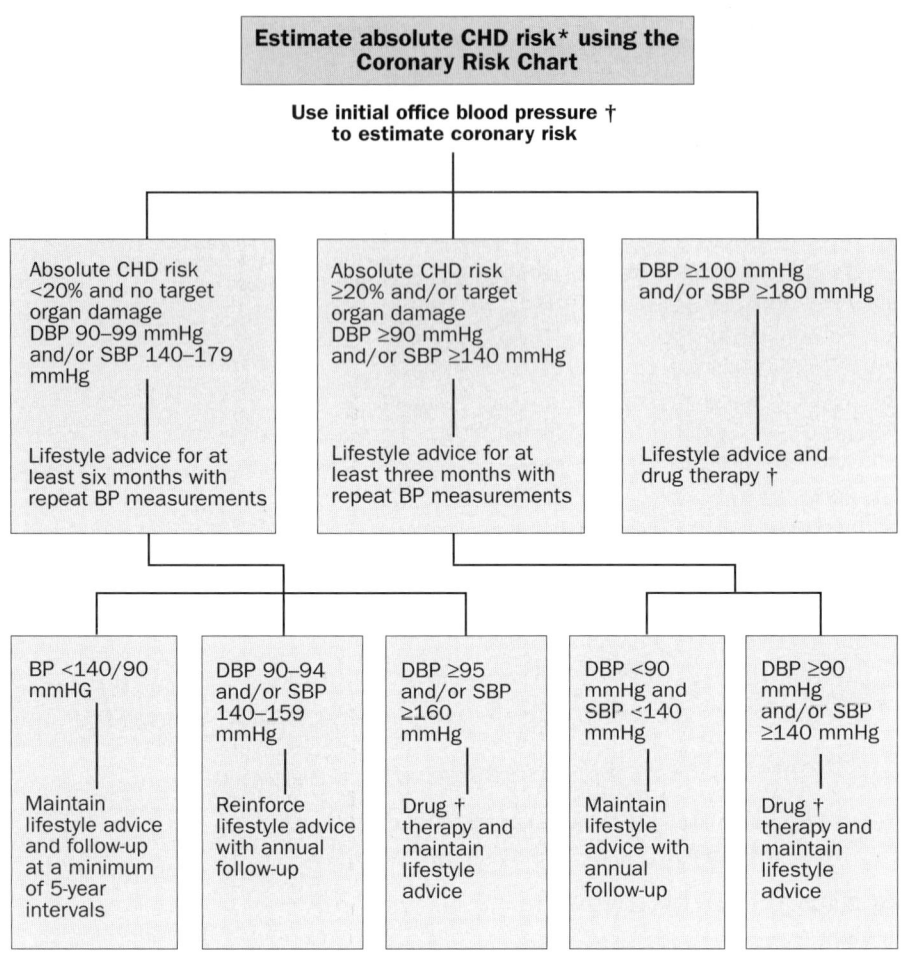

Fig. 2.11 Guide to blood pressure management in primary prevention. CHD = coronary heart disease; (S/D)BP = (systolic/diastolic) blood pressures.

* Ten-year CHD risk ≥ 20% or will exceed 20% if projected to age 60 years.

† Consider causes of secondary hypertension. If appropriate, refer to a specialist.

American Heart Association/American College of Cardiology statement on risk assessment |11|

This joint statement endorses the concept of calculating CHD risk. Absolute risk should be estimated from the major RFs. Thereafter, consideration can be given

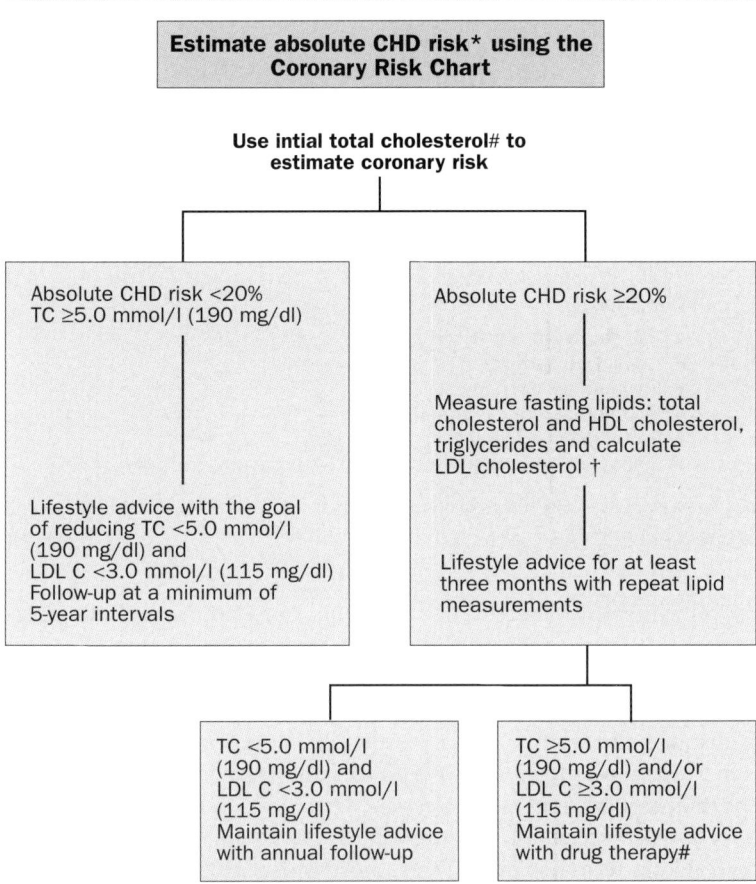

Fig. 2.12 Guide to lipid management in primary prevention. CHD = coronary heart disease; TC = total cholesterol; LDL(-C) = low-density lipoprotein (cholesterol); HDL = high-density lipoprotein.

* Ten-year CHD risk ≥ 20% or will exceed 20% if projected to age 60 years.
† HDL cholesterol < 1.0 mmol/l (40 mg/dl) and fasting triglycerides > 2.0 mmol/l (180 mg/dl) are markers for increased coronary risk.
# Consider genetically determined hyperlipidaemias (total cholesterol usually > 8.0 mmol/l (above 300 mg/dl) with stigmata of hyperlipidaemia such as obesity, diabetes, alcohol, liver and renal diseases. If appropriate, refer to a specialist.

to modifying the estimate in the presence of other RFs (Table 2.38). Clinical judgement is required to estimate the incremental risk incurred by these RFs.

Detection of patients at high risk with the aid of global risk assessment should be an important aim of routine medical evaluation of all patients. The reader is referred

Table 2.38 Other cardiovascular risk factors after consideration of major independent risk factors

Predisposing

- Obesity (Body Mass Index)
- Abdominal obesity
- Physical inactivity
- Family history of premature CHD
- Ethnic characteristics
- Psychosocial factors

Conditional

- Elevated serum triglycerides
- Small LDL particles
- Elevated serum homocysteine
- Elevated serum lipoprotein (a)
- Prothrombotic factors (e.g. fibrinogen)
- Inflammatory markers (e.g. C-reactive protein)

CHD = coronary heart disease; LDL = low-density lipoprotein. Source: AHA/ACC Statement 1999.

to JNC VI for specific therapy of hypertensive patients. Once appropriate therapies are selected, global risk scores can also be used to help instruct patients and to improve compliance with preventive interventions.

Global risk assessment is particularly useful in young and middle-aged adults for assessing both absolute and relative risk. Even though short-term risk may not be high in younger patients who have multiple RFs of only moderate severity, long-term risk can be unacceptably high. Risk assessment in those patients will highlight the need for early and prolonged intervention on RFs. In young adults, relative risk ratios help to reveal long-term risk of CHD, i.e. those within a particular age cohort who are most likely to suffer events. Although long-term prevention may not call for the use of risk-reducing drugs, it requires the introduction of lifestyle modification. Appropriate intervention, guided by risk assessment that is performed periodically in early adulthood and early middle age, has the potential to bring about a significant reduction in long-term risk.

Comment

This statement for health care professionals is long on rhetoric but short on practical advice. The method of calculating relative risk is complex and would be difficult to apply in most clinical settings. Furthermore, clear recommendations based on relative risk are not provided. Much of the advice depends on 'clinical judgement', and consistent implementation is unlikely. Again, risk projection is implicit in this statement.

Simple blood pressure guidelines for primary health care |12|

Professor Peter Sever has published a counterblast to the current epidemic of complex guidelines. He suggests four simple rules.

- **Rule 1** Abandon DBP measurement and rely on SBP values for decisions on treatment thresholds and goals.

- **Rule 2** Assess overall cardiovascular risk by history, physical examination and simple investigations (urine dipsticks, serum creatinine, glucose, lipids and ECG).

- **Rule 3** Apply a systolic threshold of 150 mmHg for the introduction of drug treatment when repeated measures of BP, following a trial of non-pharmacological treatment, remain persistently above this level. This threshold may be reduced to 140 mmHg for high-risk patients (e.g. those with TOD or diabetes) or raised to 160 mmHg for low-risk patients and the elderly.

- **Rule 4** Modify treatment if initial drug treatment is ineffective, partially effective or poorly tolerated. If BP does not fall below the pretreatment threshold, drug dosage should be increased (except that of diuretics), treatment should be changed or combinations should be used to achieve goal BP.

Comment

At first sight, these rules appear practical and refreshing, but, on closer inspection, problems appear. Apart from the elimination of DBP from the assessment, these simple guidelines are little different from a summary of the 1993 British Hypertension Society guidelines (lead author, Professor Sever). Reliance on SBP is unlikely to alter the individuals offered treatment, since very few will have DBP ≥ 100 mmHg (the 1993 guidelines threshold) and SBP < 150 mmHg.

Perhaps more importantly, it is left to the practitioner to identify high-risk patients from clinical clues. Sadly, doctors are very poor at this, as can be seen from the continued failure to identify and treat patients who are at high risk by any criteria, almost a decade after publication of the 1993 guidelines.

The goals of treatment are conservative. A target BP of 'below the treatment threshold' means that someone with a threshold SBP of 150 mmHg would be considered to have achieved satisfactory control if, on treatment, SBP was 149 mmHg. Intuitively, this makes no sense. Furthermore, the distribution of BP in the community dictates that the majority of patients who qualify for treatment will cluster around levels just above the threshold. Thus these guidelines will ensure only marginal improvement in BP in most treated patients. These guidelines may be simple, but are unlikely to result in great benefit for the individual.

Conclusions

The current guidelines all emphasize the importance of risk assessment in identifying individuals who merit treatment. Intuitive or informal assessment of risk by doctors is highly inaccurate. Without formal risk assessment, prescribing policies are very inconsistent, and are also prejudiced against certain high-risk groups such as smokers and older people. Some method of formal assessment is clearly necessary for rational prescribing.

Guidelines based on simple counting of RFs are distinctly less accurate than methods that count and weight RFs for CVD. These fail to treat individuals with high or even extremely high risk, while identifying for treatment many with a CHD risk of <0.6% per year. Provided the method of formal risk assessment is simple, it is easy to classify individuals.

Cardiovascular risk assessment has tremendous potential, but the future cannot be predicted with any real certainty for the presymptomatic individual. For 1000 adults with a 20% CVD risk, neither the 200 potential losers nor the 800 potential winners can be identified. Nevertheless, multi-variable risk equations can forecast accurately the absolute risk of future events and predict the benefit of intervention.

The challenge is to 'operationalize' the information so that patients and physicians can make informed decisions. Reaching a consensus about the threshold of absolute risk for intervention is difficult. Also, there are limitations of short-term risk assessment, which favours treatment of older individuals in whom the immediate absolute risk of disease is high. However, older individuals without symptomatic disease can be classified among the winners, since they have tolerated RFs over years. Younger patients with RFs may have short-term absolute risk below a prespecified threshold, yet gain the most benefit over the long term, and are at increased risk of premature disease.

Nonetheless, cardiovascular risk assessment is an important addition to the doctor's diagnostic and prognostic black bag. If nothing else, it provides a framework to help inform otherwise healthy individuals of increased risk and help them to make informed decisions. The poor compliance with cardioprotective drug therapy suggests that patients who start treatment are not convinced of its benefit.

Professional compliance is also poor. Despite many national and international guidelines offering evidence-based recommendations on the management of hypertension, there is little evidence that clinical practice has improved. Guidelines are widely acknowledged but largely ignored.

It appears to be assumed that recommendations will filter down to the local level; but the flow is unlikely to be successful without efforts to improve implementation. Implementation depends on availability, accessibility, audit and education. For education to be successful it must be authoritative, simple, short, practical, attractive and repeated.

Practitioners value management guidelines, but consider those available to be too scientific, excessively demanding of resources, and of impractical complexity, of limited local applicability, and also to have a short shelf-life. Guidelines appear to be updated every few years to follow current fashion rather than to respond to important new evidence. Useful guidelines would be simple, practical, consider local resources and priorities, and incorporate local experience, opinion and judgement. Guidelines are likely to be implemented if they are clear and evidence-based, but not if they are vague, controversial, or demand change in practice or practice routines.

Interventions to promote implementation have met with varied success. The most consistently successful approaches include educational outreach with an interactive component and repeated reminders of key priorities. A multifactorial targeted approach involving audit, reminders and consensus is often particularly useful. The techniques usually employed, such as dissemination of summary guidelines, have no effect.

If management of hypertension is to improve, a much more practical approach is needed. Evidence and evidence-based guidelines are still necessary, but more attention must be paid to generation, dissemination and implementation. Only then can professional non-compliance with recommendations on best practice be corrected.

References

1. Joint National Committee on Prevention, Detection, Evaluation and Treatment of High Blood Pressure. The sixth report of the Joint National Committee on Prevention, Detection, Evaluation and Treatment of High Blood Pressure. *Arch Intern Med* 1997; **157**: 2413–46.

2. Joint National Committee on Detection, Evaluation and Treatment of High Blood Pressure. Fifth report of the Joint National Committee on Detection, Evaluation and Treatment of High Blood Pressure. *Arch Intern Med* 1993; **153**: 154–83.

3. Coope JN, Warrender TS. Randomised trial of hypertension in elderly patients in primary care. *BMJ* 1986; **293**: 1148–51.

4. Guidelines Subcommittee. 1999 World Health Organisation–International Society of Hypertension guidelines for the management of hypertension. *J Hypertens* 1999; **17**: 151–83.

5. Ramsay LE, Williams B, Johnston GD, MacGregor GA, Poston L, Potter JF, *et al.* Guidelines for management of hypertension: report of the third working party of the British Hypertension Society. *J Hum Hypertens* 1999; **13**: 569–92.

6. Ramsay LE, Williams B, Johnston GD, MacGregor GA, Poston L, Potter JF, *et al.* British Hypertension Society guidelines for hypertension management 1999: summary. *BMJ* 1999; **319**: 630–5.

7. Swales JD, Ramsay LE, Coope JR, *et al.* Treating mild hypertension. Report of the British Hypertension Society working party. *BMJ* 1989; **298**: 694–8.

8. Sever P, Beevers G, Bulpitt C, Lever A, Ramsay L, Reid J, *et al.* Management guidelines in essential hypertension. Report of the second working party of the British Hypertension Society. *BMJ* 1993; **306**: 983–7.

9. Wood D, Durrington P, McInnes G, Poulter N, Rees A, Wray A. Joint British recommendations on prevention of coronary heart disease in clinical practice. *Heart* 1998; **80** Suppl 2: S1–S29.

10. Wood D, De Backer G, Faergeman O, Graham I, Mancia G, Pyörälä K. Prevention of coronary heart disease in clinical practice. Summary of recommendations of the Second Joint Task Force of European and other Societies on Coronary Prevention. *J Hypertens* 1998; **16**: 1407–14.

11. Grundy SM, Pasternak R, Greenland P, Smith S, Fuster V. Assessment of cardiovascular risk by use of multiple-risk-factor assessment equations. A statement for healthcare professionals from the American Heart Association and the American College of Cardiology. *Circulation* 1999; **100**: 1481–92.

12. Sever PS. Simple blood pressure guidelines for primary health care. *J Hum Hypertens* 1999; **13**: 725–7.

3

Ongoing trials

Introduction

The combined results of previous randomized controlled trials, involving a total of about 47 000 patients with hypertension, have demonstrated that diuretic- and beta-blocker-based regimens produce much of the epidemiologically expected benefit of the blood pressure (BP) reduction achieved [1]. The proportional reductions in the risks of strokes and coronary heart disease (CHD) events appeared to be broadly similar for patients with mild, moderate and more severe hypertension, for older and young patients, and for patients with and without a history of cerebrovascular disease. Thus the magnitude of the absolute benefit of treatment varied in direct proportion to the background level of risk (i.e., patients with the highest absolute risk of stroke or CHD experienced the largest absolute reduction of risk).

Data from four direct randomized comparisons of diuretic- and beta-blocker-based regimes collectively demonstrated no evidence of a difference between these treatments on stroke or CHD outcomes. However, although a total of 24 000 patients was studied, even in combination these studies lacked adequate statistical power to determine reliably modest but potentially important treatment differences (e.g. a 10–15% difference in the relative risk of CHD).

Even less information is available concerning the effects of newer classes of antihypertensive agents. The SYST-EUR study [2] and the Shanghai Trial of Nifedipine in the Elderly (STONE) [3] indicated a significant reduction in stroke risk of about 40–50% compared with placebo in patients treated with nitrendipine and nifedipine, respectively. In comparison with conventional therapy (diuretics, beta-blockers), long-acting calcium antagonists showed no advantage in elderly hypertensive patients [4]. Likewise, angiotensin-converting enzyme (ACE) inhibitors and conventional agents had similar effects in STOP-Hypertension–2 [4] and in CAPPP [5], although relative advantages of captopril were reported in the diabetic subset of CAPPP [5]. Unfortunately, deficiencies in the conduct of CAPPP make its results unreliable.

Ongoing randomized controlled trials have been designed primarily to provide more reliable data about the effects of newer drug classes on cardiovascular (CV) mortality and morbidity in various patient populations. The trials fall into two categories:

- comparison of newer and older drug classes for the treatment of patients with high BP; and
- evaluation of newer drugs in patients with high risk (e.g. established cardiac disease, cerebrovascular disease, diabetes, renal disease, the elderly).

At usual doses, most of the newer agents produce reductions in blood pressure (BP) of similar magnitude to those produced by diuretics and beta-blockers |6|. Hence, any differences between the effects on stroke risk and CHD risk of regimens based on the older and the newer agents would have to be due to properties of the drugs that are independent of their BP-lowering effects. Many such properties have been postulated. However, it is unknown whether these influences augment the benefits of lowering BP, and any independent effects are unlikely to be large. Detection of plausible differences in relative risk (of 15% or less) between various antihypertensive regimens on stroke and CHD will require evidence from randomized trials involving many thousands of patients and 1000 or more outcome events. Fewer events are required to detect the effect of the same treatment compared with placebo, since the likely effects of treatment will be larger; but such studies are ethically acceptable in only a few clinical circumstances.

This chapter will review the design and current status of a selection of the more important ongoing trials. Examples from both the main categories of outcome trials will be discussed. However, a clear distinction between comparisons between newer drugs and older drugs in hypertensive patients and those between various newer drugs in patients at high risk of CV events is not always easy, since patients with multiple risk factors are targeted in most trials to increase the probability of achieving the necessary event rates. In addition, in many studies, the influence of other cardioprotective strategies (such as lipid-lowering therapy) is often incorporated.

Comparison of older and newer drug classes

Antihypertensive therapy and Lipid-Lowering Heart Attack prevention Trial (ALLHAT)

Rationale and design for the Antihypertensive and Lipid-Lowering to prevent Heart Attack Trial (ALLHAT).
B R Davis, J A Cutler, D J Gordon, C D Furberg, J T Wright, W C Cushman, *et al. Am J Hypertens* 1996; **9**: 342–60.

BACKGROUND. **ALLHAT is a randomized double-blind trial in high-risk hypertensive patients. It compares a calcium channel blocker (amlodipine), an ACE inhibitor (lisinopril), and an alpha-blocker (doxazosin) with the thiazide diuretic chlorthalidone. The main eligibility criteria are systolic and diastolic hypertension in patients aged $\geq$ 55 years who have at least one further CHD risk factor, e.g. left ventricular hypertrophy (LVH), known atherosclerotic CV disease, cigarette smoking or type II diabetes mellitus.**

INTERPRETATION. ALLHAT is the only clinical trial of this nature with sufficient statistical power to assess the impact on CHD events separately from that on other CV events. It is designed to assess whether or not newer antihypertensive drugs can provide greater reductions in CV events relative to treatment with thiazide diuretics.

Outline

Patients: 42 448
Planned follow-up: 6 years
Factorial assignment: Lipid-lowering therapy
Completion date: 2002
Entry criteria: Hypertension + CV disease risk
Age: ≥ 55 years
Diastolic BP: 90–109 mmHg
Systolic BP: 140–179 mmHg
Projected events:
CHD: 2580
Strokes: 2790

ALLHAT is the largest hypertension outcome trial ever undertaken. It is a randomized, double-blind study in men and women aged ≥ 55 years. Representatives of four major classes of antihypertensive agents are compared: a diuretic (chlorthalidone), a calcium channel blocker (amlodipine), an ACE inhibitor (lisinopril) and an alpha-blocker (doxazosin). The study duration is 6–8 years.

The principal question addressed by ALLHAT is whether different antihypertensive agents differ in the prevention of CHD mortality and morbidity, independent of BP lowering—in particular whether newer agents do so when compared with a diuretic. ALLHAT also examines the question of whether lowering low-density lipoprotein (LDL) cholesterol with an HMG-CoA (3-hydroxy-3-methyl-glutaryl coenzyme A) reductase inhibitor (pravastatin) prevents CV disease and all-cause mortality better than with usual care (diet alone).

The primary endpoint is CHD death or non-fatal myocardial infarction (MI). Secondary endpoints include all-cause mortality, combined CV disease, stroke and LVH. Recruitment at 623 community centres and Veterans Administration sites throughout the US, Canada, Puerto Rico and the US Virgin Islands was completed in 1998, and results are expected in 2002. Patient follow-up is 4–8 years (average 6 years).

Participants are high-risk patients with BP ≥ 140/90 mmHg and one or more of the following risk factors: MI (not recent), stroke, coronary artery bypass graft or angioplasty, major ST segment depression or T-wave inversion on electrocardiogram (ECG), known atherosclerotic CV disease, type II diabetes, high-density lipoprotein (HDL) cholesterol ≤ 35 mg/dl, LVH and cigarette smoking. Exclusion criteria include symptomatic ischaemic heart disease (angina), left ventricular systolic dysfunction (ejection fraction < 35%) and renal impairment (serum creatinine > 2 g/dl).

Preliminary data on patient characteristics indicate that 53% are men, 35% are Afro-Americans, 16% are Hispanic and 36% have type II diabetes mellitus. ECG evidence of LVH was present at randomization in > 15% of participants. Average age is about 70 years and around 20% are cigarette smokers. About 25% of patients are enrolled in the lipid-lowering segment of the trial, which involves patients with

Table 3.1 Cardiovascular (CV) events in ALLHAT. Relative risk (RR), doxazosin versus chlorthalidone

	RR	95% CI	P-value
Combined CV disease events	1.25	1.17, 2.32	$10^{\times 10}$
Congestive heart failure	2.04	1.71, 2.35	$10^{\times 26}$
Combined CV disease events (excluding congestive heart failure)	1.13	1.06, 1.21	< 0.001
Stroke	1.19	1.01, 1.40	0.04
CHD events	1.03	0.90, 1.17	0.71

95% CI = 95% confidence interval; CHD = coronary heart disease.

mild to moderately elevated total cholesterol. Patient characteristics are evenly distributed between the treatment groups.

It is projected that ALLHAT will accumulate 2580 CHD events and 2790 strokes. This makes it the only trial of this nature with sufficient statistical power to assess the impact on CHD events separately from that on all other CV events.

One part of ALLHAT was stopped prematurely in early 2000. Users of doxazosin had 25% more CV events and were twice as likely to be hospitalized for congestive heart failure as users of chlorthalidone (Table 3.1). The drugs were similarly effective in preventing heart attacks and in reducing the risk of death from all causes. Those in the doxazosin group had slightly higher systolic BP than those in the chlorthalidone group, although diastolic BPs were the same (137/76 mmHg versus 135/76 mmHg, respectively). The doxazosin group also had poorer compliance with therapy; only 75% were still taking the drug or another alpha-blocker after 4 years, compared with 86% still taking chlorthalidone or another diuretic. Another reason for discontinuation was futility—the study had < 1% chance of detecting an advantage of doxazosin over chlorthalidone for CHD events.

It was advised that patients taking an alpha-blocker should consult their doctor about alternative therapy. An alpha-blocker may not be the best choice for initial therapy. It cannot be concluded that doxazosin is harmful, but it is less effective than chlorthalidone in reducing CV disease.

Comment

ALLHAT is a formidable scientific and logistical undertaking. Its findings will have far-reaching consequences. However, ALLHAT has limitations that may cloud interpretation. Many patients are likely to require more than one antihypertensive agent in combination, and many will have established CV disease. Since beta-blockers, with known secondary protective properties, are likely to be added as a second-step agent, producing a clear and unequivocal interpretation of the results is likely to present some difficulties. Findings in high-risk patients may also not be easy to extrapolate to the majority of hypertensive patients with much lower CV risk.

Early findings suggest that not all antihypertensive agents are created equal, and that BP reduction alone cannot be considered as a valid surrogate endpoint that reflects real outcomes (MI, stroke and death). The fact that the reassuring concept of the primacy of BP reduction has been shattered by the discovery that doxazosin is associated with poorer outcomes than chlorthalidone is ironic, since alpha-blockers have been widely advocated on the basis that their metabolic influence affords advantages over diuretics. Thus there has been much hope (or hype) that doxazosin would have benefits beyond BP reduction over diuretics by improving the surrogate marker, hypertensive metabolic syndrome. The outcome of the doxazosin arm of ALLHAT is a warning to those who advocate management decisions based on surrogate (or intermediate) endpoints. Such optimism should not have been allowed to distract from the lack of outcome data concerning this drug class and from its known relatively moderate antihypertensive efficacy, certainly in the supine posture (where we spend one-third of our lives), and relatively poor tolerability, which inevitably leads to poor compliance.

The Anglo-Scandinavian Cardiac Outcomes Trial (ASCOT)

The Anglo Scandinavian Cardiac Outcomes Trial (ASCOT).

B Dahlöf, P S Sever, N R Poulter. Proceedings of the 17th Meeting of the International Society of Hypertension, Amsterdam, 1998 (abstract).

BACKGROUND. ASCOT addresses directly two important practical issues as its primary aims:

- A comparison of the effects of conventional antihypertensive drug regimens based on beta-blocker and thiazide diuretic and contemporary antihypertensive drug regimens based on dihydropyridine calcium channel blocker and ACE inhibitor; and
- A prospective assessment of combined lipid-lowering (with atorvastatin) and antihypertensive treatment in hypertensive patients with total cholesterol ≤ 6.5 mmol/l.

INTERPRETATION. The primary endpoints in ASCOT are reductions in fatal and non-fatal CHD; secondary endpoints include other CV events and total mortality. The factorial study design allows the benefits of BP reduction and cholesterol reduction to be analysed separately.

Outline

Patients: 18 000
Planned follow-up: 5 years
Randomized treatment: Dihydropyridine calcium antagonist ± ACE inhibitor, beta-blocker ± diuretic
Factorial assignment: Atorvastatin, placebo
Completion: 2003
Entry criteria: Hypertension + CV disease risk
Age: 40–79 years

Diastolic BP: ≥ 90 mmHg
Systolic BP: ≥ 140 mmHg
Projected events:
CHD: 1150
Strokes: 400

ASCOT has a 2×2 factorial design, with an antihypertensive and a lipid-lowering wing. In the antihypertensive limb, standard therapy based on atenolol $\pm$ bendrofluazide is compared with contemporary therapy based on amlodipine $\pm$ perindopril in a Prospective Randomized Open Blinded Endpoint (PROBE) evaluation. Supplementary therapy in both regimens is with doxazosin (GITS, Gastro Intestinal Therapeutic System) $\pm$ moxonidine $\pm$ free choice, but avoiding drug classes in the comparator regimens. The lipid-lowering arm consists of a double-blind comparison of atorvastatin 10 mg daily and placebo in participants with a serum total cholesterol ≤ 6.5 mmol/l. In those subjects with higher serum total-cholesterol levels, lipid-lowering management should be according to local guidelines.

It is planned to recruit 18 000 eligible subjects in the UK, Ireland, Denmark, Finland, Iceland, Norway and Sweden. Participants are randomized to standard or contemporary antihypertensive regimens and subjects eligible for the lipid-lowering arm are secondarily randomized to atorvastatin or placebo. It is anticipated that 9000 patients will participate in the lipid-lowering arm (Fig. 3.1). Patient recruit-

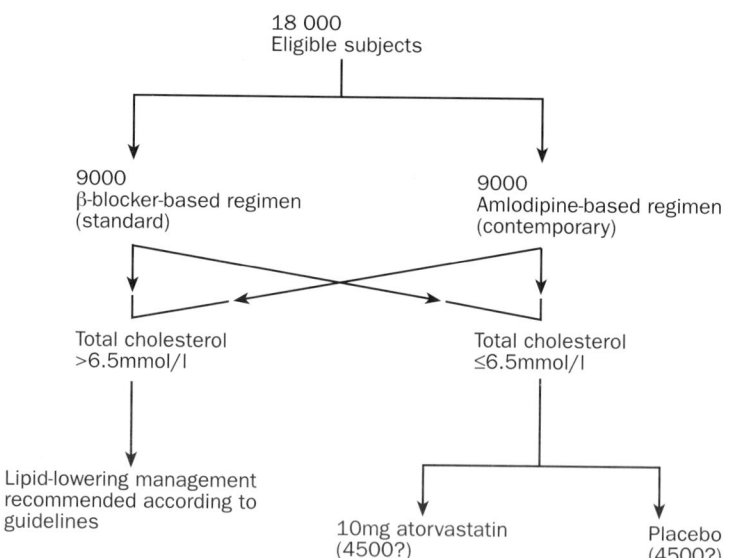

Fig. 3.1 Treatment allocation in the Anglo-Scandinavian Cardiac Outcomes Trial (ASCOT).

Table 3.2 Antihypertensive drug regimens in ASCOT

	Group A	Group B
Step 1	Amlodipine 5 mg	Atenolol 50 mg
Step 2	Amlodipine 10 mg	Atenolol 100 mg
Step 3	Amlodipine 10 mg	Atenolol 100 mg
	Perindopril 4 mg	BFZ 1.25 mg + K$^+$
Step 4	Amlodipine10 mg	Atenolol 100 mg
	Perindopril 8 mg (2 × 4 mg)	BFZ 2.5 mg + K$^+$
Step 5	Amlodipine 10 mg	Atenolol 100 mg
	Perindopril 8 mg (2 × 4 mg)	BFZ 2.5 mg + K$^+$
	Doxazosin GITS 4 mg	Doxazosin GITS 4 mg
Step 6	Amlodipine 10 mg	Atenolol 100 mg
	Perindopril 8 mg (2 × 4 mg)	BFZ 2.5 mg + K$^+$
	Doxazosin GITS 8 mg	Doxazosin GITS 8 mg

BFZ = bendrofluazide; GITS = Gastrointestinal Therapeutic System.

ment will be completed in 2000 and the study should end in 2003. Average planned follow-up is 5 years.

The primary objectives of ASCOT are to compare the effects of the two anti-hypertensive regimens on non-fatal acute MI plus total CHD events, and to compare the effects of atorvastatin and placebo on the same outcomes. There are 16 further secondary and tertiary objectives, including effects on total (fatal and non-fatal) stroke, all-cause mortality and heart failure.

Eligible patients must satisfy the following criteria: untreated systolic BP ≥ 160 mmHg or untreated diastolic BP ≥ 100 mmHg *or* treated systolic BP ≥ 140 mmHg or treated diastolic BP ≥ 90 mmHg; age 40–79 years; and ≥ 3 of 11 stipulated risk factors, *viz.* male sex, age ≥ 55 years, smoking, non-insulin-dependent diabetes mellitus, ECG changes indicative of LVH or ischaemia, peripheral vascular disease, past history of stroke (≥ 3 months previously), microalbuminuria/proteinuria, total cholesterol: HDL cholesterol ratio > 6, or a family history of premature CHD. For inclusion in the lipid-lowering limb, patients must also have serum total cholesterol ≤ 6.5 mmol/l (total cholesterol: HDL cholesterol ratio ≤ 4.5) and not be currently taking a statin or fibrate. Exclusion criteria include heart failure, drug treatment of angina, a history of acute MI and serum triglycerides > 4.5 mmol/l.

The drug treatment regimens are outlined in Table 3.2. Target BP levels are systolic BP < 140 mmHg and diastolic BP < 90 mmHg (< 130 mmHg and < 80 mmHg in diabetics).

Comment

At least 50% of high-risk hypertensive patients require two or more drugs to provide adequate BP control. Previous trials have allowed a wide range of possible drug combinations to be used, making it impossible to make recommendations about specific combinations. In ASCOT, the allowed combinations are clearly specified, as are any subsequent add-on drugs, which are common to both limbs of the trial and the agents used have been established as producing effective 24-hour BP control.

The design of ASCOT supplements that of ALLHAT. In the latter study, the allowed add-on drugs are very mixed and largely outdated (reserpine, clonidine and atenolol, with hydralazine as third-line therapy). However, the choice of doxazosin as third-line therapy in ASCOT poses problems in view of the premature discontinuation of that arm in ALLHAT. It remains unclear whether the relative disadvantage of alpha-blockade as first-line therapy can be extrapolated to the use of doxazosin in combination with other drugs. Nevertheless, in ALLHAT, it is likely that the majority of doxazosin-treated patients were also receiving atenolol, clonidine or reserpine. Further analyses of ALLHAT and other databases will be essential before firm conclusions can be reached.

The lipid-lowering arm of ASCOT is also important. Although hypertensive individuals have been included in earlier lipid-lowering trials, no trials of lipid-lowering carried out specifically in hypertensives have been reported. In particular, there is little information on lipid-lowering in hypertensive patients with total cholesterol ≤ 6.5 mmol/l and total cholesterol:HDL cholesterol ≤ 4.5. Again, the results of ASCOT will complement those of ALLHAT.

International Nifedipine GITS Study: Intervention as a Goal in Hypertension Treatment (INSIGHT)

 Study population and treatment titration in the International Nifedipine GITS Study: Intervention as a Goal in Hypertension Treatment (INSIGHT).
M J Brown, A Castaigne, P W de Leeuw, G Mancia, T Rosenthal, L M Ruilope. *J Hypertens* 1998; **16**: 2113–6.

BACKGROUND. INSIGHT seeks to establish the relative efficacy of a calcium channel blocker and a thiazide-based regimen in preventing the major cardiovascular complications of hypertension. To provide sufficient statistical power to differentiate between treatments, patients at high cardiovascular risk have been recruited.

INTERPRETATION. The main interest in this trial will be the initial answer it will provide to the question of whether 'newer' drugs show a substantial improvement in efficacy when compared to conventional therapy for the prevention of cardiovascular morbidity.

Outline

Patients: 6592
Planned follow-up: 3 years
Randomized treatment: Dihydropyridine calcium antagonist, diuretic
Completion date: 1999
Entry criteria: Hypertension + CV disease risk
Age: 55–80 years

Diastolic BP: $\geq$ 95 mmHg
Systolic BP: $\geq$ 150 mmHg
Projected events:
CHD: 246
Strokes: 123

INSIGHT is a double-blind, prospective outcome trial comparing the efficacy of the calcium channel blocker nifedipine GITS and the diuretic co-amilozide in preventing MI and stroke. The study recruited 2996 men and 3454 women, aged 55–80 years, with a BP during placebo run-in of $\geq$ 150/95 mmHg or isolated systolic BP $\geq$ 160 mmHg, from nine countries (Israel, France, Italy, Spain, the Netherlands, the UK, Norway, Sweden and Finland).

To be eligible, patients had to have one or more other additional CV risk factors. Treatment allocation to nifedipine GITS 30 mg daily or co-amilozide (hydrochlorothiazide 25 mg plus amiloride 5 mg) once daily was performed by minimization rather than randomization to balance additional risk factors. Optimal increases in treatment by dose-doubling and/or addition of atenolol or enalapril, and then by other antihypertensive drugs excluding calcium channel blockers or diuretics, was allowed to achieve a target BP $\leq$ 140/90 mmHg or a fall $\geq$ 20/10 mmHg.

Mean ages of participants were 64.9 years in men and 66.3 years in women. BP at randomization was 172/99 mmHg. The proportions of additional risk factors were: smoking > 10/day, 29%; total cholesterol > 6.43 mmol/l, 52%; family history of premature MI or stroke, 20%; LVH, 10%; previous MI, CHD and peripheral vascular disease, each 6%; proteinuria, 3%. Proportions of patients with one, two, three or more additional risk factors were 55%, 33%, 9% and 3%, respectively. BP 1 year after minimization was 139/82 mmHg in the 5226 patients still on randomized therapy. Almost 70% of these patients were receiving the primary drugs. At 1 year, 69% of patients had BP $\leq$ 140/90 mmHg.

Comment

INSIGHT is one of the first double-blind comparisons of active antihypertensive treatments requiring high-risk patients to achieve sufficient power. Despite this requirement, it appears possible to achieve good BP control in most patients without the addition of multiple treatments that may dilute any differences between the primary agents.

Of concern is the large loss of patients from randomized therapy. Some 1224 patients (almost 20%) were withdrawn from randomized therapy in the first year, the majority during the first 18 weeks. This may reflect lack of antihypertensive efficacy or more probably unacceptable tolerability in one or both of the treatment regimens. Only 55% of the 6450 patients originally randomized were well controlled.

The status of INSIGHT after 1 year suggested that the patients recruited were of sufficient CV risk to achieve or even exceed the predicted 369 endpoints required to give the study sufficient statistical power to differentiate between the treatments. However, INSIGHT was scheduled to terminate in May 1999. The delay in reporting (now expected in June 2000) suggests that the accrual rate of events was less than anticipated.

Studies to determine any possible advantage of angiotensin receptor blockers over conventional or other treatments

Several studies are investigating the potential advantage of the newly introduced angiotensin receptor blockers over conventional or other contemporary treatment. Two of the more important trials in this series are described here.

The Losartan Intervention for Endpoint Reduction (LIFE) in Hypertension Study

The Losartan Intervention For Endpoint reduction (LIFE) in hypertension study. Rationale, design, and methods.
B Dahlöf, R Devereux, U de Faire, F Fyhrquist, T Hedney, H Ibsen, *et al.* for the LIFE Study Group. *Am J Hypertens* 1997; **10**: 705–13.

BACKGROUND. The higher cardiovascular complication rate in treated hypertensive patients compared with normotensives is particularly evident in patients with LVH. Angiotensin II is an important growth factor stimulating cardiac hypertrophy, and therefore selective angiotensin receptor blockade may reduce LVH more effectively than conventional therapy, and thus improve prognosis.

INTERPRETATION. The LIFE study is a double-blind, prospective, parallel group study designed to compare the effects of an angiotensin receptor blocker, losartan, with those of the beta-blocker atenolol in the reduction of CV morbidity and mortality in hypertensive patients with LVH. It is the first prospective study with adequate power to link reversal of LVH to reduction in major CV events. Inclusion of patients was stopped on 30 April 1997.

Outline

Patients: 9194
Planned follow-up: 4 years
Randomized treatment: Angiotensin receptor blocker, beta-blocker
Completion date: 2001
Entry criteria: Hypertension + LVH
Age: 55–80 years
Diastolic BP: 95–115 mmHg
Systolic BP: 160–200 mmHg
Projected events:
CHD: 693
Strokes: 347

Although LVH is a major risk factor for all types of CV disease in hypertensive patients, the effect of regression of LVH on prognosis has not been tested in a prospective study design. The renin–angiotensin system appears to play a major role in the establishment and maintenance of LVH. Reversal of LVH with anti-hypertensive treatment may be related not only to the degree of BP reduction but also to changes in the components of the renin–angiotensin system. A definitive study is needed to determine whether or not antihypertensive therapy that interrupts the effects of the renin–angiotensin system more fully has a greater effect than conventional therapy on reversal of LVH, independent of BP reduction. An optimal study would also determine whether reversal of LVH is associated with a reduction in CV events.

It is postulated that losartan, by blocking the action of angiotensin II, will reduce cardiac morbidity and mortality to a greater extent than conventional drugs in hypertensive patients with LVH. A rigorous test of this hypothesis requires a comparison with an antihypertensive agent from a class that has been shown to reduce CV events, i.e. a diuretic or a beta-blocker. The beta-blocker atenolol was selected, since a beta-blocker might be better able to control the arrhythmias and coronary disease often associated with LVH and because of the established secondary prevention in high-risk patients. Thus the major hypothesis in the LIFE study is that, in patients with hypertension and LVH, losartan will be associated with reduction in CV outcomes superior to that of atenolol, through a greater effect on the regression of LVH.

LIFE is a prospective, double-blind, double-dummy, randomized, parallel group study. The primary objective is to compare the long-term effects of losartan and atenolol in hypertensive patients with LVH on the combined incidence of CV morbidity and mortality—fatal and non-fatal MI, fatal and non-fatal stroke, sudden death and death due to progressive heart failure or other CV causes. Secondary and tertiary endpoints include all-cause mortality, regression of ECG LVH and healthcare resource utilization.

Hypertensive patients (sitting diastolic BP 95–115 mmHg or sitting systolic BP 160–200 mmHg after 1–2 weeks placebo), aged 55–80 years and with LVH diagnosed from a standard 12-lead ECG by the core laboratory are eligible for inclusion. Exclusion criteria include conditions that may limit long-term survival or decrease the likelihood of adherence to study medication.

Approximately 830 centres in the United States, United Kingdom and Scandinavia are participating in LIFE. The first patient was enrolled in June 1995, and by 30 April 1997, when inclusion was stopped, 9194 patients had been randomized. Active treatment will continue for 4 years after the last patient was enrolled and until 1040 patients experience primary CV events.

Once-daily antihypertensive therapy will be adjusted to achieve a goal BP of ≤ 140/90 mmHg at trough (24 hours post-dose, range 22–24 hours). The treatment regimens are based on losartan 50–100 mg or atenolol 50–100 mg supplemented by hydrochlorothiazide and other drugs (but not ACE inhibitors, angiotensin receptor blockers or beta-blockers) as necessary to achieve target BP.

With a sample size of 8300 patients, this study has 80% power to detect $\geq 15\%$ reduction (15% to 12.75%) in the combined incidence of CV morbidity and mortality when 1040 patients experience primary endpoints. Interim analyses were planned after $^1/_3$ and $^2/_3$ of the expected events had occurred. The effects of regression of LVH and BP control on the incidence of CV events and the interactions between regression of LVH and BP control and treatment groups and this incidence will be compared using Cox regression models.

Comment

The LIFE study is the first to evaluate the effect of angiotensin receptor blockade in the prevention of complications of hypertension. The study will also have the power to address prospectively the issue of whether reversal of LVH in hypertensive patients is associated with reduction of CV morbidity and mortality, as well as with a decreased CV risk independent of BP lowering *per se*. The use of simple ECG criteria for LVH will make the results readily applicable to clinical practice.

The Valsartan Antihypertensive Long-term Use Evaluation (VALUE) trial

The Valsartan Antihypertensive Long-term Use Evaluation (VALUE) trial of cardiovascular events in hypertension. Rationale and design.

J Mann, S Julius for the VALUE Trial Group. *Blood Press* 1998; **7**: 176–83.

BACKGROUND. The role of angiotensin II in LVH, vascular hypertrophy, endothelial dysfunction and congestive heart failure is well recognized. VALUE explores whether antihypertensive therapy based on the angiotensin receptor blocker valsartan has advantages over therapy that does not include inhibition of angiotensin II.

INTERPRETATION. VALUE is the only ongoing trial that compares an angiotensin receptor blocker with treatment based on a contemporary drug (amlodipine). The main hypothesis is that, for an equivalent decrease in BP, valsartan will be more effective than amlodipine in decreasing cardiac mortality and morbidity. The VALUE study population consists of hypertensive patients at relatively high risk of sustaining CV events on the bases of age, gender, risk factors and disease factors. A unique feature is the assessment of the predictive power of the risk factor scale in a large population of treated hypertensives.

Outline

Patients: Over 15 000
Planned follow-up: 4 years
Randomized treatment: Angiotensin receptor blockers, dihydropyridine calcium antagonist
Completion date: 2004

Entry criteria: Hypertension + CV disease risk
Age: ≥ 50 years
Diastolic BP: 95–115 mmHg
Systolic BP: 160–210 mmHg
Projected events:
CHD: 967
Strokes: 483

The driving scientific hypothesis is that antagonizing the renin–angiotensin system may offer clinical advantages over equivalent BP control with a long-acting calcium channel blocker, which may itself have beneficial CV protective properties. Blockade of the renin–angiotensin system by ACE inhibitors (and in some cases angiotensin receptor blockers) has a beneficial action on vascular hypertrophy and LVH, atherosclerosis, endothelial dysfunction and cardiac failure. Differences in outcomes between the drug types might be expressed in rates of acute MI, congestive heart failure and cardiac deaths.

VALUE is a prospective, double-blind, randomized, parallel group comparison with a response-dependent dose titration scheme. The treatment schedule is shown in Fig. 3.2. Free add-on antihypertensive drugs exclude ACE inhibitors and drugs from the classes under study.

Eligible patients must have essential hypertension, be aged ≥ 50 years and have a high CV risk profile. Hypertension is defined as systolic BP 160–210 mmHg and/or diastolic BP 95–115 mmHg in the untreated state.

VALUE assesses CV risk by risk factors and predisposing conditions, and by disease factors, which may be documented by invasive and/or non-invasive

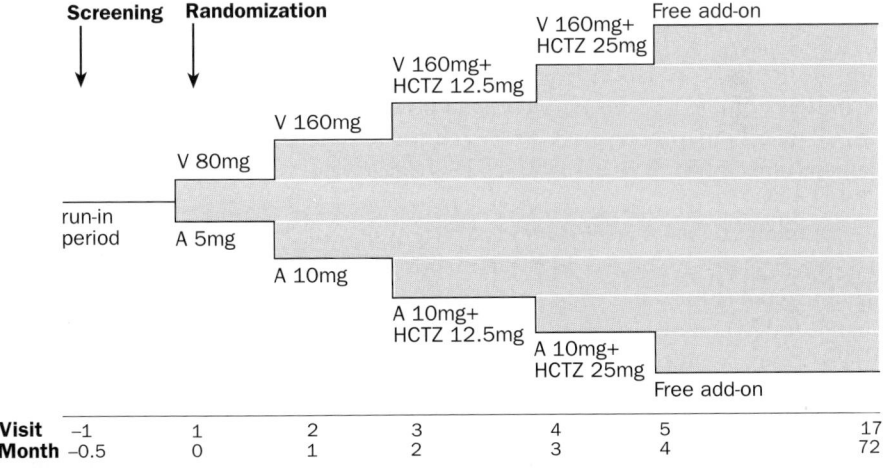

Fig. 3.2 Treatment allocation in the VALUE trial. HCTZ = hydrochlorothiazide.

Table 3.3 Risk factors and disease factors in the VALUE trial

Risk factors
- Diabetes mellitus (defined as overnight fasting plasma glucose concentration > 7.8 mmol (140 mg/l) on at least two separate occasions or as chronic intake of hypoglycaemic agents with or without occasional intake of insulin)
- Current smoking (defined as smoking 'at least 10 cigarettes/day on a regular basis for at least 5 years prior to inclusion in the study; if the patient has quit smoking, he/she will be considered a smoker if he/she stopped less than 12 months before inclusion')
- High total cholesterol (> 240 mg/dl)
- Left ventricular hypertrophy (LVH) as per ECG (Sokolow–Lyon criteria or Cornell criteria)
- Proteinuria (I+ or more on dipstick in a morning urine specimen)
- Serum creatinine > 1.7 mg/dl

Disease factors
- History of MI verified by Q-wave ECG and/or hospital records, and/or cardiovascular revascularization
- CHD verified by angiography and/or hospital records
- History of peripheral arterial occlusive disease, verified by angiography or Doppler or hospital records or statement of angiologist
- History of stroke, TIA, verified by angiography or Doppler or PET or Cat-scan or LVH with strain pattern (ST segment depression)

ECG = electrocardiogram; MI = myocarial infarction; CHD = coronary heart disease; TIA = transient ischaemic attack; PET = positron emission tomography.

Table 3.4 Risk assessment in the VALUE trial. Stratification according to age

Age 50–59 years	
Male	≥ 3 risk factors or 1 disease
Female	≥ 2 risk factors and 1 disease
Age 60–69 years	≥ 2 risk factors or 1 disease
Age > 70 years	≥ 1 risk factor or 1 disease

techniques (Table 3.3). Using these data it will be possible to assess the predictive power of a contemporary CV risk scale in a large population of hypertensive patients considered to be at high risk. Risk assessment is stratified according to age (Table 3.4).

The main exclusion criteria are renal artery stenosis, pregnancy, acute MI, coronary angioplasty or bypass in the previous 3 months, severe hepatic disease or chronic renal failure, and congestive heart failure. Patients taking beta-blockers for angina and hypertension are also excluded.

The primary outcome variable is time to first cardiac morbidity and mortality event. Secondary variables include all-cause mortality, cardiac mortality, cardiac morbidity (including silent MI), serious arrhythmias, stroke and end-stage renal failure.

A total of 14 400 patients equally allocated to each treatment is required to provide endpoints in 1450 patients, giving a power of 90% to detect a 15% difference between the groups with a two-sided P-value of 0.05. When randomization was completed in September 1999, over 15 000 patients had been randomized world-wide. VALUE is a maximum information trial, which means that it will end when 1450 patients have reached the primary endpoint.

Follow-up is expected to continue for an average of 4–5 years per patient. Two equally spaced interim analyses of the primary endpoint are planned.

Comment

VALUE compares outcomes in high-risk hypertensive patients treated with two different contemporary antihypertensive strategies. Although there are few outcome data with either angiotensin receptor blockers or calcium channel blockers in hypertension, the latter class and particularly amlodipine is rapidly becoming the most widely prescribed class of antihypertensive agents. Hence, amlodipine is a valid pragmatic comparator for the new agent, valsartan.

The study will provide important and overdue data on how well amlodipine performs against an alternative therapy in the long term. As well as comparing cardiac outcomes, it will be of clinical relevance to examine how these strategies compare with regard to tolerability.

Evaluation of newer drugs in patients at high risk

Perindopril Protection against Recurrent Stroke Study (PROGRESS)

PROGRESS: Perindopril Protection against Recurrent Stroke Study: status in July 1996.
PROGRESS Management Committee. *J Hypertens* 1996; **14** (Suppl 6): S47–S51.

BACKGROUND. **Among individuals with a history of cerebrovascular disease, the association between BP and secondary stroke is steep and continuous. Small trials of BP-lowering in patients with a history of cerebrovascular disease suggest a reduction of stroke risk. Although the proportional reduction on stroke risk appears to be similar in patients with and without cerebrovascular disease, further large prospective studies are required in patients with a history of stroke or transient ischaemic attacks.**

INTERPRETATION. PROGRESS is designed to resolve the persisting clinical uncertainty about the benefits of lowering BP in patients who have suffered a cerebrovascular event, a population with a very high risk of stroke. The primary aim is to determine precisely the balance of benefits and risks of treatment with an ACE inhibitor-based BP-lowering regimen. Since epidemiological data suggest there should be worthwhile benefits across a wide range of BP, from as low as 75 mmHg (diastolic), PROGRESS is being conducted in both normotensive and hypertensive subjects with a history of cerebrovascular disease.

Outline

Patients: 6000
Projected follow-up: 5 years
Randomized treatment: ACE inhibitor, placebo
Completion date: 2000
Entry criteria: Stroke or transient ischaemic attack
Age: Any
Diastolic BP: Any
Systolic BP: Any
Projected events:
CHD: 600
Strokes: 300

The primary objective of PROGRESS is to determine reliably the efficacy of lowering BP for the prevention of stroke in patients with a history of cerebrovascular disease. PROGRESS is a randomized, double-blind, placebo-controlled trial investigating the effects on the incidence of stroke and other major CV events and dementia of treatment with the ACE inhibitor perindopril alone and in combination with the diuretic indapamide.

The study population comprises 6000 normotensive or hypertensive patients with a history of stroke or transient ischaemic attack within the previous 5 years. The study is being conducted in over 160 centres in seven regions: Australia and New Zealand, The People's Republic of China, France and Belgium, Italy, Japan, Sweden and the United Kingdom. Recruitment is managed so that approximately one-half of the patients have a history of hypertension; and about one-half of the patients randomized to active therapy receive combination treatment with perindopril (4 mg daily) and indapamide (2.5 mg daily or 2 mg daily in Japan).

The primary study outcome is fatal and non-fatal stroke. Secondary study outcomes include fatal and total CV events (stroke, MI, CV death), cognitive function and dementia, and disability and dependency. Treatment and follow-up is scheduled to continue for a minimum of 4 years after randomization.

The study sample size of 6000 was estimated on the basis of a 1.5–2.0% annual stroke rate among control patients over 4 years of follow-up and on average difference in diastolic BP between active treatment and placebo of ≥ 4 mmHg throughout the follow-up. The projected event rate will provide at least 200 strokes among patients assigned to the placebo group and $\geq 90\%$ power to detect a 30% reduction in total stroke incidence (at 2 $P=0.05$).

Comment

PROGRESS addresses the important clinical issue of whether symptomatic reduction of BP in survivors of cerebrovascular events confers benefits. The protocol requires all subjects to be challenged with perindopril, and only those who tolerate the drug can proceed to randomization. Although intended to identify before randomization patients who might be likely to withdraw, this introduces a bias in favour of ACE inhibition. This weakness, together with the absence of a positive control group, means that PROGRESS can only provide information on the benefits (or otherwise) of BP reduction rather than those to be derived from a particular therapeutic regimen.

The Hypertension in the Very Elderly Trial (HYVET)

The Hypertension in the Very Elderly Trial: the importance of the pilot trial and modifications to the protocol.
C J Bulpitt on behalf of the HYVET Investigators. *Eur Heart J* 1999; **1** (Suppl P): 9–12.

The rationale for the Hypertension in the Very Elderly Trial (HYVET).
N S Beckett, A E Fletcher, C J Bulpitt. *Eur Heart J* 1999; **1** (Suppl P): 13–6.

BACKGROUND. **BP increases with age and elevated levels of BP are common in the elderly. The elderly are a high-risk group for CV disease, which is the leading cause of death in European countries for individuals aged ≥ 80 years. Major outcome trials have either excluded specifically those over the age of 80 years or recruited too few subjects to establish the benefits or risks of treatment in this group. Deaths from non-vascular disease and the inability of the very old to gain many extra years of life may lessen or negate any reduction in mortality. However, a reduction in morbidity and improvement in quality of life would be worthwhile, although this might not be achieved if adverse events limit the benefit or if the benefits are not large.**

INTERPRETATION. Outcome trials in elderly patients with hypertension have consistently found a reduction in cardiac mortality greater than that expected from the results of trials in middle-aged subjects. This may be due to the elderly being particularly at risk of dying from congestive heart failure as a consequence of hypertension. If this hypothesis is true, the very elderly should similarly experience a fall in cardiac mortality with antihypertensive treatment. The benefit–risk comparison from active treatment needs to be determined in the very elderly, and the Hypertension in the Very Elderly Trial (HYVET) has been designed to address this issue.

Outline

Patients: 2100
Planned follow-up: 5 years
Randomized treatment: ACE inhibitor, diuretic, placebo
Completion date: 2003

Entry criteria: Hypertension
Age: > 80 years
Diastolic BP: 90–109 mmHg
Systolic BP: 160–179 mmHg
Projected events:
CHD: 683
Strokes: 341

It may well be that treatment of hypertensive patients > 80 years is a balance between benefit in terms of a reduction in stroke and heart failure, each a major cause of disability in this age group, and the possible adverse effect of an increase in mortality. The over-80s are survivors, and are unlikely to benefit significantly from a gain in life-years. However, a reduction in disability, maintenance of independence and quality of life would clearly be of benefit. There is a need for a well-designed, randomized, controlled trial in this age group to assess the benefits of treatment and the level of risk.

HYVET is a randomized, double-blind, placebo-controlled trial. The main objective is to investigate the primary and secondary prevention of fatal and non-fatal strokes. It is designed to determine whether or not a 35% difference in stroke events (fatal and non-fatal) occurs between placebo and active treatment in hypertensive patients aged > 80 years; this is consistent with results from previous trials in hypertension in the elderly. The trial has 90% power to detect such a difference at the 1% level of significance. Secondary outcome measures include total mortality, CV mortality and stroke mortality.

A total of 2100 patients > 80 years is to be recruited from centres in the UK, Bulgaria, Finland, Romania, Spain, Lithuania, Ireland, Poland, Greece and Serbia. Follow-up will be for 5 years. Patients will be eligible for the trial if, while on single-blind placebo treatment, sustained systolic BP is 160–199 mmHg and/or diastolic BP is 90–109 mmHg. The active treatment group will receive sustained release indapamide 1.5 mg daily with perindopril 2–4 mg daily being added to achieve the target BP < 150/80 mmHg.

A pilot study in 1284 patients demonstrated the feasibility of HYVET. Recruitment started in January 1999 and the trial will end late in 2003.

Comment

Information from HYVET should aid clinicians in assessing the benefits and risks of treating hypertensive patients aged > 80 years. Subgroup analyses of earlier trials have suggested that with patients in this age range, treatment reduces stroke events (fatal and non-fatal) but may increase all-cause mortality. Thus, further reliable data are needed.

Overview of ongoing trials

 Protocol for prospective collaborative overviews of major randomized trials of blood-pressure-lowering treatments.
World Health Organization–International Society of Hypertension Blood Pressure Lowering Treatment Trialists' Collaboration. *J Hypertens* 1998; **16**: 127–37.

BACKGROUND. Prospectively planned overviews (meta-analyses) of the ongoing randomized trials of BP-lowering drugs should facilitate the generation of reliable data on the effects of newer classes of drugs on major causes of CV mortality and morbidity for a variety of patient groups. A registry has been established to collate information from over 30 trials. By 2003, data from at least 195 000 patients and 899 000 patient-years of follow-up should be available. An estimated 8000 strokes, 12 000 CHD events and 23 000 CV events should provide sufficient statistical power to detect even modest cause-specific differences in the incidence of the main study outcomes.

INTERPRETATION. This project should provide more reliable information about the effects of newer BP-lowering drugs than would any one study alone. The use of data from individual patients in the overviews will facilitate the investigation of the separate effects of various drug regimens in treating members of the major patient subgroups.

Individually, the ongoing trials are not likely to resolve all the current uncertainties about the effects of regimens based on the various agents. Systematic overviews should provide more reliable information about any differences in CV outcomes with different regimens than that from any one trial alone.

Trials are potentially eligible for inclusion if they satisfy one of the following criteria: random allocation of patients between antihypertensive regimens based on various BP-lowering agents; random allocation between a BP-lowering treatment and placebo (or other inactive control condition); or randomization of patients between various BP goals. In addition, eligible trials must have a planned minimum of 1000 patient-years of follow-up for patients in each randomly allocated treatment group.

A registry has been established to identify all major ongoing and planned randomized trials of BP-lowering agents. Data requested from each participating trial will include baseline characteristics, selected measurements performed during follow-up and details of the occurrence of all pre-defined study outcomes during the scheduled follow-up period (Table 3.5).

The study outcomes chosen for inclusion in these overviews represent the main CV disease outcomes likely to be affected by BP-lowering treatment regimens and the main non-CV disease outcomes for which questions about the safety of some newer agents have arisen, for example, cancer with calcium channel blockers. Two sets of primary comparisons have been specified in advance.

Table 3.5 Treatment Trialists' Collaboration. Baseline, follow-up and outcome data from each patient

Baseline (at or before randomization)	Follow-up (at annual or similar intervals)	Outcomes (all events in each category recorded during scheduled follow-up period)
Patient identifier	Systolic blood pressure	Ischaemic stroke
Date of randomization	Diastolic blood pressure	Cerebral haemorrhage
Treatment allocation	Weight	Subarachnoid haemorrhage
Date of birth/age	Serum cholesterol level	Other stroke (including unknown)
Sex	Serum creatinine level	Myocardial infarction
Ethnicity	Smoking status	Hospitalization for heart failure
Systolic blood pressure	Compliance	Hospitalization for renal disease
Weight		Hospitalization or transfusion for non-cerebral haemorrhage
Height		Arterial revascularization procedure
Smoking status		Bone fracture
Serum total cholesterol level		Major cancer (site-specific)
Serum creatinine level		Admission to hospital for any other cause
Regular use of aspirin/anti-platelet drug		Death (cause-specific)
Use of other blood pressure-lowering drug		Date for each event
		Date of last follow-up for fatal events
History of		Date of last follow-up for non-fatal events
Diabetes		
Left ventricular hypertrophy		
Heart failure		
Cerebrovascular disease		
Coronary heart disease		
Peripheral vascular disease		
Planned end of scheduled treatment and follow-up		

The first concerns the overview of trials comparing regimens based on newer (ACE inhibitor or calcium channel blocker) and older (diuretic or beta-blocker) forms of BP-lowering treatments that produce similar reductions in BP. In addition, comparisons of ACE inhibitor-based treatment versus calcium antagonist-based treatment will be performed. The second set of primary comparisons concerns the overview of trials comparing BP-lowering regimens (ACE inhibitor- or calcium antagonist-based) versus control.

Ongoing trials eligible for inclusion in the overviews are listed in Table 3.6. These include 17 trials comparing various drug regimens and 17 trials comparing at least one regimen with an untreated or less treated control condition. Eighteen trials are exclusively in hypertension and 18 in selected patients with coronary disease, CV disease, renal disease or diabetes.

The total planned recruitment is 194 701 patients, the mean projected follow-up is 4.6 years and the total projected number of patient-years of follow-up is 898 643. The total number of patients planned in the trials comparing various treatment regimens is 132 177, of whom 67 876 will be randomly allocated between ACE inhibitor-based treatments and diuretic or beta-blocker-based treatments, 81 421 between dihydropyridine calcium antagonist-based treatments and diuretic or beta-blocker-based treatments, and 27 414 between verapamil or diltiazem-based treatments and diuretic or beta-blocker-based treatments. The total number of patients planned in trials comparing a BP-lowering treatment with an untreated condition is less: treated control condition in 62 022, of whom 28 006 will be randomly allocated between ACE inhibitor-based therapy and control, and 9570 will be randomly allocated between calcium antagonist-based therapy and control.

Estimates of the statistical power for the principal comparisons of treatments' effects on stroke incidence, major CHD events and total CV events are given in Table 3.7. For comparisons of newer versus older treatment regimens (and ACE inhibitors versus calcium antagonist regimens), all calculations assume minimum detectable differences of 15% (relative risk 0.85), and for comparisons between treatment and untreated or less actively treated control conditions, the calculations assume minimum detectable differences of 20% (relative risk 0.80). By 2003, the estimated number of events accrued will be about 8000 strokes, 12 000 CHD events and 23 000 CV events. The available data should provide sufficient power to detect modest differences in the incidence of each of the principal outcomes for the main treatment comparisons.

Comment

This project should provide reliable data about the effects of newer classes of antihypertensive agents on major classes of CV morbidity and mortality for a variety of groups of patients who have a high risk of CV disease events. The prospective overview approach should reduce random errors and avoid bias.

The Trialists' Collaboration will accumulate a formidable body of data in terms of patient numbers and events. It is sobering to appreciate the size of comparisons required to provide adequate power to detect important differences between active treatments reliably. The limitations of individual trials, even when appropriately designed and adequately powered, are manifest.

Conclusions

As we move into the new millennium, the emphasis in the management of hypertension has moved decisively towards evidence-based medicine. It is no longer sufficient to demonstrate that an antihypertensive agent reduces BP. Now, evidence must be provided that the drug reduces real outcome measures such as CHD events. Furthermore, new drugs have to demonstrate at least equivalence to, and

Table 3.6 Characteristics of trials identified as eligible for inclusion in overviews

Title	Acronym	Patients (n)	Planned follow-up (years)	Randomized treatments (factorial assignments)	Completion date	Entry criteria	Age (years)	Diastolic blood pressure	Systolic blood pressure	Projected events CHD	Strokes
African American Study of Kidney Disease and Hypertension	AASK	1200	5	ACE, β-blocker, DCA (more, less)	2001	HBP plus renal disease	18-70	≥95	Any	144	72
Appropriate Blood Pressure Control in Diabetes Trial	ABCD	950	5	ACE, DCA	1998	Diabetes	40-74	Any	No ISH	119	59
Antihypertensive Therapy and Lipid-Lowering Heart Attack Prevention Trial	ALLHAT	40 000	6	ACE, α-blocker, DCA diuretic (CHOL, open)	2002	HBP plus CVD risk	>55	90-109	140-179	2580	2790
Australian National Blood Pressure Study 2	ANBP2	6000	5	ACE, diuretic	2002	HBP	65-84	≥90	≥160	300	150
Anglo-Scandinavian Cardiac Outcomes Trial	ASCOT	18 000	5	DCA with/without ACE, β-blocker with/without diuretic (CHOL, placebo)	2003	HBP plus CVD risk	40-79	≥90	≥140	1150	400
Bergamo Nephrology Diabetes Complication Trial	BENEDICT	2400	3	ACE, NCA, placebo	2001	Diabetes	≥40	≥90	≥140	200	100
Captopril Prevention Project	CAPPP	10 800	5	ACE, β-blocker/diuretic	1998	HBP	25-66	≥100	Any	324	162
Controlled Onset Verapamil Investigation for Cardiovascular Endpoints	CONVINCE	15 000	5	NCA, β-blocker/diuretic	2001	HBP plus CVD risk	≥55	90-109	140-189	1250	750
Collaborative Study Group Trial on Effect of Irbesartan	CSGTEI	1650	3	AIIA, DCA, placebo	2000	Diabetes plus proteinuria	30-70	≥85	≥135	124	62
Diabetes Hypertension Cardiovascular Morbidity – Mortality and Ramipril	DIAB-HYCAR	4000	3	ACE, placebo	1999	Diabetes plus proteinuria	>50	Any	Any	300	150
European Lacidipine Study of Atherosclerosis	ELSA	2251	4	DCA, β9-blocker	2000	HBP	45-75	95-115	150-209	89	44
Hypertension in Diabetes Study	HDS	1148	8.2	ACE, β-blocker, open (insulin, sulphonamide, diet)	1998	HBP plus diabetes	25-75	≥85	≥150	244	122
Heart Outcomes Prevention Evaluation Study	HOPE	9541	4.7	ACE, placebo (vitamin E, placebo)	2000	CVD risk	≥55	Any	Any	1200	550
Hypertension Optimal Treatment study	HOT	19 196	3.5	More, less (aspirin, placebo)	1997	HBP	50-80	100-115	Any	552	276
Hypertension in the Very Elderly Trial	HYVET	2100	5	ACE, diuretic, placebo	2001	HBP	>80	90-109	160-219	683	341

International Nifedipine Gastrointestinal Therapeutic System Study Intervention as a Goal in Hypertension Treatment	INSIGHT	6592	3	DCA, diuretic	1999	HBP plus CVD risk	55–80	≥95	≥150	246	123
Losartan Intervention for Endpoint Reduction in Hypertension	LIFE	9194	4	AIIA, β-blocker	2001	HBP plus LVH	55–80	95–115	160–200	693	347
National Intervention Cooperative Study in Elderly Hypertensive	NICS-EH	1000	5	DCA, diuretic	1997	HBP	≥60	<115	160–219	30	15
Nordic Diltiazem Study	NORDIL	11 000	5	NCA, β-blocker/diuretic	2002	HBP	50–69	≥100	Any	360	180
Prevention of Atherosclerosis with Ramipril	PART2	617	4	ACE, placebo	1998	Atherosclerosis	18–75	Any	Any	40	14
Plaque Hypertension Lipid-Lowering Italian Study	PHYLLIS	450	3	ACE, placebo (CHOL, placebo)	2000	CIT	45–70	95–115	151–210	7	4
Prospective Randomized Evaluation of Vascular Effects of Norvasc	PREVENT	825	5	DCA, placebo	1997	ACHD	30–80	Any	Any	20	6
Perindopril Protection Against Recurrent Stroke Study	PROGRESS	6000	5	ACE, placebo	2000	Stroke or TIA	Any	Any	Any	600	300
Quinapril Ischaemia Event Trial	QUIET	1750	3	ACE, placebo	1996	ACHD	18–75	Any	Any	500	350
Randomized Evaluation of Non-insulin-dependent Diabetes Mellitus with the Angiotensin II Antagonist Losartan	RENAAL	1500	4	AIIA, placebo	2002	Diabetes	31–70	<110	<200	100	50
Study of Cognition and Prognosis in Elderly Patients with Hypertension	SCOPE	4000	2.5	AIIA, placebo	2003	HBP	70–89	90–99	160–179	60	30
Systolic Hypertension in the Elderly Lacidipine Long-Term Study	SHELL	4800	3.5	DCA, diuretic	1999	HBP	≥60	<95	161–219	101	50
Swedish Trial in Old Patients with Hypertension	STOP-2	6628	4	ACE, β-blocker/diuretic, DCA	1998	HBP	70–84	≥105	≥180	318	167
Systolic Hypertension in Europe Multicentre Trial	SYST-EUR	4695	1.6	DCA, placebo	1997	ISH	≥60	<95	160–219	500	250
Verapamil in Hypertension Atherosclerosis Study	VHAS	1414	2	NCA, diuretic	1996	HBP	40–65	≥95	≥160	40	20

ACE = angiotensin-converting enzyme inhibitor; AIIA = angiotensin II antagonist; ACHD = angiographic coronary heart disease; CHOL = cholesterol lowering; CIT = carotid intimal thickness; CVD = cardiovascular disease; DCA = dihydropyridine calcium antagonist; HBP = high blood pressure; ISH = isolated systolic hypertension; less = less intensive blood pressure lowering; LVH = left ventricular hypertrophy; more = more intensive blood pressure lowering; NCA = non-dihydropyridine calcium antagonist; open = open control; TIA = transient ischaemic attack.

Table 3.7 Estimates of statistical power* for principal pre-specified comparisons

Comparison	n	Estimated number of events			Estimated power (%) (α = 0.05)		
		CHD	Strokes	CVD	CHD	Strokes	CVD
Data available in 1999							
Newer versus older regimens							
ACE versus β-blocker/diuretic	15 977	697	354	1156	54	30	77
Calcium antagonists versus β-blocker/diuretic	19 174	748	378	1239	57	32	80
DCA versus β-blocker/diuretic	17 760	708	358	1173	55	30	78
NCA versus β-blocker/diuretic	1414	40	20	66	5	1	7
ACE versus calcium antagonist	4419	212	111	356	19	11	31
More versus less or none							
Active versus placebo/control	33 181	1875	1077	3247	100	93	100
ACE versus placebo	7157	1008	598	1766	94	75	100
Calcium antagonist versus placebo	5520	120	106	249	19	16	37
Data available in 2003							
Newer versus older regimens							
ACE versus β-blocker/diuretic	47 407	3055	2398	5998	99	97	100
Calcium antagonist versus β-blocker/diuretic	89 230	5173	3406	9436	100	100	100
DCA versus β-blocker/diuretic	61 816	3523	2456	6576	100	98	100
NCA versus β-blocker/diuretic	27 414	1650	950	2860	90	68	99
ACE versus calcium antagonist	23 644	1524	1402	3218	87	84	100
More versus less or none							
Active versus placebo/control	62 022	4893	3286	8997	100	100	100
ACE versus placebo	26 148	3304	2466	3242	100	100	100
Calcium antagonist versus placebo	8220	336	214	605	48	32	75

ACE = angiotensin-converting enzyme; DCA = dihydropyridine calcium antagonist; NCA = non-dihydropyridine calcium antagonist; CHD = non-fatal myocardial infarctions plus deaths from coronary heart disease; Strokes = non-fatal strokes plus deaths from cerebrovascular disease; CVD = 1.1 × (CHD plus Strokes). *Calculations assume minimum detectable differences of 15% (relative risk 0.85) for comparisons between newer versus older (and ACE inhibitor versus calcium antagonist) treatment regimens, and of 20% (relative risk 0.80) for comparisons between treatment and an untreated or less actively treated control condition.

preferably superiority over, conventional therapy. In response, there is an epidemic of ongoing outcome trials.

This is a welcome development. However, even large, well-designed individual trials are unlikely to answer all the outstanding relevant questions reliably and decisively. Thus, meta-analyses of the available outcome data will be required. It is encouraging that overviews have been planned prospectively. At the conclusion of the current round of ongoing trials the management of hypertension should have a much more secure base.

References

1. Collins R, MacMahon S. Blood pressure, antihypertensive drug treatment and the risks of stroke and of coronary heart disease. *Br Med Bull* 1994; **50**: 272–98.

2. Staessen JA, Fagard R, Thijs L, Celis H, Arabidze GG, Birkenhager WH, *et al.* Randomised double-blind comparison of placebo and active treatment for older patients with isolated systolic hypertension. *Lancet* 1997; **350**: 757–64.

3. Gong L, Zhang W, Zhu Y, Zhu J, Kong D, Page V, *et al.* Shanghai trial of nifedipine in the elderly (STONE). *J Hypertens* 1996; **14**: 1237–45.

4. Hansson L, Lindholm LH, Ekbom T, Dahlöf B, Lanke J, Schersten B, *et al.* Randomised trial of old and new antihypertensive drugs in elderly patients: cardiovascular mortality and morbidity. The Swedish Trial in Old Patients with Hypertension-2 Study. *Lancet* 1999; **354**: 1751–6.

5. Hansson L, Lindholm LH, Niskanen L, Lanke J, Hedner T, Niklasson A, *et al.* Effect of angiotensin-converting enzyme inhibition compared with conventional therapy on cardiovascular morbidity and mortality in hypertension: the Captopril Prevention Project (CAPPP) randomized trial. *Lancet* 1999; **353**: 611–6.

6. Neaton JD, Grimm RH, Prineas RJ, Stamler J, Grandits GA, Elmer PJ, *et al.* Treatment of Mild Hypertension Study. Final results. *JAMA* 1993; **270**: 713–24.

Part II

Interface: hypertension and other cardiovascular risk factors

4

Management of hypertension in patients with diabetes

Introduction

Hypertension and diabetes mellitus are independent risk factors for the development of cardiovascular disease. Frequently the two conditions co-exist and hypertension is twice as prevalent in diabetic patients as it is in the general population. However, the evolution of hypertension differs slightly in type I compared with type II diabetes mellitus. In type I diabetes, hypertension is closely associated with the development of diabetic nephropathy, whereas in type II diabetes, although hypertension may again indicate an evolving diabetic nephropathy, it may also be part of the metabolic syndrome ('insulin resistance'). In either case there is also the possibility of a chance association between diabetes mellitus and essential hypertension, especially in those with a family history of hypertension.

In past years, 'tight' glycaemic control was invariably emphasized in both type I and type II diabetes mellitus with relatively little attention being directed towards blood pressure reduction or lipid modification. It is interesting to note, however, that it is only relatively recently that the benefits of tight glycaemic control have been confirmed by clinical outcome. The landmark study by the Diabetes Control and Complications Trial Research Group (DCCT) confirmed these benefits in type I, particularly in relation to microvascular complications, and a smaller-scale study produced corresponding evidence in type II diabetes mellitus, albeit with an intensified insulin regimen rather than oral hypoglycaemic drugs [1, 2].

However, the recent results of clinical outcome trials, particularly in hypertension, have provoked a significant shift in therapeutic emphasis for current practice. These results, and the current focus on the treatment of high-risk patients, has directed the treatment strategy towards blood pressure control and overall risk factor management.

Blood pressure control

Several important clinical trials have reported in the recent past. These have all involved cohorts of patients with hypertension and diabetes mellitus:

1. UK Prospective Diabetes Study (UKPDS)
2. Captopril Prevention Project (CAPPP)
3. SYST-EUR
4. HOT
5. SHEP

UK Prospective Diabetes Study

The United Kingdom Prospective Diabetes Study (UKPDS) was a long-running (about 20 years from its inception) clinical outcome trial designed to address issues relating to the optimal treatment of type II diabetes. The principal objectives of the original study design focused on glycaemic targets and the selection of the most appropriate therapeutic strategy, but a number of other issues of practical importance and clinical relevance were also addressed.

Between 1977 and 1991, 5102 newly diagnosed type II diabetic patients (58% male) were recruited into the main study, which was designed to address the following issues:

1. Does intensive treatment with oral antidiabetic agents or insulin reduce the risk of microvascular and macrovascular disease relative to less intensive, conventional measures, i.e. diet?
2. Is any particular treatment advantageous? Or disadvantageous?

In 1987 a sub-group was identified for the Hypertension in Diabetes Study and this was incorporated into the main study via a factorial design to compare 'tight' blood pressure control (target < 150/85 mmHg) compared with 'less tight' blood pressure control (target < 180/105 mmHg). In total, 1148 patients were randomized in this study, with a further subdivision in the 'tight' control group to a treatment regimen based either on an angiotensin-converting enzyme (ACE) inhibitor (captopril) or on a beta-blocker (atenolol). The principal results were as follows:

Main study—UKPDS 33: intensive glycaemic control

Intensive blood-glucose control with sulphonylureas or insulin compared with conventional treatment and risk of complications in patients with type II diabetes: UKPDS 33.

United Kingdom Prospective Diabetes Study Group. *Lancet* 1998; **352**: 837–53.

BACKGROUND. Improved blood glucose control decreases the progression of diabetic microvascular disease, but the effect on macrovascular complications is unknown. There is concern that sulphonylureas may increase cardiovascular mortality in patients with type II diabetes and that high insulin concentrations may enhance atheroma formation. We compared the effects of intensive blood glucose control with either sulphonylurea or insulin and conventional treatment on the risk of microvascular

and macrovascular complications in patients with type II diabetes in a randomized controlled trial.

INTERPRETATION. Intensive blood glucose control by either sulphonylureas or insulin substantially decreases the risk of microvascular complications, but not macrovascular disease, in patients with type II diabetes. None of the individual drugs had an adverse effect on cardiovascular outcomes. All intensive treatment increased the risk of hypoglycaemia.

Comment

Over 10 years the mean HbA_{1C} was significantly less at 7% in the intensive treatment group versus 7.9% for the diet group ($P<0.0001$), but there was no difference between the different intensive treatment subgroups. This improvement in glycaemic control was associated with a 12% risk reduction for any diabetes-related endpoint, and this was mainly attributable to a 25% reduction in microvascular endpoints ($P<0.005$). Although there was a 16% reduction in fatal and non-fatal myocardial infarction in the intensive group, this failed to achieve conventional statistical significance ($P=0.052$), but sudden death was significantly reduced ($P<0.05$). No differences were attributable to the three principal agents—chlorpropamide, glybenclamide and insulin—although, interestingly, the reduction in the risk of progression of retinopathy was less pronounced for chlorpropamide. However, blood pressure was significantly higher throughout the study in the chlorpropamide-treated patients.

Overweight subgroup—UKPDS 34: diet versus metformin

Effect of intensive blood glucose control with metformin on complications in overweight patients with type II diabetes: UKPDS 34.

United Kingdom Prospective Diabetes Study Group. *Lancet* 1998; **352:** 854–65.

BACKGROUND. **In patients with type II diabetes, intensive blood glucose control with insulin or sulphonylurea therapy decreases the progression of microvascular disease and may also reduce the risk of heart attacks. This study investigated whether intensive glucose control with metformin has any specific advantage or disadvantage.**

INTERPRETATION. Since intensive glucose control with metformin appears to decrease the risk of diabetes-related endpoints in overweight diabetic patients, and is associated with less weight gain and fewer hypoglycaemic attacks than are insulin and sulphonylureas, it may be the first-line pharmacological therapy of choice in these patients.

Comment

HbA_{1C} was significantly lower at 7.4% in the metformin group compared to 8% in the diet-only group. Significant risk reductions were observed for all-cause mortality, diabetes-related death and all diabetes-related endpoints. For all macrovascular events, there was a 30% risk reduction for metformin compared to conventional dietary treatment ($P=0.02$), with a 30% risk reduction for myocardial infarction ($P=0.01$).

Blood pressure study—UKPDS 38: 'tight' versus 'less tight' BP control

Tight blood pressure control and risk of macrovascular and microvascular complications in type II diabetes: UKPDS 38.

United Kingdom Prospective Diabetes Study Group. *BMJ* 1998; **317**: 703–13.

BACKGROUND. The objective of this study was to determine whether tight control of blood pressure (BP) prevents macrovascular and microvascular complications in patients with type II diabetes.

INTERPRETATION. Tight BP control in patients with hypertension and type II diabetes achieves a clinically important reduction in the risk of deaths related to diabetes, complications related to diabetes, progression of diabetic retinopathy and deterioration in visual acuity.

Comment

The mean achieved BP was significantly less at 144/82 mmHg in the 'tight' control group compared to 154/87 mmHg in the 'less tight' BP control group ($P<0.0001$). This difference of 10/5 mmHg was associated with significant reductions in macrovascular and microvascular events (Table 4.1): all diabetes endpoints were significantly reduced by 24%, and so also were stroke by 44% and microvascular disease by 37%.

The reduction in microvascular complications was predominantly attributable to a reduced risk of retinopathy and its progression.

Table 4.1 Tight blood pressure (BP) control in type II diabetes: events per 1000 patient-years

| | BP control | | Relative risk | |
	Tight	Less	Reduction	
Any diabetes-related endpoint	50.9	67.4	−24%	$P<0.005$
All-cause mortality	22.4	27.2	−18%	
Myocardial infarction	18.6	23.5	−21%	
Stroke	6.5	11.6	−44%	$P<0.02$
Microvascular disease	12.0	19.2	−37%	$P<0.01$

Source: UKPDS 38 (1998).

BP control—UKPDS 39: atenolol versus captopril

Efficacy of atenolol and captopril in reducing risk of macrovascular and microvascular complications in type II diabetes: UKPDS 39.

United Kingdom Prospective Diabetes Study Group. *BMJ* 1998; **317:** 713–20.

BACKGROUND. **The objective of this study was to determine whether tight control of BP with either a beta-blocker or an angiotensin-converting enzyme inhibitor has a specific advantage or disadvantage in preventing the macrovascular and microvascular complications of type II diabetes.**

INTERPRETATION. BP lowering with captopril or atenolol was similarly effective in reducing the incidence of diabetic complications. This study provided no evidence that either drug has any specific beneficial or deleterious effect, suggesting that BP reduction in itself may be more important than the treatment used.

Comment

Unfortunately, this aspect of the UKPDS was not statistically empowered to address a very important issue relating to potential additional benefits that might be attributable to an individual drug treatment. In this substudy, treatment regimens based on captopril 25–50 mg twice daily (400 patients) or on atenolol 50–100 mg daily (358 patients) were compared: there were no significant differences, but the overall trends consistently favoured atenolol (Table 4.2 and Fig. 4.1). Thus captopril and atenolol were equally effective in reducing the incidence of diabetic complications in the 'tight' BP control group. It is important to recognize, however, that single drug therapy was capable of providing 'tight' control in less

Table 4.2 Captopril versus atenolol diabetes-related endpoints

Clinical endpoint	Patients with aggregate endpoints		P	Relative risk for captopril
	Captopril (n=400)	Atenolol (n=358)		
Any endpoint	141	118	0.43	1.10
Deaths	48	34	0.28	1.27
Acute myocardial infarction	61	46	0.35	1.20
Stroke	21	17	0.74	1.12
Peripheral vascular disease	5	3	0.59	1.48
Microvascular disease	40	28	0.30	1.29

Source: UKPDS 39 (1998).

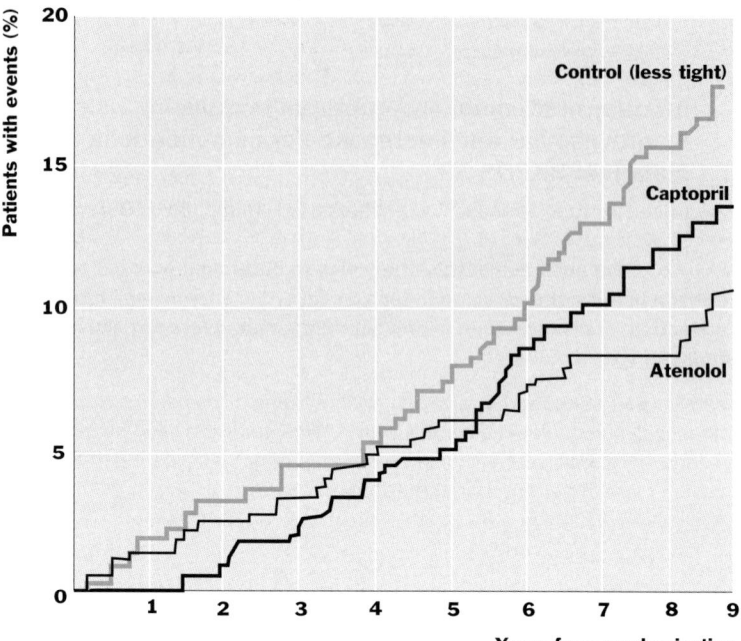

Fig. 4.1 Captopril versus atenolol diabetes-related endpoints. Cumulative event rates (%) in patients randomized to 'less tight' control and to 'tight' control with either captopril or atenolol (UKPDS).

than half the patients and that multiple drug treatments (three or more agents) were required in 29% of patients. Furthermore, after 9 years of treatment, only just over half the 'tight' control group (56%) had attained the target BP of < 150/85 mmHg.

Incidentally, in the light of reports suggesting that ACE inhibitors may predispose to hypoglycaemia while beta-blockers may delay recovery from hypoglycaemia, there were no differences in the rates for hypoglycaemic episodes in this study.

Captopril prevention project (CAPPP)

Effect of angiotensin-converting enzyme inhibition compared with conventional therapy on cardiovascular morbidity and mortality in hypertension: the Captopril Prevention Project (CAPPP) randomized trial.

L Hansson, L H Lindholm, L Niskanen, J Lanke, T Hedner, A Niklasson, et al. for the Captopril Prevention Project (CAPPP) Study Group.
Lancet 1999; **353**: 611–6.

BACKGROUND. Angiotensin-converting enzyme (ACE) inhibitors have been used for more than a decade to treat high BP, despite the lack of data from randomized intervention trials to show that such treatment affects cardiovascular morbidity and mortality. The Captopril Prevention Project (CAPPP) is a randomized intervention trial to compare the effects of ACE inhibition and conventional therapy on cardiovascular morbidity and mortality in patients with hypertension.

INTERPRETATION. Captopril and conventional treatment did not differ in efficacy in preventing cardiovascular morbidity and mortality. The difference in stroke risk is probably due to the lower levels of BP obtained initially in previously treated patients randomized to conventional therapy.

Comment

This was a prospective, randomized, open, blinded-endpoint trial in 10 985 hypertensive patients allocated to a treatment regimen based upon an ACE inhibitor (captopril) or on traditional antihypertensive drugs (thiazide diuretics or beta-blockers). Overall, for the primary endpoint, which was a composite of fatal and non-fatal myocardial infarction, stroke and other cardiovascular deaths, there was no difference between the treatment groups.

However, the most controversial finding was derived from the subgroup analysis of the patients with hypertension and diabetes mellitus. Firstly, and not surprisingly, the treatment regimen based upon the thiazides or beta-blockers was more likely to result in new cases of diabetes, albeit in small numbers, with 43 cases arising during 30 000 patient-years of treatment. Thus the well-recognized adverse effects of these traditional agents on carbohydrate metabolism were confirmed.

In the subgroup of patients with diabetes mellitus prior to entry into the study there was no difference between treatment based on the traditional treatments and captopril. Thus there was no evidence of any benefit beyond BP reduction in the captopril-treated patient group. It must be recognized, however, that only 572 patients were included in this study and it is therefore completely under-powered in statistical terms to draw any definitive conclusions. Furthermore, captopril was administered only once daily in about 50% of patients, and this regimen is unlikely to provide full 24-hour blood pressure control. Thus the captopril-treated patients may not have had the full benefit of intensive BP reduction.

SYST-EUR: diabetic cohort

Effects of calcium channel blockade in older patients with diabetes and systolic hypertension.

J Tuomilehto, D Rastenyte, W H Berkenhäger, L Thijs, R Antikainen, C J Bulpitt, *et al.* for the Systolic Hypertension in Europe Trial Investigators. *N Engl J Med* 1999; **340**: 677–84.

BACKGROUND. **Recent reports suggest that calcium channel blockers may be harmful in patients with diabetes and hypertension. These authors previously reported that antihypertensive treatment with the calcium channel blocker nitrendipine reduced the risk of cardiovascular events. This** *post hoc* **analysis compared the outcome of treatment with nitrendipine in diabetic and non-diabetic patients.**

INTERPRETATION. Nitrendipine-based antihypertensive therapy is particularly beneficial in older patients with diabetes and isolated systolic hypertension. Thus our findings do not support the hypothesis that the use of long-acting calcium channel blockers may be harmful in diabetic patients.

Comment

Increasingly, the message for intensive BP control in diabetic hypertensives is being reinforced through the sub-group analyses of clinical outcome trials. An important additional component to this basic message is the emphasis on BP control through drug treatment combinations rather than monotherapy and, while an ACE inhibitor would undoubtedly be incorporated into the treatment regimen, the balance of evidence favours aggressive BP reduction rather than reliance upon the pharmacological characteristics of any individual drug or drug class. For example, in the SYST-EUR study of 4695 patients aged 60 years or older, an antihypertensive treatment regimen based on a calcium antagonist was found to be particularly beneficial. These were older patients with systolic BP between 160 and 219 mmHg and diastolic BP < 95 mmHg. The diabetic cohort in this study comprised 492 patients, and after 2 years of follow-up systolic and diastolic BPs had been reduced by 8.6/3.9 mmHg in the treatment group relative to the patient group. The treatment group received the dihydropyridine derivative nitrendipine; but ultimately more than half the patients were on drug combination treatments to produce this BP reduction. After adjusting for confounding factors, the treated group had a 76% reduction in overall mortality from cardiovascular disease, a 73% reduction in fatal and non-fatal strokes and a 63% reduction in all cardiac events combined (Table 4.3). The benefits were significantly

Table 4.3 Reduction in mortality and CV events in diabetics versus non-diabetics

Mortality/CV events	Diabetic patients (n=492)	Non-diabetic patients (n=4203)
All strokes	−73%	−38%
All cardiac endpoints	−63%	−21%
All CV endpoints	−69%*	−26%
Total mortality	−55%	−6%
CV mortality	−76%*	−13%

* $P<0.05$ for diabetic versus non-diabetic patients. CV = cardiovascular.
Source: Tuomilheto (1999).

greater in the diabetic versus the non-diabetic patients for all cardiovascular events and for cardiovascular mortality. This emphasizes the benefits of BP reductions in high-risk patients.

HOT Study: diabetic cohort

Effects of intensive blood pressure lowering and low-dose aspirin in patients with hypertension: principal results of the Hypertension Optimal Treatment (HOT) randomized trial.

L Hansson, A Zanchetti, S G Carruthers, B Dahlöf, D Elmfeldt, S Julius, *et al.* for the HOT Study Group. *Lancet* 1998; **351:** 1755–62.

BACKGROUND. Despite treatment, there is often a higher incidence of cardiovascular complications in patients with hypertension than in normotensive individuals. Inadequate reduction of their BP is a likely cause, but the optimum target BP is not known. The impact of acetylsalicylic acid (aspirin) has never been investigated in patients with hypertension. This study aimed to assess the optimum target diastolic BP and the potential benefit of a low dose of acetylsalicylic acid in the treatment of hypertension.

INTERPRETATION. Intensive lowering of BP in patients with hypertension was associated with a low rate of cardiovascular events. The HOT study shows the benefits of lowering the diastolic blood pressure down to 82.6 mmHg. Acetylsalicylic acid significantly reduced major cardiovascular events, with the greatest benefit seen in myocardial infarction. There was no effect on the incidence of stroke or fatal bleeds, but non-fatal major bleeds were twice as common.

Comment

A cohort of 1501 patients with diabetes mellitus was identified within the 18 790 patients who participated in the HOT study, with treatment based on another dihydropyridine calcium channel blocker, felodipine. Overall, there was a significant reduction in major cardiovascular events in relation to the 'tightness' of the blood pressure control. In the group randomized to a target of < 80 mmHg the risk of major cardiovascular events was halved in comparison with that of the group randomized to a target of < 90 mmHg (Fig. 4.2). The cardiovascular event rates were generally reduced in the group targeted for < 80 mmHg relative to the group targeted for < 90 mmHg, although conventional statistical significance was not always achieved in each category.

Once again, multiple drug treatments were required, with only 26% of patients targeted to < 80 mmHg continuing with the single drug treatment. Interestingly, although reported adverse events increased with the number of administered drugs, there was no difference in relation to the BP target. In other words, 'tight' control caused no excess of side-effects.

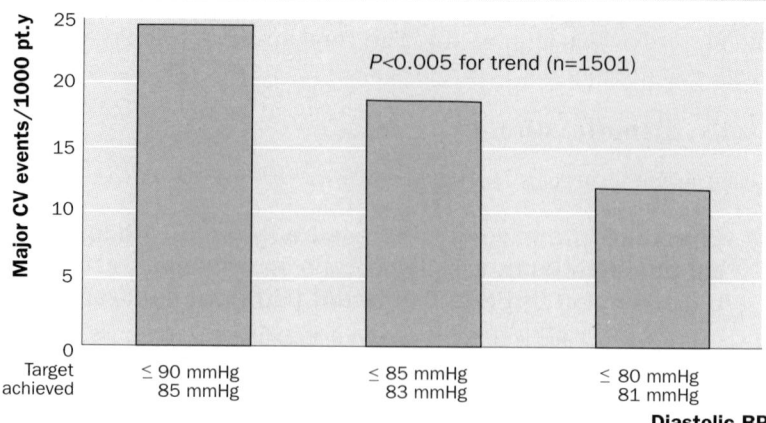

Fig. 4.2 The HOT study: cardiovascular (CV) risk reduction in diabetics. Major cardiovascular event rates according to the target BP category in the HOT study (Hansson *et al.*, 1998). pt.y = patient-year.

SHEP study: diabetic cohort

Effect of diuretic-based antihypertensive treatment on cardiovascular disease risk in older diabetic patients with isolated systolic hypertension.

D Curb, S L Pressel, J A Cutler, P J Savage, W B Applegate, H Black, *et al.* for the Systolic Hypertension in the Elderly Program Cooperative Research Group. *JAMA* 1996; **276:** 1886–92.

BACKGROUND. **The objective of this study was to assess the effect of low-dose, diuretic-based antihypertensive treatment on major cardiovascular disease (CVD) event rates in older, non-insulin-treated diabetic patients with isolated systolic hypertension (ISH), compared with non-diabetic patients.**

INTERPRETATION. Low-dose diuretic-based (chlorthalidone) treatment is effective in preventing major CVD events, cerebral and cardiac, in both non-insulin-treated diabetic and non-diabetic older patients with ISH.

Comment

The results of the studies published within the past 12 months or so are entirely confirmatory to those first identified in hypertensive patients with type II diabetes mellitus. A total of 4736 men and women aged 60 years and older with isolated systolic hypertension participated in this clinical outcome trial based on a low-dose thiazide diuretic (chlorthalidone). Within this study there were 583 non-insulin-dependent diabetic patients who were randomly assigned to receive either placebo or an active antihypertensive treatment regimen based on low-dose (12.5 or 25 mg) chlorthalidone. For both diabetic and non-diabetic patients there was a similar (34%) reduction in major cardiovascular events for active treatment compared with placebo. However, the absolute risk reduction was twice as great for diabetic versus non-diabetic patients (101 per 1000 participants versus 51 per 1000 participants at the 5-year follow-up), reflecting the higher risk of diabetic patients.

In retrospect, this study highlighted two important points. Firstly, antihypertensive treatment and significant BP reductions lead to improved cardiovascular outcomes in high-risk patients, who attained the greatest absolute benefits. Secondly, although thiazide diuretics have been implicated in causing adverse metabolic effects, including the precipitation of diabetes mellitus, there was no suggestion that the cardiovascular benefits were compromised.

Summary

Since hypertension is common in patients with diabetes, particularly type II diabetes mellitus, and is a major contributor to the development and progression of microvascular and macrovascular complications, the results of the UKPDS have clearly demonstrated the importance of intensive antihypertensive treatment and 'tight' BP control. These results accord with the findings from recently published trials involving diabetic hypertensive patients, with clear outcome benefits in such high-risk patients. However, these benefits have been obtained, with regimens based on different types of antihypertensive drug, and there is no clear evidence that any individual drug or drug class is superior. The primary target is to attain BP control with values of 140/90 mmHg or less (135/85 mmHg or less has also been recommended). Frequently this will require multiple drug treatments.

Cholesterol reduction

Dyslipidaemia tends to occur more frequently in patients with diabetes mellitus, although their total and LDL cholesterol levels are often similar to those of people without diabetes. However, these apparent similarities may mask underlying differences in lipid particle size and lipid composition, which, in turn, are influenced by the type of diabetes and the adequacy of the glycaemic control. In type II diabetes mellitus, even with adequate metabolic control, triglyceride levels tend to be elevated and HDL levels reduced.

The extent to which cardiovascular complications can be modified by conventional risk factor interventions (other than BP reduction) has also been confirmed through cholesterol reduction in the CARE study.

CARE : diabetic subgroup

 Cardiovascular events and their reduction with pravastatin in diabetic and glucose-intolerant myocardial infarction survivors with average cholesterol levels: subgroup analyses in the Cholesterol and Recurrent Events (CARE) trial.

R B Goldberg, M J Mellies, F M Sacks, L A Moyé, B V Howard, W J Howard, *et al.* for the CARE Investigators. *Circulation* 1998; **98:** 2513–9.

BACKGROUND. Although diabetes is a major risk factor for coronary heart disease (CHD), little information is available on the effects of lipid-lowering in diabetic patients. We determined whether lipid-lowering treatment with pravastatin prevents recurrent cardiovascular events in diabetic patients with CHD and average cholesterol levels.

INTERPRETATION. Diabetic patients and non-diabetic patients with impaired fasting glucose are at high risk of recurrent coronary events that can be substantially reduced by pravastatin treatment.

Comment

A subgroup of 586 patients was identified among the 4159 patients participating in the Cholesterol And Recurrent Events (CARE) trial, which was a secondary prevention trial investigating the impact of cholesterol reduction (with pravastatin) over a 5-year follow-up period. The diabetic patients were older, more obese and more hypertensive, but their baseline lipid concentrations were similar to those of the non-diabetic group. Similarly, the reductions in LDL cholesterol were similar, at 27 and 28% in the diabetic and non-diabetic groups, respectively.

In the diabetic cohort there was a 25% relative risk reduction for all major coronary events (death from coronary heart disease, non-fatal myocardial infarction or revascularization procedure) in the pravastatin-treated group compared to the placebo group. The relative risk of coronary artery bypass or percutaneous transluminal coronary angioplasty was reduced by 32%. Overall, cholesterol reduction with pravastatin treatment reduced the absolute risk of coronary events by 8.1% in the diabetic patients and by 5.2% in the non-diabetic patients: the relative risk reductions were 25% ($P=0.05$) and 23% ($P<0.001$), respectively. Of additional interest were the 342 patients who had impaired fasting glucose on entry to the study (out of the 3553 patients who were not categorized as diabetic). These patients had a higher rate of recurrent coronary events than those with normal fasting glucose; for example, 13% compared to 10% suffered a non-fatal myocardial infarction.

Summary

This *post hoc* subgroup analysis supports the general view that lipid-lowering treatment is beneficial for patients who fall into high-risk categories, and particularly for those with evidence of pre-existing cardiovascular disease with prior myocardial infarction or angina. Whether or not it is necessary to prescribe lipid-lowering drug treatment for diabetics who have no evidence of clinical cardiovascular disease remains undetermined.

Intensified multifactorial intervention

The evidence that BP reduction and cholesterol reduction can independently improve outcome was extended through the findings of a smaller study that explored the multiple risk factor approach, whereby hypertension was targeted in conjunction with intensive treatment for hyperglycaemia, dyslipidaemia and microalbuminuria.

Steno

Intensified multifactorial intervention in patients with type II diabetes mellitus and microalbuminuria: the Steno type II randomized study.

P Gaede, P Vedel, H-H Parving, O Pedersen. *Lancet* 1999; **353:** 617–22.

BACKGROUND. In type II diabetes mellitus the aetiology of long-term complications is multifactorial. The authors carried out a randomized trial of stepwise intensive treatment or standard treatment of risk factors in patients with microalbuminuria.

INTERPRETATION. Intensified multifactorial intervention in patients with type II diabetes and microalbuminuria slows progression to nephropathy, and progression of retinopathy and autonomic neuropathy. However, further studies are needed to establish the effect of intensified multifactorial treatment on macrovascular complications and mortality.

Comment

Eighty patients were randomized to standard treatment and 80 patients were randomized to intensive treatment to assess the impact on the primary endpoint of development/progression of nephropathy. The mean age of these patients was 55 years, and they were followed up for an average of 3.8 years. Patients receiving intensive treatment had significantly lower rates for progression to nephropathy, with a reduction by 73% for this primary endpoint and similar reductions in the secondary endpoints with progression of retinopathy reduced by 55% and progression of autonomic neuropathy reduced by 68%. To achieve these benefits 48 of 76 patients received antihypertensive treatment in the standard group compared to 71 of 73 patients in the intensive group who finished the study. Correspondingly, lipid-lowering drugs were administered to 33 of 73 patients in the intensive group compared to only 2 in the standard group. Furthermore, aspirin was administered to 31 in the intensive group but only 17 in the standard group. Overall, the results for the major risk factors were as follows. There was a significantly greater reduction in BP in the intensive group by 8/7 mmHg compared to 4/5 mmHg, but there were also significant reductions in cholesterol, by 0.6 mmol/l compared to 0.2 mmol/l; in glycated haemoglobin, with a reduction by 0.8% in the intensive group compared to an increase of 0.2% in the standard group; and a reduction in fasting glucose, by 2.7 mmol compared to 0.3 mmol/l.

Although these were not primary endpoints of the study, it is interesting to note that these multifactorial interventions were also associated with a trend towards improved outcomes, with mortality and major macrovascular events numbering 26 in the intensive group compared to 42 in the standard group.

Summary

Preservation of renal function remains an important component of the treatment strategy in diabetic hypertensives. As with atherosclerotic cardiovascular disease itself, improvement in all the major cardiovascular risk factors produces the greatest overall benefit.

Microalbuminuria and diabetic nephropathy

It is well recognized that BP reduction is necessary for the preservation of renal function in most types of renal impairment, particularly diabetic nephropathy. Diabetes, usually complicated by hypertension, continues to be statistically the most important cause of end-stage renal failure; and much recent research has focused attention on how best to maintain renal function and improve patient outcome. There remains considerable debate, however, about the 'best' treatment regimen, and whether or not different drug types have specifically beneficial or adverse properties. Despite the evidence from the UKPDS that BP reduction is beneficial in these high-risk patients, there also remain questions about the optimal BP targets and the most effective drug treatment strategies not only for preserving renal function, but also for improving patient outcome in terms of reducing cardiovascular morbidity and mortality.

The overall treatment emphasis in both type I and type II diabetes mellitus remains good BP control, but the debate continues as to whether or not ACE inhibitors have benefits beyond the haemodynamic. It has been suggested that this is particularly important in type I diabetes and of potential importance even in patients who are normotensive. This concept of preserving kidney function and delaying the progression from microalbuminuria to frank diabetic nephropathy has recently been further studied with captopril.

Randomized control trial of long-term efficacy of captopril on preservation of kidney function

Randomized controlled trial of long-term efficacy of captopril on preservation of kidney function in normotensive patients with insulin-dependent diabetes and microalbuminuria.

E R Mathiesen, E Hommel, H P Hansen, U M Smidt, H-H Parving.
BMJ 1999; **319:** 24–5.

BACKGROUND. In patients with insulin-dependent diabetes, angiotensin-converting enzyme inhibition delays the progression from microalbuminuria to diabetic nephropathy, but previous studies have been too short to show a preservation of kidney function.

INTERPRETATION. This study assessed the effectiveness of angiotensin-converting enzyme inhibition on preservation of kidney function in an 8-year prospective, randomized controlled trial.

Comment

This is a small-scale but well-conducted study of 44 normotensive patients with type I diabetes who were followed up for a period of 8 years. The treatment group (n=21) received captopril (100 mg per 24 hours) and bendrofluazide (2.5 mg per 24 hours), whereas the untreated group (n=23) continued without antihypertensive medication. The glomerular filtration rate declined by 11.8 ml/min in the untreated group and by 1.4 ml/min in the captopril group ($P=0.09$) and the proportion of patients who progressed to diabetic nephropathy was 40% in the control group and 10% in the captopril group ($P=0.019$). These authors concluded that the ACE inhibitor had a clinically significant effect on the preservation of a normal glomerular filtration rate by virtue of the prevention of progression from microalbuminuria to diabetic nephropathy. Unfortunately, the question as to whether or not there are benefits beyond the haemodynamic cannot be clearly answered by this study. In particular, although the patients were defined as normotensive, no information is provided about the baseline and achieved blood pressure values in either group.

Summary

The established facts are that intensive antihypertensive treatment and 'tight' BP control improve both renal and cardiovascular outcome in patients with diabetic nephropathy. It is assumed that similar 'tight' BP control will also improve outcome in other forms of renal disease. On the basis of the available evidence it appears that an appropriate treatment target is a BP of $< 135/85$ mmHg.

The choice of antihypertensive drug

An ACE inhibitor is generally regarded as the first-choice antihypertensive agent for a patient with diabetes and hypertension. In contrast, there has been considerable controversy about the role of calcium channel blockers, with some reports of adverse outcomes, particularly in two recent small-scale clinical trials:

1. FACET
2. ABCD

FACET

Outcome results of the Fosinopril versus Amlodipine Cardiovascular Events randomized Trial (FACET) in patients with hypertension and NIDDM.

P Tatti, M Pahor, R P Byington, P Di Mauro, R Guarisco, G Strollo, *et al.*
Diabetes Care 1999; **21:** 597–603.

BACKGROUND. ACE inhibitors and calcium antagonists may favourably affect serum lipids and glucose metabolism. The primary aim of the Fosinopril versus Amlodipine Cardiovascular Events randomized Trial (FACET) was to compare the effects of fosinopril and amlodipine on serum lipids and diabetes control in non-insulin-dependent diabetes mellitus patients with hypertension.

INTERPRETATION. Fosinopril and amlodipine had similar effects on biochemical measures, but the patients randomized to fosinopril had a significantly lower risk of major vascular events, compared with the patients randomized to amlodipine.

Comment

The Fosinopril versus Amlodipine Cardiovascular Events randomized Trial was not designed or statistically empowered to assess treatment-related differences in cardiovascular outcomes. The salient result was that the ACE inhibitor treatment (fosinopril) was associated with a significantly lower cardiovascular event rate than the calcium channel blocker group (amlodipine) (Table 4.4). However, this combined endpoint was a secondary endpoint, and, once the data were correctly adjusted for multiple statistical comparisons, this difference lost its statistical significance.

Interestingly, and importantly, the combination of the calcium channel blocker and the ACE inhibitor, in relation to the effectiveness of either agent alone, appeared to be most effective in reducing cardiovascular events. Overall, therefore, it seems unlikely that this long-acting calcium channel blocker was inherently dangerous for diabetic hypertensives.

Table 4.4 FACET: post-randomization analysis

	Amlodipine n=141	Fosinopril n=131	Combination n=108
Myocardial infarction	13	7	3
Stroke	10	3	1
Hospitalized angina	4	0	0
All major events	27*	10	4

* $P<0.01$ versus fosinopril. $P<0.01$ versus combination. Source: Tatti *et al.* (1998).

ABCD

The effect of nisoldipine as compared with enalapril on cardiovascular outcomes in patients with non-insulin-dependent diabetes and hypertension.

R O Estacio, B W Jeffers, W R Hiatt, S L Biggerstaff, N Gifford, R W Schrier.
N Engl J Med 1998; **338**: 645–52.

BACKGROUND. **It has recently been reported that the use of calcium channel blockers for hypertension may be associated with an increased risk of cardiovascular complications. Because this issue remains controversial, the authors studied the incidence of such complications in patients with non-insulin-dependent diabetes mellitus and hypertension who were randomly assigned to treatment with either the calcium channel blocker nisoldipine or the angiotensin-converting enzyme inhibitor enalapril as part of a larger study.**

INTERPRETATION. In this population of patients with diabetes and hypertension, there was a significantly higher incidence of fatal and non-fatal myocardial infarction among those assigned to therapy with the calcium channel blocker nisoldipine than among those assigned to receive enalapril. Since these findings are based on a secondary endpoint, they will require confirmation.

Comment

The Appropriate Blood Pressure Control in Diabetes trial contained a hypertensive cohort and a normotensive cohort. The hypertensive study was terminated prematurely on the basis of apparently adverse outcomes in the patients receiving a calcium channel blocker (nisoldipine) rather than an ACE inhibitor (enalapril). However, a close scrutiny of the statistical analysis reveals that two significant differences had been identified between the two treatments in respect of the primary and secondary endpoints. Since this represented two differences out of 36 endpoints tested, this is precisely what would be expected to occur by chance.

Summary

These two trials must be interpreted with caution. The results are certainly compatible with the prevailing view that ACE inhibitors are probably to be preferred as first-line antihypertensive agents for the hypertensive diabetic. However, there is no convincing evidence that calcium channel blockers are actually harmful, and, since 'tight' BP control will require multiple drug treatment, there is some evidence that the combination of an ACE inhibitor and a calcium channel blocker is effective and beneficial. Furthermore, the effectiveness of treatment regimens based upon dihydropyridine calcium channel blockers has already been confirmed in the subgroup analyses of large-scale prospective clinical outcome trials such as SYST-EUR and HOT.

Insulin responsiveness and treatment effects

Insulin resistance is recognized as a feature of type II diabetes mellitus and also of untreated essential hypertension, and it is generally accepted that conventional doses of thiazide diuretics and beta-blockers may further worsen this problem and amplify the underlying metabolic disturbances of lipid and glucose metabolism. In contrast, there is a popular belief that angiotensin-converting enzyme inhibitors have beneficial effects on insulin responsiveness. Although numerous studies in the literature have reported beneficial effects of ACE inhibition on aspects of glucose metabolism, only one published trial has incorporated all the following features:

1. A double-blind, placebo-controlled, cross-over design;

2. Assessment of insulin responsiveness (sensitivity) using a highly reproducible technique;

3. Adequate statistical power for avoiding clinically important type II error; and

4. Reliable exclusion of potentially confounding carry-over effects.

Captopril does not improve insulin action in essential hypertension

Captopril does not improve insulin action in essential hypertension: a double-blind placebo-controlled study.

M I Wiggam, S J Hunter, A B Atkinson, C N Ennis, J S Henry, J N Browne, *et al. J Hypertens* 1998; **16**; 1651–7.

BACKGROUND. The objective of this study was to compare the effect of captopril with that of placebo on peripheral and hepatic insulin action in essential hypertension, in the light of evidence that insulin resistance is associated with cardiovascular risk.

INTERPRETATION. Captopril therapy in uncomplicated essential hypertension has no effect on peripheral or hepatic insulin sensitivity.

Comment

This was a double-blind, placebo-controlled study designed to evaluate the effect of captopril on peripheral and hepatic insulin action in patients with essential hypertension. Eighteen hypertensive, non-diabetic patients, aged < 65 years, received captopril 50 mg twice a day or placebo for two 8-week treatment periods separated by a 6-week washout phase. For the 14 patients who completed the study there were no differences in fasting levels of glucose and insulin, and postabsorptive hepatic glucose production was similar. During the hyperinsulinaemic euglycaemic clamp it was shown that hepatic glucose production was suppressed to comparable levels after captopril and after placebo, and the glucose uptake rates were also similar at 30.0 ± 2.6 mmol/kg/min with captopril and 30.3 ± 2.6 mmol/kg/min with a placebo. These authors concluded that captopril treatment had no effect on peripheral or hepatic insulin sensitivity.

Summary

Despite the early reports that ACE inhibitor drugs improve insulin responsiveness, the accumulated evidence suggests that this is not the case. Most of these studies have had methodological shortcomings, and there are more negative or neutral reports than positive reports. Furthermore in UKPDS, glycaemic control and hypoglycaemic episodes were no different in the captopril group than in the atenolol group.

Conclusions

In the light of recent reports, there has been a clear change in emphasis in the treatment of hypertensive diabetic patients in so far as 'tight' BP control is considered to be essential and the benefits of BP reduction have now been confirmed in a number of clinical outcome trials. Of additional interest is the emerging concept that, while ACE inhibition will remain the cornerstone of antihypertensive drug treatment in this patient group, the maximum benefits may be achieved through 'tight' BP control and pronounced blood pressure reductions independently of the pharmacological characteristics of any particular antihypertensive drug. However, it is not only BP control that is important. Intensive management of all risk factors safely and effectively reduces the risk of the chronic complications of diabetes.

References

1. DCCT Research Group. The effect of intensive treatment of diabetes on the development and progression of long-term complications in insulin-dependent diabetes mellitus. *N Engl J Med* 1993; **329**: 977–86.

2. Ohkubo Y, Kishikawa H, Araki E, Miyata T, Isami S, Motoyoshi S, *et al.* Intensive insulin therapy prevents the progression of diabetic microvascular complications in Japanese patients with non-insulin-dependent diabetes mellitus: a randomized prospective 6-year study. *Diabetes Res Clin Pract* 1995; **28**: 103–17.

5

Lipid-lowering treatment

Introduction

There is now clear evidence that lipid-lowering drug treatment (particularly with statins) is of benefit in the primary and secondary prevention of coronary heart disease. Since the publication of the 'landmark' Scandinavian Simvastatin Survival Study (4S) in 1994 |1| there have been two further primary and two further secondary prevention studies:

Primary prevention: WOSCOPS (1995)
                     AFCAPS/TexCAPS (1998)

Secondary prevention: CARE (1996)
                       LIPID (1998)

Recent clinical outcome trials

Primary prevention

Primary prevention of acute coronary events with lovastatin in men and women with average cholesterol levels.

J R Downs, M Clearfield, S Weis, E Whitney, D R Shapiro, F A Beere, *et al.*
JAMA 1998; **279**: 1615–22.

BACKGROUND. Although cholesterol-reducing treatment has been shown to reduce fatal and non-fatal coronary disease in patients with coronary heart disease (CHD), it is unknown whether benefit from the reduction of low-density lipoprotein cholesterol (LDL-C) in patients without CHD extends to individuals with average serum cholesterol levels, women and older persons.

AIM. To compare lovastatin with placebo for prevention of the first acute major coronary event in men and women without clinically evident atherosclerotic cardiovascular disease with *average* total cholesterol (TC) and LDL-C levels and *below-average* high-density lipoprotein cholesterol (HDL-C) levels.

INTERPRETATION. Lovastatin reduces the risk for the first acute major coronary event in men and women with average TC and LDL-C levels and below-average HDL-C levels. These findings support the inclusion of HDL-C in risk factor assessment, confirm the benefit of LDL-C reduction to a target level, and suggest the need for reassessment of the National Cholesterol Education Program guidelines regarding pharmacological intervention.

The Airforce/Texas Coronary Atherosclerosis Prevention Study (AFCAPS/TexCAPS) was a randomized, double-blind, placebo-controlled trial involving 6605 subjects (of whom 997 were women) who had 'average' lipid levels. The average age of the participants was 58 years, with 22% aged 65 years or more. All subjects were advised to continue with a low-saturated-fat, low-cholesterol diet, and then they were randomly assigned to lovastatin (20–40 mg daily) or placebo. After an average follow-up of 5.2 years there were significant reductions in all the major endpoints, both primary and secondary (Table 5.1).

Overall, the reductions in CHD events and coronary intervention procedures by respectively 40% and 33% in AFCAPS/TexCAPS were remarkably similar to the corresponding reductions of 31% and 37% in the WOSCOPS (West of Scotland Coronary Prevention) study. Also remarkably similar were the percentage changes in lipid fractions (see Fig. 5.1) even though the average pre-treatment cholesterol values were different: 7.0 mmol/l in WOSCOPS and 5.7 mmol/l in AFCAPS/TexCAPS.

Comment

The results of this study are confirmatory and reassuring. Firstly, this is the first primary prevention study to include women (albeit in the minority), and it is important to note that women benefited from treatment to at least as great an extent as men. Secondly, benefit was apparent across all baseline levels (tertiles) of cholesterol (2.33–6.0 mmol per litre), with no evidence to suggest a threshold level. Finally, absolute benefit was greatest in those at greatest risk, for example, in those with concomitant hypertension. The event rate was approximately twice as great in those

Table 5.1 Airforce/Texas Coronary Atherosclerosis Prevention Study (AFCAPS/TexCAPS): reductions in major endpoints after lovastatin treatment after an average follow-up of 5.2 years (Downs *et al.*, 1998)

Endpoints	Event rate (per 1000 patient-years)		Relative risk reduction	$P<$
	Placebo	Lovastatin		
Primary	10.9	6.8	37%	0.001

(Fatal/non-fatal myocardial infarction, unstable angina, sudden cardiac death)

Endpoints	Placebo	Lovastatin	Relative risk reduction	$P<$
Secondary				
CV events	15.3	11.5	25%	0.003
CHD events	12.8	9.6	25%	0.006
Revascularization	9.3	6.2	33%	0.001
Myocardial infarction	5.6	3.3	40%	0.002
Unstable angina	5.1	3.5	32%	0.02
Fatal CV events	1.4	1.0	–	–
Fatal CHD events	0.9	0.6	–	–

CV = cardiovascular; CHD = coronary heart disease.

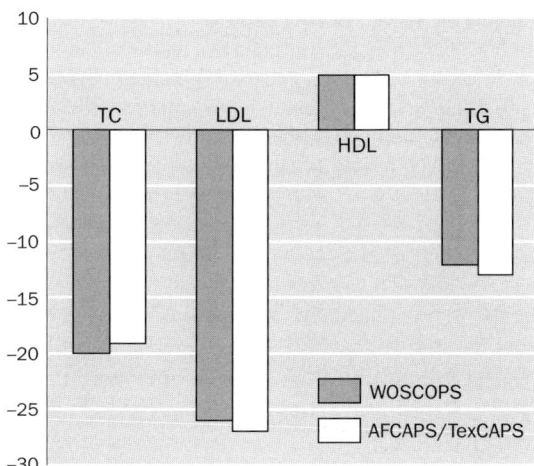

Fig. 5.1 Comparison of percentage changes in lipid fractions in WOSCOPS and AFCAPS/TexCAPs. TC = total serum cholesterol; LDL = low-density lipoprotein; HDL = high-density lipoprotein; TG = triglyceride.

with hypertension, and the relative risk reduction for a first primary endpoint event tended to be greater, at 39% in the hypertensives compared to 27% in the normotensive subjects.

Secondary prevention

Prevention of cardiovascular events and death with pravastatin in patients with coronary heart disease and a broad range of initial cholesterol levels.
The Longterm Intervention with Pravastatin in Ischaemic Disease (LIPID) Study Group. *N Engl J Med* 1998; **339**: 1349–57.

BACKGROUND. In patients with CHD and a broad range of cholesterol levels, cholesterol-lowering therapy reduces the risk of coronary events, but the effects on mortality from CHD and overall mortality have remained uncertain.

INTERPRETATION. Pravastatin therapy reduced mortality from CHD and overall mortality, as compared with the rates in the placebo group, as well as the incidence of all pre-specified cardiovascular events in patients with a history of myocardial infarction or unstable angina who had a broad range of initial cholesterol levels.

LIPID was a double-blind, randomized comparison of the effects of pravastatin (40 mg daily) and placebo in 9014 patients, aged 31–75 years, with a past history of myocardial infarction or hospitalization for unstable angina. The mean pretreatment cholesterol was approximately 5.6 mmol/l, the mean follow-up period was 6.1 years and mortality from CHD was the primary outcome measure. In the pravastatin group there was a highly significant risk reduction in death by 24% due to CHD and significant reductions in other outcome measures, including a 19% reduction in stroke events. Once again, there was a reassuring consistency in these findings relative to the results of 4S and CARE, which led the authors to conclude that 'cholesterol-lowering therapy should now be considered for virtually all patients presenting with CHD'.

Comment

These findings should be considered to have placed the 'final seal of approval' on lipid-lowering treatment in patients known to have CHD. The only significant medical issues that remain the subject of debate are 'What is the optimal target concentration for total and/or LDL cholesterol?' and 'How important are the concentrations of HDL cholesterol and trigyclerides?'

Conclusion

These recent studies have confirmed that improved lipid profiles, particularly in response to treatment with statins, lead to cardiovascular benefits. The current 'obsession', however, does not relate to optimal medical treatment but instead is focused on 'cost-effectiveness', i.e. politics rather than medicine.

From clinical trials to clinical practice

Despite the progressive accumulation of evidence that lipid-lowering drug treatment is particularly beneficial in high-risk patients, and especially in secondary prevention in patients known to have CHD, there continues to be a discrepancy between 'recommendation' and 'implementation' with respect to the prescription of lipid-lowering drugs in routine clinical practice. This not only applies in the USA, but is also apparent in Western Europe and Asia.

EUROASPIRE: A European Society of Cardiology survey of secondary prevention of coronary heart disease: principal results.
EUROASPIRE Study Group. *Eur Heart J* 1997; **18**: 1569–82.

BACKGROUND. The three main European scientific societies in cardiovascular medicine—the European Society of Cardiology (ESC), the European Atherosclerosis Society and the European Society of Hypertension—published in October 1994 joint recommendations on prevention of CHD in clinical practice. Patients with established

CHD, or other major atherosclerotic disease, were deemed to be the top priority for prevention. A European survey (EUROASPIRE) was therefore conducted under the auspices of the European Society of Cardiology to describe current clinical practice in relation to secondary prevention of CHD.

The aims of EUROASPIRE were:

1. to determine whether the major risk factors for coronary heart disease are recorded in patients' medical records;
2. to measure the modifiable risk factors and describe their current management following hospitalization; and
3. to determine whether first-degree blood relatives have been screened.

INTERPRETATION. This European survey has demonstrated a high prevalence of modifiable risk factors in CHD patients. There is considerable potential for cardiologists and physicians to reduce CHD further in addition to morbidity and mortality and improve patient chances of survival.

This survey explored the medical records of 4863 patients known to have CHD or other major atherosclerotic disease. Although 44% of these patients had raised total plasma cholesterol > 5.5 mmol/l, only 32% were receiving lipid-lowering drugs. Of those receiving lipid-lowering drugs, 49% continued with a TC > 5.5 mmol/l and 13% with one > 6.5 mmol/l. These disappointing findings in relation to cholesterol were matched by equally disappointing findings relating to other cardiovascular risk factors: for example, of the patients receiving antihypertensive drugs, 50% had a systolic blood pressure > 140 mmHg and 21% one > 160 mmHg.

Comment

The high and persisting prevalence of modifiable risk factors in CHD patients is disappointing. However, a probably even greater disappointment is that the introduction of drug treatment was not pursued to its full extent, and poor control of both elevated cholesterol and blood pressure was widely tolerated. The effective management of hypertension and dyslipidaemia (together with hyperglycaemia) is well justified by current scientific evidence, and there would be clear benefits in terms of reduced needs for revascularization procedures, fewer hospitalizations, and lower CHD morbidities and mortality. For patients, these outcomes would be perceived as a better quality of life and a longer life expectancy.

Practical aspects of lipid-lowering strategies

The volume and consistency of the evidence derived from studies of different 'statin' drugs underlies their position as the most commonly prescribed lipid-lowering medication. In contrast, the early clinical outcome trials with bile acid sequestrant resins (cholestyramine) and fibrates (clofibrate and gemfibrozil) created a confused picture. Nevertheless, despite the recent positive evidence with statins, a number of important practical issues remain to be resolved and clarified definitively. For example, although the magnitude of the reductions in total and LDL cholesterol achieved with statins is generally greater than that obtained through dietary efforts, dietary modifications or lifestyle interventions continue to be recommended as the initial and cornerstone approach to improving lipid profiles. At present, the major practical issues relate to the following:

1. The role of dietary modification;

2. The relevance of hypertriglyceridaemia and other lipid-lowering treatments;

3. The threshold and target levels for total and LDL cholesterol treatment; and

4. The choice of the optimal, or most cost-effective, statin treatment.

Dietary modifications

 Systematic review of dietary intervention trials to lower blood total cholesterol in free-living subjects.
J L Tang, J M Armitage, T Lancaster, C A Silagy, G H Fowler, H A W Neil.
BMJ 1998; **316**: 1213–20.

BACKGROUND. This study aimed to estimate the efficacy of dietary advice to lower blood and TC concentration in free-living subjects and to investigate the efficacy of different dietary recommendations.

INTERPRETATION. Individualized dietary advice for reducing cholesterol concentration is modestly effective in free-living subjects. More intensive diets achieve a greater reduction in serum cholesterol concentrations. Failure to comply fully with dietary recommendations is the likely explanation for this limited efficacy.

This analysis indicates that the effectiveness of dietary intervention, in the patient with 'average' motivation, is of modest effectiveness, with TC reductions in the range of 5–10%, at best. This result does not negate the value of dietary modification, but places it in a practical perspective.

Comment

Dietary change is likely to be useful but not definitive for reducing cholesterol in the majority of 'at-risk' patients. Nevertheless, the result in any single (motivated) individual may be sufficiently effective to avoid the need for drug treatment. The role of dietary modification, therefore, may be more important as a mechanism for 'involving' the patient in the overall risk-reduction strategy.

 Despite good compliance, very low-fat diet alone does not achieve recommended cholesterol goals in outpatients with coronary heart disease.
R Aquilani, R Tramarin, R F E Pedretti, G Bertolotti, M Sommaruga,
P Mariani, *et al. Eur Heart J* 1999; **20**: 1020–9.

BACKGROUND. **A low-saturated-fat, low-cholesterol diet is important in the treatment of hypercholesterolaemia in patients with CHD. The aim of this study was to investigate the efficacy of a very low-fat diet to achieve a targeted serum LDL cholesterol level ≤ 2.59 mmol/1) in outpatients with coronary heart disease.**

INTERPRETATION. Diet alone does not allow patients with CHD to achieve the recommended blood cholesterol levels, even if its fat content is highly reduced.

This is an interesting study in 126 male patients who were all ex-smokers and with known CHD. They were carefully assessed in terms of energy expenditure and then assigned to four different treatment groups: group A were instructed in a low-fat diet (related to their energy expenditure); group B were on a standard low-fat diet as described by the National Cholesterol Education Programme (Step 2 diet); and groups C and D had the corresponding diets augmented by simvastatin 10 mg daily. All patients were set a target LDL cholesterol of < 2.59 mmol/l, and the effectiveness of the different treatment regimens was assessed after 6 months.

The average decrease in serum LDL cholesterol did not differ between group A and group B; but neither of these dietary regimens proved capable of reaching the target. The only significant difference between the two diets was that there was a significant increase (by 29%) in HDL cholesterol in group A, which obviously led to a significant reduction in the LDL/HDL cholesterol ratio. Obviously the drug treatments were more effective in reducing total and LDL cholesterol than dietary intervention alone.

Comment

The target of LDL cholesterol < 2.59 mmol/l set a very demanding test for the efficacy of dietary modification in reducing cholesterol. The average changes in total and LDL cholesterol were modest in the two dietary regimens, –13 and –18%, respectively, in the more rigorous diet and –5 and –6% respectively on the standard Step 2 diet. None of these patients with dietary restriction alone achieved the primary target of LDL cholesterol < 2.59 mmol/l. The Step 2 diet corresponds approximately to the 'usual' lipid-lowering diets that are widely applied, and the reduction of 5% for total cholesterol and 6% for LDL cholesterol is typical of what has been reported elsewhere. For the target LDL cholesterol of < 3.37 mmol/l in this study, only 26% achieved target with the rigorous diet and 0% (again) reached target with the standard Step 2 diet.

Conclusion

In an apparently well-conducted study in a relatively well-motivated patient group, the effectiveness of standard dietary intervention was modest at best. The overall conclusion from each of these publications is that dietary modification may be sufficient in an individual patient to produce a worthwhile reduction in cholesterol but, and especially if rigorous targets are set, drug treatment will inevitably be required for the great majority of patients.

Other lipid-lowering drugs

The fibrate drugs principally decrease serum triglycerides (often by about 30–40%) by several mechanisms, one of which involves enhanced triglyceride clearance from the circulation by a process involving interaction of the fibrate with hepatic and adipocyte peroxisomal proliferator activator receptors. The effect on cholesterol is less than the effect on triglycerides, and less than that obtained with statins. The results of further trials to define patients who may benefit more from a fibrate than a statin are awaited. In the meantime, the principal indication is in the treatment of severe hypertriglyceridaemia and in combination with a statin in some patients who are at particularly high coronary risk through elevations of both cholesterol and triglycerides. Combination treatment, however, must be closely monitored, because of potential problems with adverse effects and the increased risk of myositis.

Gemfibrozil for the secondary prevention of coronary heart disease in men with low levels of high-density lipoprotein cholesterol.

H Bloomfield Rubins, S J Robins, D Collins, C L Fye, J W Anderson, M B Elam, *et al. N Engl J Med* 1999; **341**: 410–8.

BACKGROUND. Although it is generally accepted that lowering elevated serum levels of LDL cholesterol in patients with coronary heart disease is beneficial, there are few data to guide decisions about therapy for patients whose primary lipid abnormality is a low level of HDL cholesterol.

INTERPRETATION. Gemfibrozil therapy resulted in a significant reduction in the risk of major cardiovascular events in patients with CHD whose primary lipid abnormality was a low HDL cholesterol level. The findings suggest that the rate of coronary events is reduced by raising HDL cholesterol levels and lowering levels of triglycerides without lowering LDL cholesterol levels.

Comment

Fibrates retain a role in the management of these patients with 'mixed' or severe dyslipidaemia, particularly where low HDL cholesterol concentrations are featured.

Treatment targets

There is strong evidence to support the use of lipid-lowering drugs, and statins in particular, in those patients at high absolute risk of CHD. Once the treatment decision has been made, the target should be a cholesterol of < 5 mmol/l in both primary and secondary prevention.

The evidence of benefit is strongest in secondary prevention in those patients known to have CHD and a TC value of > 5 mmol/l or an LDL cholesterol value of > 3 mmol/l.

Patients with other major atherosclerotic disease (in the absence of overt coronary disease), for example, those with peripheral vascular disease or cerebrovascular disease, should be managed in the same way as those with overt CHD (i.e. through secondary prevention), although there is no direct clinical trial evidence of benefit. Thus the benefits in high-risk CHD patients, which *are* supported by evidence, are extrapolated to other high-risk patients with established atherosclerotic cardiovascular disease.

Lipid drug treatment of disorders.
R H Knopp. *N Engl J Med* 1999; **341**: 498–510.

BACKGROUND. Arteriosclerosis of the coronary and peripheral vasculature is the leading cause of death among men and women in the United States and worldwide.

INTERPRETATION. Cardiovascular disease accounts for nearly 50% of all deaths in the United States. Clinical trials and pathophysiological evidence support the use of aggressive therapy in patients with arteriosclerotic vascular disease and in those with several risk factors for the disease. Combination therapy with lipid-lowering drugs is advisable, especially in patients with combined hyperlipidemia.

Comment

This review article summarizes the evidence to date and recommends treatment according to the thresholds shown in Table 5.2. It is likely that these thresholds will be revised to lower values in the near future, although there are not yet prospective studies from which targets can be clearly defined; but the general view is 'the lower the better'.

Table 5.2 Drug thresholds for treatment of lipid disorders as recommended in Knopp (1999)

Cardiovascular risk factor	Threshold for initiation of dietary therapy, mg/dl (mmol/l)		Threshold for initiation of drug therapy, mg/dl (mmol/1)	
	Total cholesterol	LDL cholesterol	Total cholesterol	LDL cholesterol
No or one risk factor(s)	240 (6.24)	160 (4.16)	275 (7.15)	190 (4.94)
Two or more risk factors	200 (5.2)	130 (3.38)	240 (6.24)	160 (4.16)
Established cardiovascular disease	160 (4.16)	100 (2.6)	200 (5.2)	130 (3.38)

LDL = low-density lipoprotein.

Which statin? The choice of the optimal, or most cost-effective, statin treatment

This is a topical issue because of the potential cost implications if all at-risk patients are prescribed lipid-lowering drug treatment. Unfortunately, there are no definitive comparative studies, although the balance of evidence suggests that, across the recommended dose ranges, atorvastatin is the most effective.

 Comparative dose efficacy study of atorvastatin, lovastatin, and fluvastatin in patients with hypercholesterolaemia (the CURVES study).
P Jones, S Kafonek, I Laurora, D Hunninghake. *Am J Cardiol* 1998; **81**: 582–7.

BACKGROUND. The objective of this multicentre, randomized, open-label, parallel group, 8 week study was to evaluate the comparative dose efficacy of the 3-hydroxy-3-methyl-glutaryl coenzyme A (HMG-CoA) reductase inhibitor atorvastatin 10, 20, 40 and 80 mg compared with simvastatin 10, 20 and 40 mg, pravastatin 10, 20 and 40 mg, lovastatin 20, 40 and 80 mg, and fluvastatin 20 and 40 mg.

INTERPRETATION. Atorvastatin 10, 20 and 40 mg produced greater ($P \leq 0.01$) reductions in LDL cholesterol, –38%, –46% and –51%, respectively, than the milligram equivalent doses of simvastatin, pravastatin, lovastatin and fluvastatin. Atorvastatin 10 mg produced LDL cholesterol reductions comparable to or greater than simvastatin 10, 20 and 40 mg ($P < 0.02$), pravastatin 10, 20 and 40 mg, lovastatin 20 and 40 mg and fluvastatin 20 and 40 mg. Atorvastatin 10, 20 and 40 mg produced greater reductions in total cholesterol ($P < 0.01$) than the milligram equivalent doses of simvastatin, pravastatin, lovastatin and fluvastatin. All reductase inhibitors studied had similar tolerability. There was no incidence of persistent elevations in serum transaminases or myositis.

Comment

This study evaluated the responses to five different agents in a total of 534 hyper-cholesterolaemic patients. The principal results are shown in Fig. 5.2, where it can be seen that fluvastatin consistently produced the smallest reductions in LDL cholesterol whereas atorvastatin consistently produced the greatest reductions in LDL cholesterol.

While it might be assumed from this that atorvastatin is the most powerful lipid-lowering agent, it is necessary to modify this conclusion with the rider of 'at the doses studied'. Thus it may simply be a reflection of the fact that the recommended dose range for atorvastatin appears to have encompassed the lipid-lowering potential of this agent, whereas the dose ranges of most of the other agents may be at relatively and inappropriately low points on their dose–response curves.

 Atorvastatin compared with simvastatin-based therapies in the management of severe familial hyperlipidaemias.
A S Wierzbicki, P J Lumb, Y Semra, G Chik, E R Christ, M A Crook. *Q J Med* 1999; **92**: 387–94.

BACKGROUND. This study compared atorvastatin with simvastatin-based therapies in a prospective observational study of 201 patients with severe hyperlipidaemia.

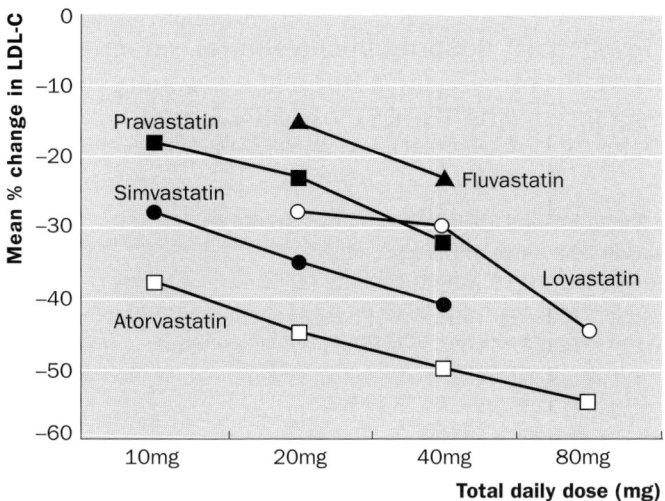

Fig. 5.2 Comparative dose efficacy of atorvastatin, fluvastatin, lovastatin, pravastatin and simvastatin in patients with hypercholesterolaemia (data from CURVES study, Jones *et al.*, 1998). LDL-C = low-density lipoprotein cholesterol.

INTERPRETATION. These data suggest that atorvastatin is more effective than current simvastatin-based therapies in achieving treatment targets in patients with familial hypercholesterolaemia, but at the expense of a possible increase in side-effects. This issue needs further study in randomized controlled trials.

Comment

It is well recognized that patients with severe hyperlipidaemias, and typically those with familial hypercholesterolaemia or combined hyperlipidaemia, have a poor prognosis because of the difficulties of achieving aggressive and effective cholesterol reductions. In this study, treatment based on atorvastatin (10–20 mg daily) proved superior to simvastatin (20–40 mg) treatment in so far as it reduced LDL cholesterol by more than twice as much as simvastatin, with or without the addition of cholestyramine. However, although atorvastatin is generally considered to be similar to other statins in respect of its profile of adverse effects, the results in this study indicated a slightly greater incidence. Depending upon the dose, 10–36% of patients reported adverse effects with atorvastatin. These authors concluded that although atorvastatin was more effective, and particularly more effective at lower doses than simvastatin, there is an increased likelihood of adverse effects, particularly with the highest dose of 80 mg.

Safety of low-density lipoprotein cholesterol reduction with atorvastatin versus simvastatin in a coronary heart disease population (the TARGET TANGIBLE trial).

W März, H Wollschläger, G Klein, A Neiß, M Wehling. *Am J Cardiol* 1999; **84**: 7–13.

BACKGROUND. Reduction in plasma lipids has been recognized as one of the primary cardiovascular risk reduction strategies in the secondary prevention of CHD. The primary endpoints of TARGET TANGIBLE were the safety (adverse events and laboratory measurements) and efficacy (responder rates) of therapy with atorvastatin versus simvastatin, with the aim of achieving LDL cholesterol lowering to ≤ 100 mg/dl (2.6 mmol/l).

INTERPRETATION. Atorvastatin resulted in a significantly greater number of patients reaching the LDL cholesterol goal than simvastatin, with 67% of atorvastatin patients and 53% of simvastatin patients reaching the target LDL cholesterol level of ≤ 100 mg/dl (2.6 mmol/l) (*P*<0.001).

Some 2856 patients (out of 3748 screened) with LDL cholesterol > 3.4 mmol/l were randomly assigned to treatment with atorvastatin or simvastatin for 14 weeks. These were patients with known coronary heart disease, and treatment was generally well tolerated, with only 2% of the atorvastatin patients and 3% of the simvastatin patients reporting serious adverse events. Overall adverse event rates were equivalent for atorvastatin and simvastatin, at 36.3% and 35.7%, respectively. The principal efficacy measure showed that a significantly greater number of patients reached the LDL cholesterol goal with atorvastatin: 67% of atorvastatin patients compared to 53% of simvastatin reached the target LDL cholesterol level of < 2.6 mmol/l. Correspondingly, significantly fewer patients in the atorvastatin group required titration to 40 mg: 38% of atorvastatin patients versus 54% of simvastatin patients.

Comment

This is an interesting study, which again demonstrates the overall efficacy and good tolerability of the statin group of drugs. On a milligram-for-milligram basis there is accumulating evidence that atorvastatin is the most effective of the currently available drugs. However, it remains unclear whether or not atorvastatin is intrinsically more potent, or whether the results simply reflect the fact that different statins have different effective dose ranges.

Increased thrombotic vascular events after change of statin.

M Thomas, J Mann. *Lancet* 1998; **352**: 1830–1.

BACKGROUND. This study described an increase in serum lipids after the introduction of a referencing pricing for HMG-CoA reductase inhibitors in New Zealand. When patients receiving simvastatin were charged more for prescriptions, there was a

general switch to fluvastatin, the only fully subsidized statin to be made available. As a result of this policy, patients received insufficient doses of a less potent drug that predictably altered their lipid control.

INTERPRETATION. Switching patients to less potent statins and/or consequent increases in lipids may act to unleash otherwise quiescent atheroma, with plaque instability, leading to an increase in vascular events. In addition, these findings caution against sudden increases in cholesterol that may be associated with a change in or cessation of therapy.

Comment

While accepting that there are limitations in the evidence relating to drug and dose comparability, this report illustrates the potential problems when cost alone (i.e. drug acquisition cost) is the sole criterion. In terms of the outcome data there are shortcomings because of the 'before-and-after' design of the study; nevertheless, the message is compelling in so far as the cheaper drug was significantly less effective for reducing cholesterol, and this, in turn, was associated with poorer patient outcome by virtue of more arterial thrombotic events (Table 5.3).

Conclusion

These studies illustrate the difficulties inherent in making simplistic assumptions about the comparability of different drugs, especially when the doses may not be comparable on a milligram-per-milligram basis and especially when cost considerations assume an overriding importance. The observation study by Thomas and Mann is clearly not definitive, but it does create anxieties about using cost considerations to direct treatment, especially when the available evidence, although it had limitations, indicated that fluvastatin was probably the least effective of the available agents. Whether or not atorvastatin is the most effective of the available agents remains to be clearly established because, on the basis of current evidence, it may simply be that the recommended dosages for atorvastatin are more appropriately within the effective therapeutic range than the currently recommended dosages of comparator drugs.

The role of aggressive lipid-lowering treatment

Aggressive lipid-lowering therapy compared with angioplasty in stable coronary artery disease.

B Pitt, D Waters, W V Brown, J Van Boven, L Schwartz, L M Title, *et al.*
N Engl J Med 1999; **341**: 70–6.

BACKGROUND. **Percutaneous coronary revascularization is widely used in improving symptoms and exercise performance in patients with ischaemic heart disease and stable angina pectoris. This study compared percutaneous coronary revascularization with lipid-lowering treatment for reducing the incidence of ischaemic events.**

Table 5.3 Changes in lipid concentrations and event rates after substitution of fluvastatin for simvastatin

n	Simvastatin dose (mg)	Fluvastatin dose (mg)	Percentage rise (total cholesterol)	Percentage rise (LDL cholesterol)	Percentage rise (triglyceride)	Events in most recent 6 months (simvastatin)	Events in following 6 months (fluvastatin)
44	10	23.5	17.7*	46.7*	6.2	3	5
52	20	38.6	16.1*	22.6*	19.1*	3	12
30	40	54	21.5	32.9*	16.0*	3	10
126	21.8	36.8	17.8*	33.6*	13.8*	9	27*

*P = 0.05. LDL 5 low-density lipoprotein. Source: Thomas and Mann (1998).

INTERPRETATION. In low-risk patients with stable coronary artery disease, aggressive lipid-lowering therapy is at least as effective as angioplasty and usual care in reducing the incidence of ischaemic events.

Comment

This study in more than 300 patients with known coronary artery disease investigated the efficacy of medical treatment with either atorvastatin (80 mg daily) or percutaneous transluminal coronary angioplasty (PTCA) with a follow-up period of 18 months, during which 'usual care' was permitted in the intervention group, including lipid-lowering treatment. Aggressive lipid-lowering treatment led to a 46% reduction in LDL cholesterol and was accompanied by ischaemic events in 13% of patients. In contrast, 21% of patients who underwent PTCA had an ischaemic event, despite an 18% reduction in LDL cholesterol. As compared with the patients treated with angioplasty followed by usual care, the patients who received atorvastatin and obtained pronounced reductions in LDL cholesterol had a significantly longer time to the first ischaemic event.

These results support other corresponding studies that have shown that aggressive medical treatment was at least as effective as conventional cardiological intervention.

Conclusion

The evidence of benefit from lipid-lowering strategies is virtually indisputable. Treatment of patients at high cardiovascular risk is now mandatory, and the only real debate relates to the 'optimal' target levels and the 'optimal' drug treatment. While the studies are not definitive, there is evidence to suggest that, at the usually recommended doses, atorvastatin is the most effective. Elsewhere, the issues relate to cost-effectiveness because of the (potentially) huge number of patients at relatively low risk who might nevertheless benefit, in the long term, from primary prevention of cardiovascular disease through drug treatment to reduce cholesterol.

Reference

1. Scandinavian Simvastatin Survival Study Group. Randomised trial of cholesterol lowering in 4444 patients with coronary heart disease; the Scandinavian Survival Study. *Lancet* 1994; **344:** 1383–9.

6

Hormone replacement therapy and cardiovascular risk

Introduction

The incidence of atherosclerotic cardiovascular disease is low in pre-menopausal women; it increases in post-menopausal women, and, reportedly, is reduced to pre-menopausal levels in those women who receive hormone replacement therapy with oestrogen (HRT or o/estrogen replacement therapy, ERT) after the menopause. Additionally, HRT has been reported to be particularly beneficial for secondary prevention, with hormone users having between 35 and 80% fewer recurrent events than non-users. However, the lower rates of coronary heart disease (CHD) in women taking HRT have been identified in observational studies and, relative to the available evidence, two important issues arise: firstly, can the beneficial effects of HRT be clearly demonstrated in a prospective, randomized, large-scale, clinical outcome trial; and, secondly, if HRT is beneficial, can the underlying mechanisms be clearly identified?

Effects of HRT on cardiovascular disease and cancer

Observational studies have shown a reduction in cardiovascular disease risk and mortality in post-menopausal women on oestrogen replacement therapy (ERT), but to what extent this reduction results from selection bias is contested. The increased risk of endometrial cancer has been greatly decreased or almost eliminated by the addition of progestogen to ERT |**1**|, but opinions are still divided on the association between ERT and increased risk of breast cancer |**2**|.

Cardiovascular and cancer morbidity and mortality and sudden cardiac death in postmenopausal women on oestrogen replacement therapy (ERT).
L Sourander, T Rajala, I Räihä, J Mäkinen, R Erkkola, H Helenius. *Lancet* 1998; **352**: 1965–9.

B ACKGROUND . **Advantages and disadvantages of post-menopausal oestrogen replacement therapy (ERT) are still not clear. This study aimed to analyse the relation between post-menopausal ERT, cardiovascular disease, and cancer.**

INTERPRETATION. Current ERT primarily reduced sudden cardiac death and predicted reduced cardiovascular mortality, but did not reduce morbidity. ERT did not increase the risk of breast cancer, but was associated with increased risk of endometrial cancer.

This Finnish community-based prospective study investigated cardiovascular disease mortality and the associated risk of breast and endometrial cancer in post-menopausal women taking ERT. During 1987–8, 8164 women (mean age 61 years) were invited to participate in a free mammography screening programme for breast cancer. Some 7944 women participated in the study and completed detailed questionnaires about a wide range of health-related issues, including the use of HRT. At baseline, 988 women were identified as current users of HRT, 757 as former users and 5572 as never users, and all women were followed up until 1995.

Compared with never users, there was a significant reduction in cardiovascular mortality with a risk ratio of 0.21 (adjusted for other risk factors). There were significant differences in absolute risk for death from coronary artery disease, at 0 in current HRT users, 0.81 in former HRT users and 1.0 per 1000 woman-years for never users. The corresponding figures for sudden cardiac death were 0, 1.0 and 1.6 per 1000 woman-years. There was a similar trend for deaths related to acute myocardial infarction, at respectively 0.45, 1.2 and 1.1 per 1000 woman-years, but this trend did not reach statistical significance. There were, however, significant reductions in death from stroke, with figures of respectively 0.15, 1.0 and 1.2 per 1000 woman-years. However, in contrast to the mortality results there were no significant differences for morbidity from coronary artery disease or stroke.

The incidence of endometrial cancer, but not breast cancer, was increased among current users (although most use unopposed oestrogen) with values of 5.06, 1.27 and 1.0 in the current users, former users and never users, respectively.

Comment

Hormone replacement therapy reduced cardiovascular mortality but not morbidity during this period of approximately 8 years of follow-up. The conclusion was drawn that HRT might be more likely to interfere with the progression of existing coronary disease than to prevent it primarily. Although this is an important study and although the conclusions may be valid and correct, the study design cannot eliminate selection bias in relation, for example, to the reasons for taking or not taking HRT, or for responding or not to the invitation for breast screening.

HRT, cardiovascular risk factors and vascular effects

Mechanistic studies have suggested that oestrogen has a vasodilator effect on arteries, including coronary arteries, and this has been attributed to both calcium channel blockade and augmented nitric oxide mechanisms. Anti-ischaemic and anti-anginal effects have also been described. These benefits in combination with a positive effect on lipid metabolism have been proffered as the explanation for the positive cardiovascular effects of HRT. With regard to blood pressure itself, there are some inconsistencies in the published literature, but the results of most studies suggest that blood pressure is lowered by HRT.

Risk factors

A randomised trial on effects of hormone therapy on ambulatory blood pressure (ABP) and lipoprotein levels in women with coronary artery disease.

U Pripp, G Hall, G Csemiczky, S Eksborg, B M Langdren, K Gustafsson. *J Hypertens* 1999; **17**: 1379–86.

BACKGROUND. This study investigated 1-year effects of hormone replacement therapy (HRT) on ambulatory blood pressure (ABP) and lipoprotein levels in post-menopausal women with coronary artery disease (CAD).

INTERPRETATION. One year of HRT in patients with CAD does not influence ABP. Oral HRT induces beneficial effects on lipoprotein levels.

Sixty post-menopausal women, mean age 59 years, were randomized to three treatment groups to receive conjugated equine oestrogen (CEE) (n=20), transdermal oestrodiol (TTSE) (n=20) or placebo (n=20) during repeated 28-day cycles for one year. Each monotherapy was administered for 18 days and then combined with medroxyprogesterone for the remaining 10 days of each cycle. The ABP results in the three groups are summarized in Table 6.1 (see p. 145). Overall, there was a small but non-significant trend for blood pressure to reduce during 12 cycles of treatment: average daytime blood pressure was 125/78 mmHg in the 32 women receiving HRT compared to 125/75 mmHg in the 13 women assigned to placebo. After 12 months of treatment, the corresponding daytime averages were 125/76 in the HRT group and 124/72 in the placebo group. Corresponding figures for night-time blood pressure showed an overall decrease, which was statistically significant. With respect to the lipid parameters there were no changes in triglyceride levels, but the increases in high-density lipoprotein (HDL) cholesterol and decreases in low-density lipoprotein (LDL) cholesterol did achieve statistical significance.

The effects of different types and doses of oestrogen replacement therapy on clinic and ambulatory blood pressure and the renin–angiotensin system in normotensive post-menopausal women.

P J Harvey, L M Wing, P J Savage, D Molloy. *J Hypertens* 1999; **17**: 405–14.

BACKGROUND. The effect on blood pressure (BP) of oral 'replacement' doses of oestrogen may depend on the type and dose of oestrogen administered. This study was designed to compare with placebo the effect of once-daily treatment with a 'natural' oestrogen, piperazine oestrone sulphate, in two different doses, and a

semi-synthetic oestrogen, ethinyloestradiol, on clinic and ABP and the renin–angiotensin system in post-menopausal women.

INTERPRETATION. In normotensive post-menopausal women, replacement doses of natural and semi-synthetic oestrogen reduce night-time ABP, with either no change or a small reduction in clinic BP. Reduction in BP is not explained by reduced activity of the renin–angiotensin system, but could have a component of reduced central sympathetic drive consistent with the decreased heart rate.

This was a randomized, double-blind, cross-over study involving 24 normotensive post-menopausal women, aged 47–60 years, who received four different treatments, each of 4 weeks' duration. The treatments were a 'natural' oestrogen in two different doses, a semi-synthetic oestrogen and placebo. There were no significant effects on daytime ABP, but night-time BP, both systolic and diastolic, was significantly reduced by two of the oestrogen preparations. There were no significant differences between treatments for the clinic systolic BPs, but two of the oestrogen preparations were associated with significant reductions in diastolic BP relative to the placebo phase.

Transdermal oestrogen reduces daytime blood pressure in hypertensive women.
K Manhem, H Ahlm, I Milsom, A Svensson. *J Hum Hypertens* 1998;
12: 323–7.

BACKGROUND. **The aim of this study was to investigate the acute effects of transdermally administered 17-β-oestradiol on ABP in hypertensive post-menopausal women.**

INTERPRETATION. This study supports previous evidence that HRT is safe in hypertensive women. The data in the present study also imply an acute, but small reduction in daytime BP due to transdermal oestrogen in hypertensive, post-menopausal women. Furthermore, oestrogen neither blunted nor increased the dipping phenomenon during the night in these women.

Importantly, this study again involved a double-blind, randomized, cross-over design comparing transdermal oestrogen with placebo in 13 post-menopausal women who were already receiving antihypertensive treatment. There was a small but significant decrease in BP during the daytime and no change in the night-time BP, with preservation of the nocturnal dip.

Comment

These three studies, albeit with some limitations in methodology, provide reassurance that HRT does not increase BP. In fact, the published literature now shows an overall consistency in reporting a small reduction in BP and a beneficial trend in lipid measures.

Vascular effects

Oestrogen improves abnormal norepinephrine-induced vasoconstriction in post-menopausal women.

B H Sung, M Ching, J L Izzo Jr, P Dandona, M F Wilson. *J Hypertens* 1999; **17**: 523–8.

BACKGROUND. An exaggerated BP response to mental stress in post-menopausal women has been reported, but the underlying mechanism is not clear. The present study examined the role of oestrogen in the BP response to mental stress.

INTERPRETATION. Healthy, normotensive post-menopausal women showed an exaggerated BP response to norepinephrine, and loss of oestrogen-mediated vasodilation may contribute to the increased BP response to stress in post-menopausal women without oestrogen replacement therapy.

Withdrawal of hormone therapy for 4 weeks decreases arterial compliance in post-menopausal women.

T K Waddell, C Rajkumar, J D Cameron, G L Jennings, A M Dart, B Kingwell. *J Hypertens* 1999; **17**: 413–8.

BACKGROUND. A previous cross-sectional study demonstrated that arterial compliance is elevated in post-menopausal women taking oestrogen-containing hormonal therapy, which may partially account for the reduction in cardiovascular events.

INTERPRETATION. These data suggest that hormonal modulation of distal arterial vascular tone may account for short-term changes in arterial compliance associated with oestrogen-containing hormonal therapy.

Comment

The improvements in arterial compliance, in relation to oestrogen treatment, are entirely consistent with the improvements reported in the clinical BP studies.

Estrogen stimulates delayed mitogen-activated protein kinase activity in human endothelial cells via an autocrine loop that involves basic fibroblast growth factor.

S Kim-Schulze, W L Lowe, W Schnaper. *Circulation* 1998; **98**: 413–21.

BACKGROUND. Oestrogen plays a significant role in protecting pre-menopausal women from cardiovascular disease. We have found that estradiol augments endothelial cell activities related to vascular healing and that human coronary artery and umbilical vein endothelial cells (HUVEC) express oestrogen receptors (ERs). Classically, the ER functions as a transcription factor, but the cytoplasmic targets of this genomic effect have not been defined for endothelial cells. The present study examined the potential role of the mitogen-activated protein (MAP) kinases ERK1 and ERK2 as mediators of oestrogen action.

INTERPRETATION. These data describe an autocrine mechanism for E2 induction of ERK1/2 in HUVEC. Because previous studies by the same authors suggested that certain cardioprotective effects of oestrogen are genomic in nature, the results are consistent with the hypothesis that autocrine stimulation of endothelial ERK1/2 activity by bFGF (basic fibroblast growth factor) may play a role in the beneficial effects of oestrogen on cardiovascular biology.

Comment

This is an interesting experimental study that seeks to explore the mechanisms underlying the vascular effects of oestrogen. In short, the addition of oestrogen to human umbilical vein endothelial cells was associated with an improvement in endothelial cell function. These findings are consistent with the small changes in blood pressure and in arterial compliance that have been seen in clinical studies.

The protective effects of oestrogen on the cardiovascular system.

M E Mendelsohn, R H Karas. *N Engl J Med* 1999; **340**: 1801–11.

CONTENT. This review article summarizes the current research information relating to the effects on cardiovascular risk factors.

Conclusion

Overall, from molecular biology to clinical studies, there is a consistent message that oestrogen has beneficial modulating effects on endothelial function, vascular resistance and BP. These effects, and the effects on cholesterol and other risk factors, are extended in a recent research review.

HRT and cardiovascular outcomes

Randomized trial of oestrogen plus progestin for secondary prevention of coronary heart disease in post-menopausal women.

S Hulley, D Grady, T Bush, R T Furberg, D Herrington, B Riggs, *et al.* for the Heart and Estrogen/progestin Replacement Study (HERS) Research Group. JAMA 1998; **280**: 605–13.

BACKGROUND. Observational studies have found lower rates of coronary heart disease (CHD) in post-menopausal women who take oestrogen than in women who do not, but this potential benefit has not been confirmed in clinical trials. The objective was to determine if oestrogen plus progestin therapy alters the risk for CHD events in post-menopausal women with established coronary disease.

INTERPRETATION. During an average follow-up of 4.1 years, treatment with oral conjugated equine oestrogen plus medroxyprogesterone acetate did not reduce the overall rate of CHD events in post-menopausal women with established coronary disease. Based on the finding of no overall cardiovascular benefit and a pattern of early increase of risk of CHD events, we do not recommend this treatment for the purpose of secondary prevention of CHD. However, given the favourable pattern of CHD events after several years of therapy it could be appropriate for women already receiving this treatment to continue.

This was a randomized, blinded, placebo-controlled secondary prevention trial in 2763 women < 80 years (mean age 66.7 years) who were known to have CHD and who were post-menopausal with an intact uterus. Follow-up averaged 4.1 years, with 82% of those assigned to HRT taking it at the end of 1 year and 75% at the end of 3 years.

Overall, there was no significant difference between groups in the primary outcomes (non-fatal myocardial infarction or CHD death) or in any of the secondary cardiovascular outcomes. Myocardial infarction or CHD death occurred in 172 women receiving HRT and in 176 receiving placebo. The lack of any overall beneficial effect occurred despite a net reduction of 11% in LDL cholesterol and a net 10% increase in HDL cholesterol in the HRT group ($P<0.001$). Within the overall null effect, however, there was a statistically significant time trend, with more CHD events in the HRT group during year 1 and fewer events in years 4 and 5. Furthermore, the HRT group had more episodes of venous thromboembolic events (34 versus 12) and gall bladder disease (84 versus 62 events).

Comment

The Heart and Oestrogen/progestin Replacement Study (HERS) was a landmark study because it was the first (and, to date, the only) double-blind, randomized trial of HRT in women with pre-existing coronary heart disease. Unfortunately, there was a highly significant increase in CHD events during the first year of oestrogen treatment, with a relative increase for any CHD event by 2.3 in months 0–4, 1.46 in months 5–8 and 1.18 in months 9–12. This overall lack of benefit was observed despite significant and beneficial changes in both HDL and LDL cholesterol. Total mortality was similar in both groups at 131 deaths in the HRT group and 123 deaths in the placebo group.

HRT: practical issues

Ethnic differences in use of hormone replacement therapy: community-based survey.
T J Harris, D G Cook, P D Wicks, F P Cappuccio. *BMJ* 1999; **319**: 610–1.

BACKGROUND. **Hormone replacement therapy is widely promoted to prevent cardiovascular disease and osteoporosis and relieve menopausal symptoms, although concern exists that much of the cardiovascular effect may be due to its selection by healthy women. Little is known about its use by women from different ethnic groups in the United Kingdom.**

INTERPRETATION. The differences in use of hormone replacement reported here have not to our knowledge been described before in the United Kingdom.

This population-based survey was carried out in South London in women aged 40–59 years. The response rate was 60%, and 802 out of the 941 women were of Afro-Caribbean or South Asian descent. The salient result was that 25% of white women were using HRT, and this was significantly more than the 15% of Afro-Caribbean women and the 10% of South Asian women.

Comment

These authors identified an important issue that might potentially be a source of bias in observational studies, i.e. ethnic or cultural differences between those women who use HRT and those who do not. However, they also convey a potentially still more important message that the process of assessing women for HRT provides an opportunity for health promotion in general, including the assessment of conventional cardiovascular risk factors and discussion about cervical and breast cancer screening. Irrespective of the need for HRT, opportunities for such discussion with women from ethnic minority groups may be being missed, since it is also recognized that the uptake of other preventive health measures is lower, for example, in South Asian women.

The Women's Health Initiative Memory Study (WHIMS): a trial of the effect of oestrogen therapy in preventing and slowing the progression of dementia.
S Schumaker, B A Reboussin, M A Espeland, S R Rapp, W L McBee, M Dailey, *et al. Control Clin Trials* 1998; **19**: 604–21.

BACKGROUND. **Evidence from animal, human, cross-sectional, case–control, and prospective studies indicates that HRT is a promising treatment for delaying the onset of symptoms of dementia.**

INTERPRETATION. The WHIMS study is designed to provide more than 80% statistical power to detect a 40% reduction in the rate of all-cause dementia, an effect that could have profound public health implications for older women's health and functioning.

Comment

This type of prospective outcome study is conspicuously sparse in the current literature on HRT. Objective evidence of this nature is essential for defining the future role of HRT.

Hormone replacement therapy.
Clinical Synthesis Panel on HRT. *Lancet* 1999; **345**: 152–5.

BACKGROUND. **From June 23 to June 25, 1999, a conference was held at the European Institute of Oncology, Milan, Italy, with the aim of synthesizing the clinical data on HRT.**

INTERPRETATION. Although there is considerable evidence about the health effects of long-term use of HRT, on average the balance between the risks and benefits shows no overwhelming inclination in either direction. For many women the benefits of long-term HRT use will outweigh the risks; for others risks outweigh the benefits. The use of HRT has to be tailored to the needs and desires of the individual.

Comment

This is a thoughtful and well-referenced summary of the arguments relating to clinical issues. The conclusions are balanced and reasonable and the principal summarizing recommendations are shown in Tables 6.1 and 6.2.

Table 6.1 Cardiovascular disease and hormone replacement therapy (HRT)

- Although a cause-and-effect relation is not proved, evidence that HRT lowers the risk of coronary heart disease in women without a history of this disease is sufficiently strong to consider this potential benefit when deciding whether or not to use HRT.
- HRT raises the risk of venous thromboembolism, but the absolute risk is small in women without predisposing conditions.

Conclusion

Epidemiological studies have consistently shown an association between hormone (oestrogen) replacement therapy (HRT) and lower rates of cardiovascular morbidity and mortality. This is illustrated by the results of a recent meta-analysis of 20

Table 6.2 Hormone replacement therapy (HRT) and the risk of cancer

- HRT is associated with a slight increase in the risk of breast cancer that is restricted to current and recent users, the risk increasing with increasing duration of use. This effect wears off within 5 years of stopping use. Among 1000 women who use HRT continuously for 10 years starting at age 50, it is estimated that there will be an additional six breast cancers, raising the incidence from a background of 45 cases to 51 cases. Progestagens do not seem to diminish the excess risk associated with oestrogen. Use of HRT for a few years should not lead to any appreciable risk of breast cancer.

- The excess risk of endometrial cancer due to oestrogen HRT use can be substantially reduced by concurrent progestogen therapy during at least 12 days in each month. Progestogens are sometimes poorly tolerated. Doctors should inform their patients of the importance of adherence and should check adherence to progestogen therapy while oestrogen is being taken. Failure to take progestogen with oestrogen can raise the risk of endometrial cancer.

- The breast and endometrial cancers that are diagnosed in HRT users are less aggressive clinically than those in never users.

- Current and recent use of HRT may be associated with a decreased risk of colorectal cancer.

observational studies showing that women taking HRT, usually as unopposed oestrogen treatment, had a relative risk of 0.5 for developing coronary artery disease relative to non-users. However, the results of these observational studies are not supported by the only prospective randomized outcome study, and some doubts therefore remain. To put the problem in its most simplistic form, those women who are motivated to request HRT, and who have no contraindication to its use, are likely to have a healthier overall lifestyle. Although statistical adjustments have taken account of all known confounding factors in the observational studies, it remains possible that the findings were biased.

There remain many unanswered questions about the use of HRT, primarily because of the lack of well-designed prospective clinical studies. With respect to cardiovascular disease, there are several mechanisms by which HRT might be beneficial, and modest but positive changes have been demonstrated in relation to BP, vascular compliance, endothelial function and lipid parameters. Unfortunately, the only published prospective randomized study of HRT produced a mixed picture, suggesting that HRT might actually be harmful if initiated in patients at increased cardiovascular risk by virtue of pre-existing cardiac disease.

Overall, however, the balance of evidence suggests that HRT is likely to be beneficial for delaying the progression of atherosclerotic cardiovascular disease, and it may therefore be an appropriate treatment for primary prevention as part of an overall package that addresses cardiovascular risk reduction. There may be some concerns, however, about initiating HRT in women with established CHD. The results of further studies are awaited with interest to allow clarification of many important practical issues.

References

1. Lobo RA. The role of progestogens in hormone replacement therapy. *Am J Obstet Gynecol* 1992; **168**: 1997–2004.

2. Sismondi P, Biglia N, Gioi M, Campognoli C. Hormone replacement therapy and breast cancer. *Eur Menop J* 1996; **3**: 227–31.

Part III

Hypertension: emerging concepts

7

Essential hypertension: the search for specific genetic markers

Introduction

The last decade has seen significant advances in molecular genetic technology, which will result in the imminent completion of the Human Genome Mapping project early in the next millennium. This will provide a wealth of information on the biological mechanisms that influence the progression and outcome of many disease entities. To date almost 100 genes, causing various genetic diseases, have been identified by positional cloning. Most of these disorders are monogenic (for example, Huntington's chorea, glucocorticoid suppressible hyperaldosteronism and familial cardiomyopathy); the study of complex, polygenic disorders, such as hypertension, continues to present a more difficult problem.

Human essential hypertension is generally regarded as a complex, multifactorial and polygenic disorder that arises as a consequence of the interaction of environmental risk factors and genetic susceptibility. There is a substantial body of evidence that, as well as the major lifestyle-dictated environmental factors of obesity and sodium intake, *in utero* environment is also important in determining the programming of several physiological systems involved in the subsequent risk of adult cardiovascular disease [1-3]. This environmental susceptibility interacts with genetic risk, which is estimated to account for 30–40% of the variance in blood pressure within a population.

The aim of current genetic studies is, therefore, to identify the genes that predispose to this genetic susceptibility. This in turn will aid our understanding of the underlying pathophysiological basis of hypertension and provide stratification of risk and prognosis based on an individual's genotype.

Candidate gene studies in hypertension—current status

With over 100 000 genes already sequenced, it is important to consider that many of the polymorphisms identified will be irrelevant to the disease in question. A number of criteria should be met before a particular DNA change can be linked to a disease trait. In particular, the polymorphism should result in a functional alteration in gene product, and the number of individuals demonstrating a specific association between genotype and phenotype should be large enough to be convincing. In addition, the hypothesis must be biologically plausible and the phenotypes easily distinguished. Notwithstanding these concerns and the limitations of candidate gene studies, such investigations have been informative in identifying potential loci and mechanisms that may underlie the genetic basis of high blood pressure. This chapter will review the most recent candidate gene studies in the following areas:

(a) **Renin–angiotensin–aldosterone system**
   Angiotensinogen gene
   ACE gene
   Aldosterone synthase gene

(b) **Sodium handling**
   Renal: Epithelial sodium channel
   Adducin gene
   Cellular: G-protein β3-subunit polymorphism

(c) **Endothelial function**
   Nitric oxide production
   Endothelin-1 and receptors

Renin–angiotensin–aldosterone system

Angiotensinogen

The angiotensinogen (AGT) gene encodes the protein that is cleaved by renin to yield angiotensin I (see Fig. 7.1). Initial studies in families with a predisposition to

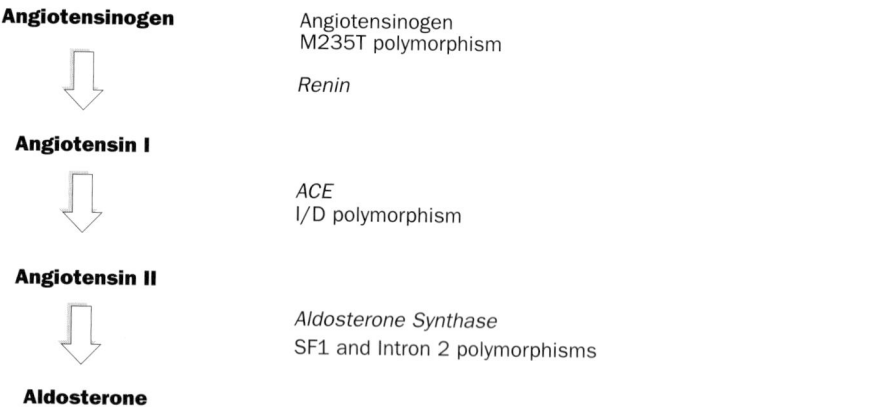

Fig. 7.1 Renin–angiotensin–aldosterone system and common polymorphisms.

developing high BP suggested that AGT levels were higher in those with a strong family history of the disorder, drawing attention to the locus |8|. Linkage studies confirmed an association between the angiotensinogen gene locus and hypertension, and to date 10 bi-allelic polymorphisms have been identified at this locus. The polymorphic variant that has generated most interest is characterized by the mutation's encoding threonine instead of methionine at amino acid position 235 (M235T). This is in turn associated with variation in plasma levels of AGT, with homozygotes for the M235 variant having the lowest levels and homozygotes for the 235T variant demonstrating the highest. Functionally, it appears that the M235T variant is in tight linkage with a proposed causal mutation in the promoter region of the gene, which is thought to affect basal transcription rates.

Several case–control studies have evaluated the association of the AGT M235T polymorphism and hypertension and assessed its influence on the response to antihypertensive therapy.

The angiotensinogen T235 variant and the use of antihypertensive drugs in a population-based cohort.

H Schunkert, H-W Hense, A Gimenez-Roqueplo, J Stieber, U Keil, G A J Riegger, *et al. Hypertension* 1997; **29**: 628–33.

BACKGROUND. Variants of the angiotensinogen gene (AGT) may increase the risk of developing arterial hypertension, but their effect on the use of antihypertensive medication in the general population remains unclear.

INTERPRETATION. This study concludes that the AGT T235 allele accounts for a substantial proportion of antihypertensive drug use in this middle-aged, population-based group of white subjects.

Comment

This population-based study aimed to assess the influence of the AGT M235T polymorphism on requirements for antihypertensive therapy. Six hundred and thirty-four middle-aged subjects were recruited from the Monitoring Trends and Determinants of Cardiovascular Disease (MONICA) Augsburg cohort, with the final endpoints taken as the need for, and number of, antihypertensive drugs.

The results confirmed the expected relationship between genotype and plasma AGT levels, as detailed above. Multivariate analysis demonstrated that individuals possessing at least one T235 allele had higher systolic and diastolic BPs than homozygotes for the M235 allele. The T235 allele was also found to be associated with a 1.6-fold increase in the likelihood of taking antihypertensive medication, although the actual numbers of drugs taken were low, at only 0.39 and 0.25 antihypertensive drugs per individual in the T235 and M235 groups, respectively.

Genotype also influenced the number of antihypertensive drugs required, with carriers of the T235 allele having a 2.1-fold increase in the need for polypharmacy, defined as two or more antihypertensive drugs.

Evaluation of the angiotensinogen locus in human essential hypertension.

E Brand, N Chatelain, B Keavney, M Caulfield, L Citterio, J M C Connell, *et al. Hypertension* 1998; **31**: 725–9.

BACKGROUND. **Different family and case–control studies support genetic linkage and association at the human angiotensinogen (AGT) locus with essential hypertension. To extend these previous observations, a European collaborative study of nine centres was set up to create a large resource of affected sibling pairs.**

INTERPRETATION. Although several arguments from association studies suggest a role of the AGT gene in essential hypertension, this large family study did not replicate the initial linkage reported in smaller studies. The results highlight the difficulty of identifying susceptibility genes by linkage analysis in complex diseases.

This large, multicentre, European collaborative study aimed to ascertain if there was support, from genetic linkage analysis, for an association of the AGT locus with essential hypertension. The cohort consisted of 350 families, comprising 630 affected sibling pairs. Linkage analysis with AGT microsatellites in hypertensive sibships failed to find any significant difference between the allele frequency in each group and overall estimated allele frequency. Further analysis, after adjusting for severity of blood pressure, age of onset and Body Mass Index, in isolation or in combination, again failed to find any evidence of linkage of the AGT locus with essential hypertension.

Comment

The MONICA study is of a case–control population design. In this type of study, patients with hypertension are matched, as carefully as possible, with controls drawn from the same base population. The frequency of allelic variants of candidate genes (or regions) within cases and controls is then compared, and when there is a significant difference between cases and controls, the role of the candidate is inferred.

This approach has significant weaknesses. Firstly, it depends on identifying suitable candidate genes in the first instance. Secondly, and more significantly, matching between cases and controls, even in relatively homogeneous populations, can be extremely difficult. In an attempt to overcome these weaknesses family-based linkage studies are performed. This type of study assesses the inheritance pattern of alleles within sibling pairs. Where a large number of affected sibling pairs with hypertension (or any other complex disorder) can be assembled, the inheritance by descent of a particular allele can be examined. Simple genetic principles dictate that siblings share, on average, no more than 50% of a single allele by descent; where the proportion of sharing is significantly increased from this, the allele is implicated in the inheritance of the phenotype. The main limitation of the affected sibling pair approach is that, although relatively simple in design, it is not particularly powerful and for this reason, large numbers of siblings are necessary to identify loci that carry, in themselves, relatively weak relative risks.

The European study detailed above utilizes this design, and the power of the study is such that, had the AGT M235T polymorphism influenced blood pressure regulation, it would have been detected. However, in view of its negative findings, this study casts doubt on the importance of the AGT locus in essential hypertension.

Angiotensin-converting enzyme (ACE)

Studies of rodent hypertension identified a Quantitative Trait Locus (QTL) for hypertension on rat chromosome 10, and this QTL was found to contain the gene encoding ACE [4]. Subsequent sequencing of the human ACE gene, on chromosome 17, demonstrated a bi-allelic polymorphism within the gene. This polymorphism is characterized by the presence (insertion) or absence (deletion) of a 287 bp fragment in intron 16 of the gene, and Rigat *et al.* demonstrated that this polymorphism accounted for approximately 50% of the variance in serum and tissue ACE levels and activity [5]. Individuals homozygous for the deletion allele have twice the level of ACE of those homozygous for the insertion allele, with heterozygotes demonstrating intermediate levels.

The most recent study assessing any association between the ACE polymorphism and hypertension has been the Framingham Heart Study.

Evidence for association and genetic linkage of the angiotensin-converting enzyme locus with hypertension and blood pressure in men but not women in the Framingham Heart Study.
C J O'Donnell, K Lindpainter, M G Larson, V S Rao, J M Ordovas, E J Schaefer, *et al. Circulation* 1998; **97**: 1766–72.

BACKGROUND. There is controversy regarding the association of the angiotensin-converting enzyme insertion-deletion (ACE I/D) polymorphism with systemic hypertension and with blood pressure. We investigated these relations in a large population-based sample of men and women using association and linkage analyses.

INTERPRETATION. In our large, population-based sample, there is evidence for association and genetic linkage of the ACE locus with hypertension and with diastolic blood pressure in men but not women. These data support the hypothesis that ACE, or a nearby gene, is a sex-specific candidate gene for hypertension. Confirmatory studies in other large population-based samples are warranted.

Background

The Framingham Heart Study started in 1948, with the initial cohort consisting of 5209 subjects. In 1971, a further 5124 cohort offspring and spouses were enrolled. Participants were invited to attend on a regular basis, and between 1987 and 1991 3095 subjects (1445 males, 1650 females) were genotyped for the ACE I/D polymorphism and found to be eligible for the study.

Aim

The aim was to assess the association of the ACE I/D polymorphism and systemic hypertension and blood pressure (BP) variation using association and linkage analysis (hypertension being defined as systolic BP >140 mmHg or diastolic > 90 mmHg or current use of antihypertensive treatment).

Results

Association study: A sex-specific association of the ACE genotype and age-adjusted diastolic BP was noted in males only (see Table 7.1), with mean diastolic BPs of 81.6 ($\pm$ 0.5), 80.9 ($\pm$ 0.4), and 79.6 ($\pm$ 0.6) for the DD, DI and II genotypes, respectively ($P=0.03$). This result was no longer statistically significant when adjusted for other co-variants (Body Mass Index, diabetes mellitus, cigarette smoking, alcohol consumption and ischaemic heart disease). No association was found for pulse pressure or systolic BP in males or diastolic or systolic BP or pulse pressure in females. Subgroup analysis of the hypertensive cohort (689 males, 705 females) indicated a similar sex-specific effect in males, with an odds ratio for hypertension of 1.67 (95% confidence interval CI 1.21–2.31) and 1.19 (95% CI 0.88–1.61) in the DD and DI groups, respectively, with the II group used as the reference. In this instance the odds ratios remained similar after adjusting for other co-variants. Again, in the female cohort no relationship between ACE genotype and hypertension was noted.

Linkage analysis: A cohort of 1044 sibling pairs was available for the linkage study. The analyses provided support for linkage of the ACE I/D polymorphism with diastolic BP in male siblings only. There was no evidence for linkage with pulse pressure in males or with either variable in females.

Table 7.1 Odds ratios for hypertension according to ACE genotype in men and women

Sex	ACE genotype	Odds ratio	95% CI
Male	DI	1.18	0.87–1.62
	DD	1.59	1.13–2.23
Female	DI	0.78	0.56–1.09
	DD	1.00	0.70–1.44

The II genotype is the reference group. ACE = angiotensin-converting enzyme; CI = confidence interval.
Source: Adapted from O'Donnell *et al.* (1998).

Aldosterone synthase

Excess production of aldosterone, such as occurs in Conn's syndrome and gluco-corticoid remediable aldosteronism (GRA), results in sodium retention, hypo-kalaemia and hypertension. Aldosterone synthase is the enzyme that regulates the terminal conversion of deoxycorticosterone to aldosterone in the zona glomerulosa of the adrenal cortex. Polymorphisms associated with the aldosterone synthase gene again make attractive candidates in essential hypertension. Polymorphisms identified to date include a single nucleotide variation, (C→T), in the 5 prime pro-moter region at position −344, known as the steroidogenic factor-1 binding site (SF-1) |6|. This polymorphism alters the binding of a steroidogenic factor, and potentially may change expression of the gene within the zona glomerulosa. It is of interest that this polymorphism is in tight linkage disequilibrium with another variation that results in conversion of intron 2 of the aldosterone synthase gene to the intron of the immediately adjacent gene encoding corticosteroid 11β-hydroxy-lase |6|.

Recent studies have examined the relevance of these polymorphisms in relation to aldosterone excretion, blood pressure and left ventricular mass and function.

Aldosterone excretion rate and blood pressure in essential hypertension are related to polymorphic differences in the aldosterone synthase gene (*CYP11B2*).
E Davies, C D Holloway, M C Ingram, G C Inglis, E C Friel, C Morrison, *et al.*
Hypertension 1999; **33**: 703–7.

BACKGROUND. Significant correlation of body sodium and potassium with BP may suggest a role for aldosterone in essential hypertension. In patients with this disease, the ratio of plasma renin to plasma aldosterone may be lower than in control subjects and plasma aldosterone levels may be more sensitive to angiotensin II infusion. Because essential hypertension is partly genetic, it is possible that altered control of aldosterone synthase gene expression or translation may be responsible.

INTERPRETATION. Urinary aldosterone excretion rate may be a useful intermediate phenotype linking these genotypes to raised BP. However, no causal relationship has yet been established, and it is possible that the polymorphisms may be in linkage with other causative mutations.

Comment

This well-matched case–control study examined the frequencies of two linked polymorphisms, one in the SF-1 binding site and the other an intronic conversion (IC) of the aldosterone synthase gene, in 138 hypertensives and 200 normotensive controls. The cases had significantly higher BP, at 154.3 (± 22)/95.8 (± 10.9) mmHg

Table 7.2 Genotype and allele frequencies of the SF-1 and intronic conversion polymorphisms of the aldosterone synthase gene in hypertensive and normotensive groups

	Genotype (%)			Allele (%)		
SF-1 site	**CC**	**CT**	**TT**	**C**	**T**	
Cases	8	65	27 ⎫	40	60 ⎫	
			$P=0.042$			$P=0.009$
Controls	20	53	26 ⎭	47	53 ⎭	
Intronic site	**WT 11**	**12**	**Con 22**	**Wild**	**Con**	
Cases	20	49	32 ⎫	44	56 ⎫	
			$P=0.02$			$P=0.016$
Controls	33	49	18 ⎭	58	42 ⎭	

Source: Adapted from Davies *et al.* (1999).

compared to 123.8 ($\pm$15)/76.8 ($\pm$8.7) mmHg in controls. Other baseline parameters, including age and sex, were individually matched.

Genetic analysis of the general population for the SF-1 binding site polymorphism indicated population frequencies for the C allele of 0.49 and 0.51 for the T allele. The allele frequencies for the IC site were 0.48 for the wild type and 0.52 for the conversion allele. There was evidence of significant linkage between the polymorphisms, with three common haplotypes observed, T/conversion (0.38), T/wild (0.13) and C/wild (0.45). In the case–control populations, both polymorphisms were in Hardy–Weinberg equilibrium in the control group, as was the IC in the hypertensive cohort. However, the SF-1 binding site polymorphism failed to demonstrate Hardy–Weinberg equilibrium ($P=0.0007$), with evidence of an excess of TT homozygotes ($P=0.042$) and T allele overall ($P=0.009$) (see Table 7.2).

In a further study of 486 subjects from the North Glasgow MONICA population, SF-1 and IC genotypes were compared with tetrahydroaldosterone (Thaldo) excretion rate. Despite both polymorphisms being in Hardy–Weinberg equilibrium, the Thaldo levels were significantly higher in those individuals with the T allele of the SF-1 binding site and conversion allele of the IC site ($P=0.021$), suggesting that urinary aldosterone excretion rates can provide an intermediate phenotype linking genotype and hypertension.

Association between human aldosterone synthase (*CYP11B2*) gene polymorphisms and left ventricular size, mass, and function.

M Kupari, A Hautanen, L Lankinenn, P Koskinen, J Virolainen, H Nikkila, *et al. Circulation* 1998; **97**: 569–75.

BACKGROUND. Aldosterone has direct and indirect effects on the heart, and genetic variations in aldosterone synthesis could therefore influence cardiac structure and function. Such variations might be associated with polymorphisms in the gene encoding aldosterone synthase (*CYP11B2*), the enzyme catalysing the last steps of aldosterone biosynthesis.

INTERPRETATION. Genetic variations in or near the aldosterone synthase (*CYP11B2*) gene strongly affect left ventricular size and and mass in young adults free of clinical heart disease. These polymorphisms may also influence the response of the left ventricle to an increase in dietary salt.

Comment

This study of 84 young Finnish subjects aimed to assess the influence of polymorphisms of the aldosterone synthase gene on left ventricular (LV) size, mass and function. Results from multiple regression analysis indicated that the polymorphism of the SF-1 binding site strongly predicts LV end-diastolic and systolic diameter, with a moderate effect on LV mass. This effect was in a gene dose-dependent manner, with each parameter increasing according to the number of −344C alleles (see Fig. 7.2). No relationship was found for the IC polymorphism. The effect of the

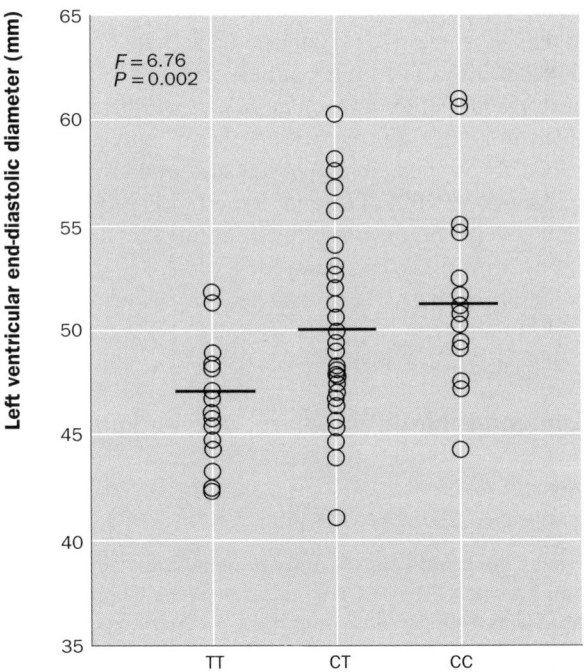

Fig. 7.2 Left ventricular end-diastolic diameter in relation to the −344 C/T polymorphism in the promoter of *CYP11B2*. Short horizontal lines indicate group mean values. Source: Kupari *et al.* (1998).

SF-1 site was unchanged when corrected for height, weight and Body Mass Index. When salt intake was added to the equation the predictive power of the model significantly increased. The CC group demonstrated a highly significant influence of sodium intake on LV mass, with the CT group showing an intermediate effect and the TT group no effect.

Summary

Both studies, although somewhat contradictory, do suggest an influence of the polymorphisms of the aldosterone synthase gene. However, the relevance of the echocardiographic data in young subjects free of hypertension and cardiovascular disease is uncertain. Further studies to ascertain the underlying physiological significance of both polymorphisms are necessary, as are case–control studies of populations with cardiovascular disease.

Sodium handling

Renal

Adducin

Adducin is a membrane cytoskeletal protein that regulates the activity of Na⁻K⁺-ATPase and subsequent sodium transport. Abnormalities of renal sodium re-absorption may be important in the initiation and maintenance of hypertension, and therefore the genes involved in renal sodium handling are of interest in this regard. The adducin gene was initially implicated in hypertension when a mutation in rat α-adducin was found to account for 50% of a major hypertensive effect in the Milan strain of rat |7|. In man, a specific point mutation at amino acid 460 in the α-adducin gene results in the substitution of tryptophan for glycine.

The significance of this polymorphism has been assessed in various different ethnic cohorts.

Human α-adducin gene, blood pressure, and sodium metabolism.
A Kamitani, Z Y H Wong, R Fraser, D L Davies, J M Connor, C J W Foy, *et al. Hypertension* 1998; **32**: 138–43.

BACKGROUND. The adducin genes contribute significantly to population variation in rat BP and cell membrane sodium transport. The 460Trp mutation of the human α-adducin gene has been associated with hypertension, in particular hypertension sensitive to sodium restriction.

INTERPRETATION. These findings suggest that in this study's Scottish population, the α-adducin 460Trp polymorphism is not related to BP and does not affect whole body or cellular sodium metabolism.

Comment

This population-based association study was performed to examine the relationship of the α-adducin 460Trp polymorphism on blood pressure variation and whole-body and cellular sodium metabolism in a Scottish cohort. A 'four corner' approach was used to select young adults with contrasting genetic predispositions to high BP. From 603 families, 151 offspring and 224 patients with BP in either the upper or lower 30% of the population were genotyped for the 460Trp α-adducin polymorphism. The influence of the polymorphism on sodium metabolism was also assessed with estimates of total exchange sodium and water, as well as cellular sodium and potassium concentrations in 79 of the offspring cohort.

No difference was detected in genotype or allele frequencies in the offspring or parents with high or low BP. The overall frequency of the 460Trp allele was 24% and 29% in the high- and low-pressure groups, respectively. Additional analysis of total exchangeable and intracellular sodium and components of the renin–angiotensin system in the offspring cohort failed to find any relationship with the 460Trp mutation.

Lack of association between the α-adducin locus and essential hypertension in the Japanese population.

N Kato, T Sugiyama, T Nabika, H Morita, H Kurihara, Y Yazaki, *et al.*
Hypertension 1998; **31**: 730–3.

BACKGROUND. Significant linkage and association of α-adducin, a cytoskeleton protein involved in transmembrane ion transport, with essential hypertension were recently shown in Caucasian populations, especially in relation to salt sensitivity. The present study investigated the relevance of this candidate gene to hypertension in a well-characterized Japanese population.

INTERPRETATION. The present study brought up an important issue concerning the pathophysiological role of α-adducin in non-Caucasian populations, given the likely variation in the nature of genetic susceptibility loci. The 460Trp variant of the α-adducin gene is unlikely to have a major effect on the susceptibility to hypertension in the Japanese population studied, although the present study does not exclude the involvement of α-adducin in the pathogenesis of hypertension.

Comment

A further study in a Japanese cohort also aimed to examine the association between the α-adducin locus and essential hypertension. Five hundred and seven subjects, 223 of whom were hypertensive, were genotyped for the 460 residue of the α-adducin gene. Results demonstrated that, despite an increased prevalence of the 460Trp variant (54–60%) in the Japanese compared to 13–20% in Caucasians, there was no difference in genotypic distribution or allele frequency between cases and controls. Even among the subset of subjects with severe hypertension, no significant association was demonstrable.

Comment

In view of the negative findings from the Japanese cohort, and given that the Scottish study had sufficient power to detect a 7% excess in frequency of the 460Trp mutation reported in hypertensives compared to controls, it would appear unlikely that the 460Trp variant of the α-adducin gene has a major effect on susceptibility to essential hypertension.

Epithelial sodium channel

The epithelial sodium channel (ESC) is responsible for regulating sodium reabsorption from the kidney. In a rare inherited form of hypertension, known as Liddle's syndrome, there is a gain of function mutation of subunits of the ESC, which results in excess sodium reabsorption in the distal renal tubule. This in turn leads to volume expansion, inhibition of renin and aldosterone secretion and hypertension. Many of the clinical features of Liddle's syndrome overlap with those of essential hypertension: hence the genes encoding the ESC have generated interest as yet further candidate genes for essential hypertension.

Association of hypertension with T594M mutation in β subunit of epithelial sodium channels in black people resident in London.

E H Baker, Y B Dong, G A Sagnella, M Rothwell, A K Onipinla, N D Markandu, *et al. Lancet* 1998; **351**: 1388–92.

BACKGROUND. Liddle's syndrome is a rare inherited form of hypertension in which mutations of the epithelial sodium channel (ESC) result in increased renal sodium reabsorption. Essential hypertension in black patients also shows clinical features of sodium retention, so this study screened black people for the T594M mutation, the most commonly identified sodium-channel mutation.

INTERPRETATION. Among black London people the T594M sodium channel β subunit mutation occurs more frequently in people with hypertension than in those without. The T594M variant may increase sodium-channel activity, and could raise BP in affected people by increasing renal tubular sodium reabsorption. These findings suggest that the T594M mutation could be the most common secondary cause of essential hypertension in black people identified to date.

Comment

The aim of this case–control study was to examine the relationship of a mutation (T594M) in the β subunit of the ESC in black subjects and hypertension. Essential hypertension in black patients often shows features of sodium retention, namely

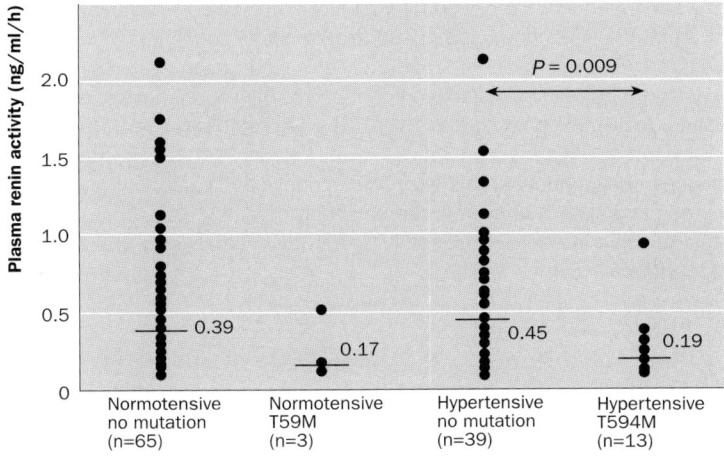

Fig. 7.3 Plasma renin activity in black normotensive and hypertensive individuals with and without T594M mutation. Individual values and median are shown. Source: Baker *et al.* (1998).

low renin activity and marked sodium sensitivity, thereby making a mutation of the ESC particularly attractive in this subgroup. Subjects were recruited from a hypertension clinic between 1995 and 1996 with age and sex-matched controls recruited randomly from GP registers in the London area. A total of 206 hypertensives and 142 controls had DNA analysis for the T594M mutation of the sodium-channel β subunit. This variant was found in 8.3% of hypertensives and 2.1% of controls, giving a crude odds ratio of 4.17 (95% confidence interval, CI 1.12–18.25). When adjusted for sex and Body Mass Index the odds ratio was similar, at 5.52. Additional analysis of those subjects with the T594M variant demonstrated lower renin activity; however, BP, serum sodium, potassium and aldosterone levels were similar to those in subjects without it (see Fig. 7.3).

Genetic linkage of β and γ subunits of epithelial sodium channel to systolic blood pressure.

Z Y H Wong, M Stebbing, J A Ellis, A Lamantia, S B Harrap. *Lancet* 1999; **353**: 1222–5.

BACKGROUND. Mutation in the genes on chromosome 16p12 that encode the β and γ subunits of the epithelial sodium channel (SCNNIB and SCNNIG, respectively) have been linked with rare sodium-dependent forms of low and high BP and the risk of CHD and stroke.

INTERPRETATION. Chromosome 16p12 and the SCNNIB and SCNNIG genes are implicated in the physiological variation of systolic BP. These findings are important in explaining individual cardiovascular risk within the general population.

A genetic linkage approach was used to analyse BP in relation to chromosome 16p12, which contain the genes that encode the β and γ subunits of the ESC, in Caucasian families in Victoria, Australia. The cohort comprised 286 families, consisting of both parents and two children. Four microsatellite markers were used to genotype chromosome 16p12 and this was correlated with phenotype. Significant linkage between systolic blood pressure (SBP) and chromosome 16p12 was noted ($P<0.001$). The mean difference in SBP between siblings identical for the locus was only 7.1 mmHg compared to 14 mmHg for siblings non-identical at this site. This is equivalent to 80% of 1 SD of the observed difference in sibling SBP overall, thereby implying that genes within the 16p12 chromosomal region contribute significantly to individual variation in SBP. No linkage was noted for diastolic BP.

Comment

The Australian linkage study indicates that the chromosomal region encoding the β and γ subunits of the ESC significantly contributes to variation in SBP. However, it is important to note that it may be other genes in this region that are responsible for this effect on blood pressure. Further collaborative evidence, from the London case–control study, implicates the β subunit of the ESC as an important predictor of essential hypertension in black subjects. Larger linkage and case–control studies in different ethnic populations are necessary to confirm these initial positive findings. This in turn may help to identify individuals whose blood pressure may be affected by manipulation of dietary salt intake.

Cellular

G-protein β3-subunit

G-proteins are important mediators of intracellular signalling for many vasoactive and proliferative stimuli. Initial reports identified a mutation (C825T) in exon 10 of the gene encoding the β3-subunit of the G-protein (*GNB3*) involved in sodium handling. This resulted in a splice variation and production of a truncated protein that appears to increase sodium-handling ability |**9**|. The functional significance of this polymorphism has yet to be established; however, several studies have examined its potential role in essential hypertension.

G-protein β3 subunit gene (*GNB3*) variant in causation of essential hypertension.

A V Benjafield, C L Jeyasingam, D R Nyholt, L R Griffiths, B J Morris. *Hypertension* 1998; **32**: 1094–7.

BACKGROUND. Essential hypertensives display enhanced signal reduction through pertussis toxin-sensitive G-proteins. The T allele of a C825T variant in exon 10 of the G-protein β3-subunit gene (*GNB3*) induces formation of a splice variant (Gβ3-s) with enhanced activity. The T allele of *GNB3* was shown recently to be associated with hypertension in unselected German patients (frequency=0.31 versus 0.25 in control).

To confirm and extend this finding in a different setting, we performed an association study in Australian white hypertensives.

INTERPRETATION. In conclusion, the present study of a group with strong family history supports a role for a genetically determined, physiologically active splice variant of the G-protein β3-subunit gene in the causation of essential hypertension.

Comment

The aim of this Australian association study was to examine the C825T variant of the *GNB3* gene in a Caucasian hypertensive cohort with a strong genetic predisposition to hypertension. Allele and genotype frequencies were examined in 110 age- and sex-matched hypertensives, each of whom was the offspring of two hypertensive parents, and 189 normotensive offspring of normotensive parents.

The T allele frequency was significantly higher in the hypertensive group, at 0.43 compared to 0.25 in the normotensive group ($P=0.00002$) (see Table 7.3). There also appeared to be a gene dose effect on pretreatment diastolic blood pressure, with homozygotes for the T allele having higher diastolic BP than the CC homozygotes, with heterozygotes showing intermediate levels.

Table 7.3 Genotype and allele frequencies of the C825T polymorphism of the GNB3 in hypertensive and normotensive groups

Group	Genotype (%)			Allele (%)	
	CC	CT	TT	C	T
Hypertensive	25	65	11 $\left.\right\}$ $P=1.7\times10^{-6}$	57	43 $\left.\right\}$ $P=1.6\times10^{-5}$
Normotensive	53	43	3	75	25

Adapted from Benjafield *et al.* (1998).

G-protein β subunit C825T variant and ambulatory blood pressure in essential hypertension.

J Beige, H Hohenbleicher, A Distler, A M Sharma. *Hypertension* 1999; **33**: 1049–51.

BACKGROUND. Recent studies have identified a novel polymorphism (C825T) of the gene encoding the β3-subunit of heterotrimetric G-proteins (Gβ3) associated with enhanced activation of G-proteins that appears to be more common in hypertensive patients. The present study examined the relationship between this genetic variant and hypertension in 479 white patients with established essential hypertension recruited from the hypertension clinic of the Universitäts klinikum Benjamin Franklin in Berlin, Germany, and 1000 normotensive gender- and age-matched controls.

INTERPRETATION. While these data confirm the association between the Gβ3-C825T variant and essential hypertension, they do not support the hypothesis that this marker is associated with more severe BP in patients with already established hypertension.

Comment

This further study in a German Caucasian cohort examined the relationship of the C825T polymorphism in 479 hypertensives and 1000 age- and sex-matched controls. There was a significant difference between cases and controls, with presence of the T allele associated with an odds ratio of 1.5 (95% confidence interval, CI 1.1–2.2) versus non-T carriers, for the presence of hypertension. However, subgroup analysis of the hypertensive cohort revealed no genotypic difference in BP level, age of onset or severity of hypertension (indicated by number of antihypertensive drugs).

The 825C/T polymorphism of the G-protein subunit β3 is not related to hypertension.

E Brand, S-M Herrmann, V Nicaud, J-B Ruidavets, A Evans, D Arveiler, *et al.*
Hypertension 1999; **33**: 1175–8.

BACKGROUND. A polymorphism at position 825 (CT) of the cDNA that encodes subunit (*GNB3*) of the pertussis toxin-sensitive GF protein was recently shown to be associated with human hypertension. To verify this finding and to investigate whether this polymorphism could also be associated with coronary heart disease, we analysed the *GNB3* variant in subjects from two previously described studies.

INTERPRETATION. There was no association of the *GNB3* polymorphism with early onset of hypertension, family history of hypertension or BP. We conclude that the 825C/T polymorphism of the *GNB3* gene did not contribute in any important way to the risk of essential hypertension or myocardial infarction (MI) in these studies.

Comment

This, the largest study to date, assessed the relationship of the *GNB3* polymorphism with essential hypertension and coronary heart disease. The Projet d'Etude des Gènes de l'Hypertension Artérielle Sévère modérée Essentielle (PEGASE) is a French case–control study of moderate–severe hypertension (681 cases and 308 controls) and the Etude Cas-Témoins de l'Infarctus du Myocarde (ECTIM) was a study of French and Northern Irish post-MI males, aged 25–64, recruited from 1988 to 1991 (564 cases and 633 controls). In both studies allele frequencies were in Hardy–Weinberg equilibrium, with no difference in allele and genotype frequencies in cases or controls.

Summary

As was pointed out above, the inherent weakness of association studies is the difficulty in accurately matching cases and controls, which in turn may lead to false-positive results. Therefore, the negative findings from the ECTIM and PEGASE studies cast doubt over the importance of the G-protein β3-subunit polymorphism as a marker for essential hypertension.

Endothelial function

Nitric oxide

Essential hypertension is associated with vascular endothelial dysfunction. Therefore, alterations in genes encoding proteins that regulate endothelial nitric oxide production are of interest as potential candidate genes in essential hypertension. The enzyme responsible for the generation of endothelial nitric oxide is endothelial nitric oxide synthase (eNOS). Several lines of evidence exist to implicate eNOS in hypertension. For example, nitric oxide production is reported to be reduced in essential hypertension; inhibition of NOS elevates BP in healthy humans, while studies of mice homozygous for the knockout of the eNOS gene show that they have a BP 15 mmHg higher than that of control mice. The gene encoding eNOS is located on human chromosome 7, and to date five polymorphic variants have been identified. Only one, a single nucleotide polymorphism on exon 7, results in an amino acid substitution (an aspartate for glutamine at amino acid residue 298 (Glu[298]Asp)). Two recent trials have assessed the importance of this polymorphism of the eNOS gene for hypertension.

Endothelial nitric oxide synthase gene is positively associated with essential hypertension.
Y Miyamoto, Y Saito, N Kajiyama, M Yoshimura, Y Shimasaki, M Nakayama, *et al. Hypertension* 1998; **32**: 3–8.

BACKGROUND. Essential hypertension has a genetic basis. Accumulating evidence, including findings of elevation of arterial BP in mice lacking the endothelial nitric oxide synthase (*eNOS*) gene, strongly suggests that alteration in NO metabolism is implicated in hypertension.

INTERPRETATION. It was concluded that the Glu[298]Asp mis-sense variant was significantly associated with essential hypertension, which suggests that it is a genetic susceptibility factor for essential hypertension.

Comment

This was a genetic association study of two independent Japanese populations, in which 218 hypertensives and 240 controls were recruited from one centre and 187 hypertensives and 223 controls from another. Not surprisingly, the hypertensive cohort had a higher baseline left ventricular mass index, plasma atrial naturetic

peptide, brain naturetic peptide and uric acid levels. All other baseline characteristics, including age, Body Mass Index, cholesterol and serum creatinine, were
similar.

Results

The Glu[298]Asp mis-sense variant demonstrated a significant effect of genotype on
hypertension, with an odds ratio of 2.3 (95% CI 1.4–3.9, $P=0.0015$). The allele
frequencies of the Glu[298]Asp variant were 5.0% in normotensives and 10.3% in
hypertensives. No significant gender difference was noted.

Lack of evidence for association between the endothelial nitric oxide synthase gene and hypertension.

N Kato, T Sugiyama, H Morita, T Nabika, H Kurihara, Y Yamori, *et al.*
Hypertension 1999; **33**: 933–6.

BACKGROUND. **Significant association between Glu[298]Asp polymorphism of the
endothelial nitric oxide synthase (*eNOS*) gene and essential hypertension was recently
reported in Japanese populations, with the [298]Asp variant showing a higher prevalence
in hypertensive patients (10.3% to 12.0%) than in normotensive subjects (5.0% to
5.8%). In contrast, another study demonstrated that the 298Glu variant was
significantly associated with hypertension in a Caucasian population.**

INTERPRETATION. Taken together, these results do not support the previous
observation that the molecular variant of the *eNOS* gene may confer the principal
susceptibility for essential hypertension, but rather suggest the existence of sampling
variation.

Comment

This association study of a larger Japanese cohort of 1062 (549 hypertensives, 513
controls) subjects aimed to establish whether there was an association between the
Glu[298]Asp variant of the *eNOS* gene and essential hypertension. Statistical analysis
was performed in two ways. Firstly, a case–control study assessing allele frequencies
between hypertensives and controls was examined, and secondly an analysis of
variance was performed in which BP was considered as a continuous variable across
the entire population. Both types of analysis failed to demonstrate any association.
The frequency of the Glu[298]Asp variant was 8.4% and 8.2% in cases and controls,
respectively.

Comment

The results from several studies assessing the Glu[298]Asp variant of the *eNOS* gene
have been inconclusive (see Fig. 7.4). The inherent weakness of small association
studies means that we will still have to wait for a more detailed linkage analysis that
is powerful enough for the task before this locus can be conclusively excluded.

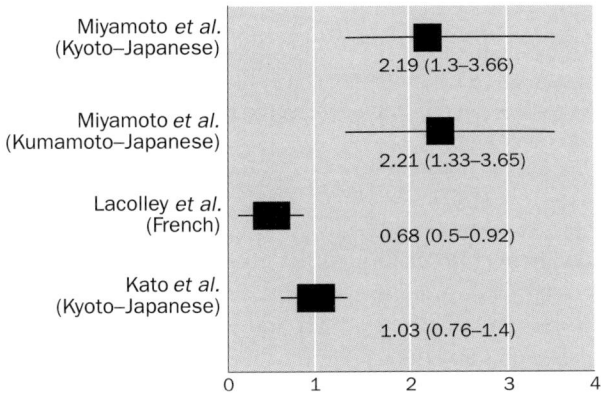

Miyamoto *et al.*
(Kyoto–Japanese)
2.19 (1.3–3.66)

Miyamoto *et al.*
(Kumamoto–Japanese)
2.21 (1.33–3.65)

Lacolley *et al.*
(French)
0.68 (0.5–0.92)

Kato *et al.*
(Kyoto–Japanese)
1.03 (0.76–1.4)

0   1   2   3   4

Fig. 7.4 Review of studies comparing the prevalence of [298]Asp with that of [298]Glu in essential hypertension. Results given as odds ratios and summary estimates with 95% confidence intervals. Adapted from Kato *et al.* (1999).

Endothelin-1 and endothelin A and B receptors

Endothelin-1 (ET1) is a potent vasoconstrictor produced by cleavage from its 38 amino acid precursor by endothelin-converting enzyme. ET1 exerts its effects by binding to the endothelin A (ETA) and B (ETB) receptors on vascular smooth muscle cells, and is thought to contribute to basal vascular tone. Therefore, the genes encoding ET1 and the ETA and B receptors again make attractive candidate genes for hypertension. To date, only one study, the ECTIM study, has examined the relationship between polymorphisms of the endothelin receptors and BP.

Polymorphisms of the endothelin-A and -B receptor genes in relation to blood pressure and myocardial infarction.
The Etude Cas-Témoins sur l'Infarctus du Myocarde (ECTIM) Study.

V Nicaud, O Poirier, I Behague, S-M Herrmann, C Mallet, A Troesch, *et al. Am J Hypertens* 1999; **12**: 304–10.

BACKGROUND. Endothelin-1 (ET-1) is a potent vasoconstrictor that also has mitogenic properties, stimulating the synthesis and secretion of several vasoactive molecules. There is much evidence to suggest that ET-1 might be involved in the pathogenesis of hypertension, atherosclerosis, and ischemic heart disease. ET-1 exerts its effects through at least two receptors, ETA and ETB, which are encoded by different genes and have separate tissue distributions and biological properties. The objective of this study was to identify polymorphisms of the ETA and ETB receptor

genes and to study their association with myocardial infarction (MI) and blood pressure.

INTERPRETATION. These results do not support an involvement of the endothelin receptor genes in a predisposition to MI or the determination of BP levels, but suggest that a polymorphism of the ETA receptor gene might influence the pulse pressure. This result will have to be confirmed in other studies.

Comment

The ECTIM study, as detailed above, also examined the genes encoding the ETA and ETB receptors and their relationship, if any, with BP. From this multicentre study, comparing 652 patients having survived an MI and 773 controls, six and three polymorphisms of the gene encoding the ETA and ETB receptors were identified, respectively. Associations between these polymorphisms, BP and MI were studied. The allele distribution for these numerous polymorphisms was similar between cases and controls, and measurements of mean systolic and diastolic BP did not vary between genotypes. One polymorphism (C→T) in exon 8 of the ETA gene was associated with pulse pressure; however, the clinical significance of this finding is unclear. Once again large multicentre studies will be required to clarify the role of this locus in essential hypertension.

Conclusions

The current status of studies into the genetics of cardiovascular disease can be considered to be unsatisfactory, since at present there are many contradictory reports on a relatively limited number of candidate genes. The most appropriate way to identify important loci would be to perform large-scale, suitably powered studies that could provide comprehensive coverage of the human genome using a genome-wide search. This type of approach is now being carried out in large-scale studies both nationally and internationally. New technological developments may be vital in this regard. For example, recent availability of DNA 'chip' technology allows the rapid and high-throughput screening of large numbers of samples for single nucleotide polymorphisms, which are frequent within the human genome. Indeed, very recent papers have used this approach to study potential genes involved in cardiovascular regulation, and have shown that such polymorphisms are frequent and alter protein sequence. The functional importance of this variability remains unclear, but the availability of this dense genetic information holds considerable promise for future identification of the important genes involved in hypertension. However, until such data are available, it would seem hazardous to speculate about the relative importance of existing candidates. The information from these large-scale studies and the dividend from the Human Genome-Mapping project may well identify new and hitherto unsuspected loci, which may be important in cardiovascular disease and which may lead, in time, to new methods of drug development and targeting of patients at high risk.

References

1. Fall CH, Osmond C, Barker DJ, Clark PM, Hales CN, Stirling Y, *et al.* Fetal and infant growth and cardiovascular risk factors in women [see comments]. *BMJ* 1995; **310**(6977): 428–32.

2. Barker DJ, Osmond C, Golding J, Kuh D, Wadsworth ME. Growth *in utero*, blood pressure in childhood and adult life, and mortality from cardiovascular disease. *BMJ* 1989; **298** (6673): 564–7.

3. Barker DJ, Osmond C, Simmonds SJ, Wield GA. The relation of small head circumference and thinness at birth to death from cardiovascular disease in adult life. *BMJ* 1993; **306** (6875): 422–6.

4. Hilbert P, Lindpaintner K, Beckmann JS, Serikawa T, Soubrier F, Dubay C, *et al.* Chromosomal mapping of two genetic loci associated with blood-pressure regulation in hereditary hypertensive rats. *Nature* 1991; **353**: 521–9.

5. Rigat B, Hubert C, Alhenc-Gelas F, Cambien F, Corvol P, Soubrier F. An insertion/deletion polymorphism in the angiotensin I-converting enzyme gene accounting for half the variance of serum enzyme levels. *J Clin Invest* 1990; **86** (4): 1343–6.

6. White PC, Slutsker L. Haplotype analysis of *CYP11B2*. *Endocr Res* 1995; **21** (1–2): 437–42.

7. Salardi S, Saccardo B, Borsani G, Modica R, Ferrandi M, Tripodi MG, *et al.* Erythrocyte adducin differential properties in the normotensive and hypertensive rats of the Milan strain. Characterization of spleen adducin m-RNA. *Am J Hypertens* 1989; **2** (4): 229–37.

8. Walker WG, Whelton PK, Saito H, Russell RP, Hermann J. Relation between blood pressure and renin, renin substrate, angiotensin II, aldosterone and urinary sodium and potassium in 574 ambulatory subjects. *Hypertension* 1979; **1** (3): 287–91.

9. Siffert W, Rosskopf D, Siffert G, Busch S, Moritz A, Erbel R, *et al.* Association of a human G-protein β3 subunit variant with hypertension. *Nat Genet* 1998; **18**: 45–8.

8

Nitric oxide and superoxide in hypertension: current research and clinical relevance

Introduction

For many years nitric oxide (NO) was regarded as a noxious pollutant in car exhaust fumes, fossil fuel smoke and cigarette smoke, responsible for acid rain and depletion of the ozone layer. However, interest in the physiological role of this simple diatomic molecule has risen exponentially in the 10 years since the endothelium-derived relaxing factor (EDRF), proposed by Furchgott and Zawadski in 1980 [1], was identified in 1987 by Palmer *et al.* as NO [2]. In 1992, interest was such that NO was voted 'molecule of the year' by *Science* and earned Robert F. Furchgott, Louis J. Ignarro and Ferid Murad the Nobel Prize in Physiology or Medicine in 1998 for their discoveries concerning 'nitric oxide as a signalling molecule in the cardiovascular system'. More recently, interest has grown in another free radical, the superoxide anion (O_2^-), and its interaction with NO in hypertension and other cardiovascular diseases. This will be discussed in more detail later. This chapter reviews the current position and highlights recent papers of particular interest.

The physiological role of NO

NO is a simple diatomic gas that is not stored and diffuses freely to its site of action, where it binds covalently to produce its effect. In biological systems, NO has an estimated half-life of only 3–5 seconds, as it interacts with superoxide anion and haem-containing proteins. Classical receptors can easily distinguish between two closely related molecules produced by distant endocrine systems (e.g. adrenaline and noradrenaline) because of subtle differences in their shape. With only two atoms, NO encodes information not by its shape, but by changes in its local concentration. If NO were more stable, the target guanylate cyclase would become saturated, thus obliterating any information being transferred.

NO diffuses from the endothelium to the vascular smooth muscle layer, where it binds to the haem moiety of guanylate cyclase and activates the enzyme. Guanylate cyclase then catalyses the production of cyclic guanosine monophosphate (cGMP) from guanosine 5'-triphosphate. Cyclic GMP causes vascular smooth muscle relaxation mainly by reducing intracellular calcium; but the precise mechanism for this remains poorly understood. Endothelium-derived NO can also diffuse into the lumen of the vessel, where it can prevent platelet aggregation and adhesion to the endothelium by a cGMP-dependent mechanism. This is thought to be one of the many mechanisms whereby NO prevents atherogenesis.

Nitric oxide synthesis

NO is synthesized from the abundant amino acid L-arginine by the actions of a family of nitric oxide synthase (NOS) enzymes, through a hitherto unrecognized pathway—namely, the L-arginine-nitric oxide pathway. One of the guanidino nitrogen atoms of L-arginine undergoes a five-electron oxidation to yield the free radical NO and L-citrulline |3| via an N^G-OH-L-arginine intermediate (Fig. 8.1). Interestingly, L-citrulline has been shown, in endothelial cell culture at least, to be

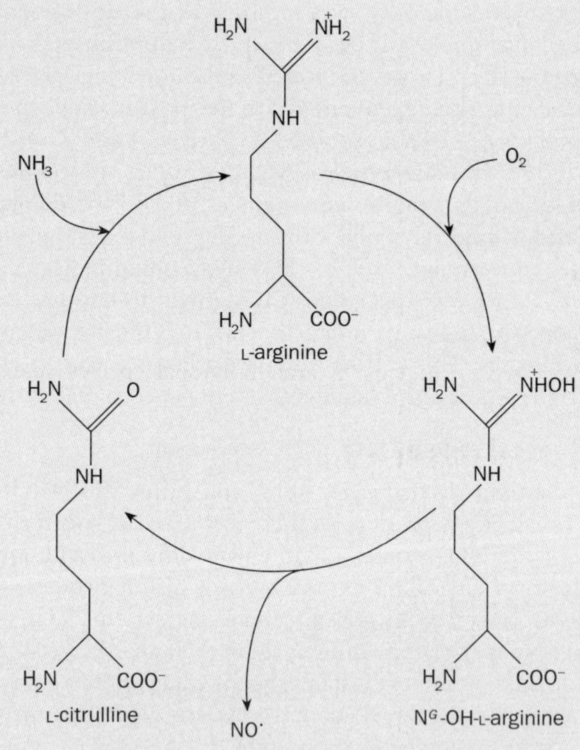

Fig. 8.1 Biosynthesis of nitric oxide (NO) from L-arginine, via N^G-OH-L-arginine, by incorporating molecular oxygen (O_2). L-citrulline can be recycled back to L-arginine by incorporation of ammonia (NH_3).

Table 8.1 Characteristics of the three human nitric oxide synthase isoforms

Gene	Enzyme nomenclature		Chromosomal expression	Localization	Gene structure	Protein M$_r$ (kDa)	Enzyme structure
	Old	**New**					
Nos1	nNOS, bNOS	NOS I	Constitutive	12q24.2 – 24.31	≈160 kb, 29 exons	155	Dimer
Nos2	iNOS, macNOS	NOS II	Inducible	17cen – q11.2	≈37 kb, 27 exons	125–135	Dimer
Nos3	eNOS, ecNOS	NOS III	Constitutive	7q35 – 36	≈21 kb, 26 exons	135	Dimer

recycled back to L-arginine by the incorporation of one nitrogen atom from urea |**4, 5**|, which not only regenerates substrate for further NO production, but also eliminates excess nitrogen created by the cell's metabolism (Fig. 8.1).

There are three known enzymatic isoforms of NOS: neuronal NOS (NOS I), inducible NOS (NOS II) and endothelial NOS (NOS III) (Table 8.1), which are products of three distinct genes. All three isoforms catalyse the same reaction; it is therefore no surprise that they share several common features. They all have binding sites for, and rely for their action on, the cofactors flavin mononucleotide, flavin adenine dinucleotide, haem, calmodulin and tetrahydrobiopterin (BH$_4$). As the NOS genes are very highly conserved, isoforms from the same tissue of different species are essentially identical to such an extent that, by way of illustration, there is 94% sequence identity between bovine and human NOS III. In contrast, the three isoforms from different tissues in any individual species share only 50–55% sequence identity with each other.

Endothelial nitric oxide synthase (NOS III)

For a long time, the endothelium had been regarded as a simple inert barrier between the blood in the lumen and the underlying vascular smooth muscle cells. However, the endothelium is now known to be a metabolically and physiologically dynamic tissue with multiple functions. The first clue that the endothelium and NO may be important in cardiovascular regulation came via the demonstration that an intact endothelium was essential for the vasodilator action of acetylcholine (ACh) in isolated arterial strips or rings |**1**|. Removal of the endothelium prevented the relaxant effects of ACh and even led to contraction. It was deduced that endothelial cells released a substance, initially called endothelium-derived relaxing factor (EDRF). It was also shown that the action of EDRF was destroyed by oxyhaemoglobin and enhanced by superoxide dismutase; and, unlike the other known endogenous vasodilator, prostacyclin, its activity was not inhibited by indomethacin.

In due course, it was shown that NO exhibited all the properties of EDRF |**2**|. For example, EDRF and NO produced identical relaxation in bioassay tissues; both substances were equally unstable; bradykinin caused the dose-dependent release of

NO from the cells in amounts sufficient to account for the biological activity of EDRF; the relaxations induced by EDRF and NO were inhibited by haemoglobin and enhanced by superoxide dismutase to a similar degree. All of this was taken as sufficient evidence that EDRF was in fact NO.

Nitric oxide in hypertension

Human essential hypertension and several animal models of hypertension are associated with increased peripheral vascular resistance |6|. The crucial structures of the circulation that determine peripheral vascular resistance are arteries of diameter < 200 μm; the so-called 'resistance arteries' |7|. As NO is accepted as an endogenous vasodilator |2| there are theoretical reasons why reduced NO production or bio-availability would lead to vasoconstriction and hence increased peripheral vascular resistance. NO has been found to regulate the tone of normal vessels |8|, including resistance vessels |9|. In addition, NO causes renal vasodilation, with consequent diuresis and natriuresis |10|. These actions would tend to lower blood pressure; therefore a reduction in this mechanism is another way in which NO deficiency may theoretically contribute to hypertension. However, there are many conflicting reports about the role of NO deficiency in experimental models of hypertension and human essential hypertension.

Nitric oxide in hypertension: conflicting results

Experimental hypertension

Since the identification of NO as an endogenous vasodilator |2|, there have been many studies examining the role of NO in experimental hypertension. These have been comprehensively reviewed recently |11|. Some studies indicate reduced NO in hypertensive animals compared to normotensive controls, while others show increased NO or no difference. On balance, it would appear that the NO system may be overactive in the spontaneously hypertensive rat (SHR) model of genetic hypertension, but depressed in the related stroke-prone spontaneously hypertensive rat (SHRSP) model and in experimental mineralocorticoid and renal hypertension. However, some studies remain contradictory.

Despite the large number of endogenous vasocontrictors and vasodilators that can potentially affect blood pressure, the importance of the L-arginine/NO system is apparent in models where the system is manipulated. Exogenous L-arginine, but not D-arginine, normalizes blood pressure in salt-sensitive Dahl/Rapp rats made hypertensive by high-salt chow |12|. Conversely, NOS can be inhibited by a variety of L-arginine analogues, including N^G-L-arginine methyl ester (L-NAME) and monomethyl-L-arginine (L-NMMA). This model will be discussed later. However, such pharmacological intervention affects all isoforms of NOS; hence their individual contribution to blood pressure control cannot be distinguished.

Very specific interruption of the endothelial L-arginine/NO system has recently become possible with the advent of mice with targeted disruption of the *Nos3* gene |**13,14**|. These so-called *Nos3* 'knock-out' mice have no NOS III protein in their endothelium, and consequently have increased blood pressure compared to control littermates, suggesting that NOS III is indeed important in blood pressure regulation.

The opposite side of the coin from 'knock-out' technology is transgenic technology, where extra copies of the gene of interest can be expressed in mice or rats, even in a tissue- or cell-specific manner. Such technology has recently provided further evidence for the role of NOS III in blood pressure control.

Hypotension and reduced nitric oxide-elicited vasorelaxation in transgenic mice overexpressing endothelial nitric oxide synthase.

Y Ohashi, S Kawashima, K Hirata, R Yamashita, T Ishida, N Inoue, *et al. J Clin Invest* 1998; **102**: 2061–71.

BACKGROUND. Nitric oxide (NO), constitutively produced by endothelial nitric oxide synthase (eNOS), plays a major role in the regulation of blood pressure and vascular tone. We generated transgenic mice overexpressing bovine eNOS in the vascular wall using murine preproendothelin-1 promoter.

INTERPRETATION. Thus this novel mouse model of chronic eNOS overexpression demonstrates that, in addition to the essential role of eNOS in blood pressure regulation, tonic NO release by eNOS in the endothelium induces reduced vascular reactivity to NO-mediated vasodilators, providing several insights into the pathogenesis of nitrate tolerance.

Comment

In this study, Ohashi *et al.* generated transgenic mice containing three to eight extra copies of the bovine *Nos3* gene driven by an endothelium-specific promoter. Bovine *Nos3*-specific mRNA was detected in the heart, lung, aorta and uterus, and to a lesser extent in the brain, liver, kidney and intestine. No bovine NOS-specific mRNA was detected in control littermates. Immunohistochemistry was used to demonstrate bovine *Nos3* protein predominantly in the endothelium of the aorta. To exclude a possible oestrogen effect on NO generation, male animals were used to assess the physiological consequences of *Nos3* overexpression. The significant differences between transgenic and control mice are detailed in Table 8.2. In addition, 2 weeks of L-NAME (1 mg/ml) in the drinking water increased the mean blood pressure in both groups of animals, but to a greater extent in the transgenic animals, with the result that there was no difference in blood pressure on L-NAME treatment. Surprisingly, relaxations of aortic rings to both the endothelium-dependent vasodilator, ACh, and the NO donor, sodium nitroprusside, were attenuated in the transgenic animals.

Table 8.2 Physiological differences between bovine *Nos3* transgenic mice and control mice

	Transgenic (n)	Control (n)	*P*
Systolic blood pressure (mmHg ± SEM)	89 ± 4 (10)	111 ± 3 (9)	< 0.01
Mean blood pressure (mmHg ± SEM)	81 ± 4 (10)	99 ± 3 (9)	< 0.01
Diastolic blood pressure (mmHg ± SEM)	73 ± 3 (10)	92 ± 3 (9)	< 0.01
Plasma nitrite + nitrate (μmol/l ± SEM)	31.6 ± 3.1 (18)	19.4 ± 3.3 (16)	< 0.05
Basal aortic cGMP levels (pmol/mg protein ± SEM)	5.21 ± 0.71 (3)	3.26 ± 0.20 (3)	< 0.05

Source: Ohashi *et al.* (1998). cGMP = cyclic guanosine monophosphate; SEM = standard error of the mean.

Conclusion

These data are further evidence that *Nos3*-derived NO regulates blood pressure. However, despite the implication from 'knock-out' and transgenic mouse studies that the *Nos3* gene is important in blood pressure regulation, genetic studies in several animal models have failed to link hypertension to the *Nos3* gene, or to either of the other two isoforms for that matter. An initial study linking hypertension to *Nos2* on rat chromosome 10 |**15**| was later shown, by the same investigators, not to be accurate |**16**|.

Human essential hypertension

The role of NO in human essential hypertension also remains controversial. There have been many studies employing forearm venous occlusion plethysmography to examine stimulated NO release in response, typically, to ACh infused into the brachial artery. When essential hypertensive patients are compared to matched normotensive controls, the majority of the studies shows a reduction in stimulated NO release |**19**|, although another study was interpreted as showing no difference |**20**|. Basal NO production, as measured by the reduced forearm blood flow in response to L-NMMA, has also been shown to be reduced in patients with hypertension compared to normotensive controls |**21**|.

The use of forearm venous occlusion plethysmography to measure endothelium-dependent vasodilation is susceptible to errors related to different basal blood flows and conduit vessel lengths |**22**|. Such effects are seldom considered in these studies, and may partly explain some of the above discrepancies. Using flow-mediated vasodilation of the brachial artery as an alternative method of quantifying stimulated NO production, Laurent *et al.* found no difference between essential hypertensives and normotensive controls |**23**|.

Basal nitric oxide synthesis in essential hypertension.
P Forte, M Copland, L M Smith, E Milne, J Sutherland, N Benjamin. *Lancet* 1997; **349**: 837–42.

BACKGROUND. There is indirect evidence that synthesis in the vascular endothelium of patients with hypertension is altered. The aim of this study was to estimate more

directly NO production in patients with untreated esssential hypertension by measurement of synthesis of inorganic nitrate, which is the end product of NO oxidation in humans. Two separate studies were undertaken in patients with hypertension and appropriate healthy controls.

INTERPRETATION. These data suggest that whole-body NO production in patients with essential hypertension is diminished under basal conditions. The origin of the NO measured in this study is not known, and we cannot tell whether the impaired synthesis is primary or secondary to a rise in blood pressure.

Comment

In this study, Forte *et al.* employed yet another method of estimating NO production, in a further attempt to circumvent the limitations of forearm venous occlusion plethysmography. They fed a group of 10 essential hypertensive patients, and a group of 13 matched normotensive controls, a fixed low-nitrate diet for 2 days. On the second day they measured 24-hour ambulatory blood pressure and 24-hour urinary nitrate excretion. In a separate study, they administered the stable isotope L-$[^{15}N]_2$-guanidino arginine intravenously to 11 hypertensives and 11 controls, then measured ^{15}N excretion over the next 36 hours.

Main results. In the first study, they found nitrate excretion (μmol/24 hours $\pm$ SEM) to be reduced in the hypertensive group (450 $\pm$ 37) compared to controls (760 $\pm$ 77; $P<0.001$). In addition, they found an inverse relation between nitrate excretion and daytime mean ambulatory blood pressure ($P=0.007$; $r^2=-0.73$). In the second study, they also found the 36-hour ^{15}N excretion (pmol $\pm$ SEM) to be significantly reduced in the hypertensive group (1313 $\pm$ 50) compared to the normotensive controls (2133 $\pm$ 142; $P<0.001$), and again there was a significant inverse correlation between mean daytime ambulatory blood pressure and ^{15}N excretion ($P=0.002$, $r^2=-0.59$).

Conclusion

This is certainly more direct evidence for reduced whole-body NO production in hypertensive patients, but the authors accept that the source of the NO is unknown. NOS II could have been induced in the controls as a result of subclinical infection or inflammation, although attempts were made to exclude such subjects from the study.

Nitric oxide activity in childhood hypertension.
C D A Goonasekera, V Shah, D D Rees, M J Dillon. *Arch Dis Childh* 1997; **77**: 11–6.

BACKGROUND. The objective of this study was to investigate NO activity in childhood hypertension using nitrite and nitrate (NOx) concentrations in plasma as an index of NO generation.

INTERPRETATION. P_{NOx} is increased in children with hypertension even after statistical elimination of the glomerular filtration rate and age influences. This suggests a normal or increased NO synthase activity in childhood hypertension in contrast with adults with hypertension, in whom it is described as reduced.

Comment

Similar nitrate studies have been conducted in children with hypertension, who represent a unique group in whom hypertension is invariably secondary. In this recent study, Goonasekera *et al.* measured plasma and urinary nitrite/nitrate (NOx) in 16 normotensive children, 13 children with renovascular hypertension and 25 children with hypertension secondary to renal parenchymal disease.

Main results. When corrected for glomerular filtration rate, they found increased plasma NOx (mmol/l ± SD) in a group with renal parenchymal disease (18.3 ± 11.4) compared to a group with renovascular hypertension (15.3 ± 11.4) and a group of normotensive children (11.9 ± 5.9; $P=0.007$ by factorial ANOVA), but found no differences in urinary NOx between any of the groups. There was no significant correlation between plasma NOx and systolic blood pressure in any of the groups (normal controls, $r=0.003$, $P=0.9$; renovascular disease, $r=0.2$, $P=0.4$; renal parenchymal disease, $r=0.1$, $P=0.5$).

Conclusion

The authors suggest that this is evidence for normal or increased NO synthesis in childhood hypertension, in contrast to adult hypertension. This study is weakened by the fact that no dietary restrictions were made, and while pyrexial patients were excluded, NOS II could have been induced in some patients with renal parenchymal disease.

As with experimental hypertension, genetic studies have tried to link human essential hypertension to the NOS genes, most notably *Nos3*. The *Nos3* gene has been associated with smoking-related coronary heart disease [24] and myocardial infarction [25]. However, with regard to human essential hypertension the situation is less clear. The first such study by Bonnardeaux *et al.* failed to find linkage between a highly polymorphic microsatellite marker (CA repeat) in the *Nos3* gene and hypertension in 145 hypertensive Caucasian pedigrees (269 sib pairs, 346 subjects) [26]. They concluded that their data did not suggest involvement of common molecular variants of the endothelial nitric oxide synthase (*eNOS*) gene in essential hypertension. This negative conclusion was confirmed by two other groups using the same marker in other Caucasian populations [27, 28]. Contrary to this, two more recent studies found a significant association between the *Nos3* gene and essential hypertension in Caucasian and Japanese populations.

Nitric oxide synthase gene polymorphisms, blood pressure and aortic stiffness in normotensive and hypertensive subjects.

P Lacolley, S Gautier, O Poirier, B Pannier, F Cambien, A Benetos.
J Hypertens 1998; **18**: 31–6.

BACKGROUND. **The objective of this study was to assess the contribution of two polymorphisms of the endothelial nitric oxide synthase (*eNOS*) gene to aortic stiffness in normotensive and hypertensive subjects in the same cohort.**

INTERPRETATION. The present results do not suggest that two common polymorphisms of the *eNOS* gene are involved in the regulation of aortic stiffness in hypertensive and normotensive individuals. The higher prevalence of the *eNOS* [298]G allele among hypertensives suggests that this gene is involved in essential hypertension, but this observation needs further confirmation.

Comment

Lacolley *et al.* studied 311 untreated hypertensive patients of European extraction (>140/90) and 128 normotensive subjects (<140/90). They studied two different polymorphisms in the *Nos3* gene from the previous studies, i.e. G^{10}-T at intron 23 ($G^{IN23}T$) and G^{298}-T at exon 7 ($Glu^{298}Asp$). They measured aortic stiffness non-invasively using carotid–femoral pulse-wave velocity.

Main results. When the frequency distribution of the different alleles of the $G^{IN23}T$ polymorphism was compared between the hypertensive and normotensive populations, there was no significant deviation from Hardy–Weinberg equilibrium. However, with regard to the $Glu^{298}Asp$ polymorphism, there was a significantly higher incidence of the G allele in the hypertensive group (χ^2=10.88, P=0.004, Table 8.3). They found no association of either polymorphism with aortic stiffness in either the hypertensive or the normotensive group.

Table 8.3 Distribution of *Nos3* $Glu^{298}Asp$ genotypes in normotensive and hypertensive subjects

$Glu^{298}Asp$ genotype	Normotensives n (%)	Hypertensives n (%)
GG	35 (28)	140 (45)*
GT	67 (55)	122 (40)
TT	21 (17)	47 (15)
G%	56	· 65

*χ^2=10.88, P=0.004.
Source: Lacolley *et al.* (1998).

Conclusions

Although this study was not designed to assess the role of *Nos3* polymorphisms in the control of blood pressure, this was the first report suggesting an association of the incidence of hypertension with *Nos3* polymorphism. Its conclusion was that *Nos3* was not involved in aortic stiffness, and that larger studies would be necessary to confirm the implication of the *Nos3* [298]G allele in human essential hypertension.

Endothelial nitric oxide synthase gene is positively associated with essential hypertension.

Y Miyamoto, Y Saito, N Kajiyama, M Yoshimura, Y Shimasaki, M Nakayama, *et al. Hypertension* 1998; **32**: 3–8.

BACKGROUND. Essential hypertension has a genetic basis. Accumulating evidence, including findings of elevation of arterial blood pressure in mice lacking the endothelial nitric oxide synthase (*eNOS*) gene, strongly suggests that alteration in NO metabolism is implicated in hypertension. There are, however, no reports indicating that polymorphism in the *eNOS* gene is associated with essential hypertension.

INTERPRETATION. The Glu[298]Asp mis-sense variant was significantly associated with essential hypertension, which suggests that it is a genetic susceptibility factor for essential hypertension.

Comment

Similarly, Miyamoto *et al.* studied four different polymorphisms of the *Nos3* gene, including the exon 7 Glu[298]Asp, in two different Japanese populations totalling 405 essential hypertensive patients and 463 normotensive subjects.

Main results. They found no significant association between essential hypertension and three of the polymorphisms, but found a significant association with the Glu[298]Asp polymorphism, with an odds ratio of 2.3 (95% confidence interval, CI 2.0–2.7, $P=0.000005$, Table 8.4).

Conclusion

This represents even stronger evidence for an association between the *Nos3* gene and essential hypertension, even if only in a Japanese population. Curiously, in this study the [298]Asp allele was more frequent in the Japanese hypertensive group, which is in contrast to the Lacolley study, where the [298]Glu allele was more common in the Caucasian hypertensive group. This would suggest that this point mutation *per se* does not cause the hypertension, which is in keeping with the fact that [298]Glu does not lie in a part of the molecule identified as a critical region.

Table 8.4 Comparison of genotype and allele frequencies for Glu^{298}Asp variants of the *Nos3* gene in a Japanese population

	Normotensives (n=463)	Hypertensives (n=405)
Genotypes		
Glu/Glu, n (%)	414 (89.4)	317 (78.3)
Glu/Asp + Asp/Asp, n (%)	49 (10.6)	88 (21.7)
Significance	P=0.000005	
Odds ratio (95% CI)	2.3 (2.0–2.7)	
Alleles		
Glu, n (%)	876 (94.6)	720 (88.9)
Asp, n (%)	50 (5.4)	90 (11.1)
Significance	P=0.000009	

Source: Miyamoto *et al.* (1998). CI = confidence interval.

Lack of evidence for association between the endothelial nitric oxide synthase gene and hypertension.

N Kato, T Sugiyama, H Morita, T Nabika, H Kurihara, Y Yamori, *et al.*
Hypertension 1999; **33**: 933–6.

BACKGROUND. **Significant association between Glu^{298}Asp polymorphism of the endothelial nitric oxide synthase (eNOS) gene and essential hypertension was recently reported in Japanese populations, with the ^{298}Asp variant showing a higher prevalence in hypertensive patients (10.3% to 12.0%) than in normotensive subjects (5.0% to 5.8%). In contrast, another study demonstrated that the ^{298}Glu variant was significantly associated with hypertension in a Caucasian population.**

INTERPRETATION. Taken together, our results do not support the previous observation that the molecular variant of the *eNOS* gene may confer the principal susceptibility for essential hypertension, but rather suggest the existence of sampling variation.

Comment

In an attempt to resolve this issue, Kato *et al.* conducted a case–control study of a relatively large Japanese population of 549 hypertensive patients and 513 normotensive controls, with the χ^2 statistic used to test the significance of an association between *Nos3* genotype and the presence of hypertension. They focused solely on the Glu^{298}Asp polymorphism, which had shown a significant association with essential hypertension as described above. In addition, they used ANOVA to test the significance of an association between the *Nos3* genotype and the level of blood pressure within the entire population, excluding 167 hypertensive patients who had been on treatment.

Main results. As shown in Table 8.5, no significant association was observed in the comparison of either genotype distribution (χ^2=0.057, df=2; P=0.97) or

Table 8.5 Glu^{298}Asp genotypes in hypertensive and normotensive groups

Residue 298 genotype	Hypertensive (n=549)	Normotensive (n=513)
Glu/Glu	461	433
Glu/Asp	84	76
Asp/Asp	4	4
Frequency of Asp allele	0.084	0.082

Genotype distribution: χ^2=0.057, df=2; P=0.97
Allele frequency: χ^2=0.026, df=1; P=0.87
Source: Kato *et al.* (1999).

Table 8.6 Clinical characteristics of participants according to genotypes at residue 298 of *Nos3*

Variable	Total	Glu/Glu	Glu/Asp	Asp/Asp	ANOVA (*P*)
n (men/women)	998 (570/428)	844 (486/358)	146 (80/66)	8 (4/4)	
Blood pressure (mmHg)					
Systolic	138.6 ± 27.2	138.4 ± 26.9	140.1 ± 28.7	142.4 ± 36.5	0.73
Diastolic	86.1 ± 15.4	85.9 ± 15.4	87.4 ± 15.6	84.4 ± 14.9	0.52
BMI (kg/m^2)	22.9 ± 3.0	22.9 ± 3.0	23.0 ± 2.8	22.5 ± 5.6	0.84
Age (years)	58.6 ± 12.2	58.5 ± 12.4	58.8 ± 11.0	65.7 ± 7.9	0.24

BMI = Body Mass Index.
Source: Kato *et al.* (1999).

allele frequency (χ^2=0.026, df=1; P=0.87) between hypertensive and normo-tensive groups. The lack of observed association was independent of age and Body Mass Index in a logistic regression analysis. When tested with ANOVA, association was still not significant between the Glu^{298}Asp polymorphism and BP measure-ments (Table 8.6). The odds ratio for ^{298}Asp versus ^{298}Glu allele frequency was 1.03 (95% confidence interval, CI 0.76–1.40) in this study.

Conclusion

The authors state that their results do not support the previous observation that the molecular variant of the *Nos3* gene confers the principal susceptibility for essential hypertension, and attribute previous associations to sampling variation. Taking all the above association studies into consideration, discrepancies between results are only likely to be resolved by finding intermediate phenotypes, e.g. NOS enzyme activity, and demonstrating an effect of genetic variants on these intermediate phenotypes.

The question of whether the endothelial dysfunction is primary or secondary to hypertension is frequently raised. This question is impossible to answer, but the fact that endothelial dysfunction is found in secondary forms of hypertension, and can be improved by treatment of hypertension with antihypertensive agents, would suggest that, at least in some cases, it is a result of hypertension rather than a cause. However, this may not always be the case, as Taddei *et al.* have recently shown a defective L-arginine-nitric oxide pathway in normotensive offspring of essential hypertensive patients compared to matched normotensive offspring of normotensive parents |**29**|. The authors conclude from this that endothelial dysfunction is primary and predates the onset of hypertension. The offspring in this study are in their 20s, so it would be interesting to determine which subjects develop hypertension in later life.

Over and above the methodological problems, another reason for the discrepancies in the above studies may be that patients with essential hypertension represent a heterogeneous group, among whom a small, as yet undefined, subgroup may have NO deficiency, while others have normal or even increased NO release as a compensatory mechanism. To distinguish those with NO deficiency from the rest of the hypertensive population in a practical way would require a simple screening test. Such a simple test may have been discovered by Jilma *et al.*, who measured NO in parts per billion (ppb) in a single breath and found it to be higher in males (34 ppb) compared to females (20 ppb) |**30**|. Such a gender difference in NO production is interesting in itself, but the point is that such a test, while subject to the vagaries of dietary nitrate and non-NOS III production, may be easily employed to screen large numbers of hypertensive patients.

Hypertension induced by inhibition of nitric oxide synthase

There have been many animal studies examining the effects of acute or chronic blockade of NOS by a variety of L-arginine analogues, but they are too numerous to describe in any detail here.

Chronic nitric oxide inhibition model six years on.
R Zatz, C Baylis. *Hypertension* 1998; **32**: 958–64.

REVIEW. The discovery in 1987 that endothelium-derived NO mediates the vasodilatory effect of certain endothelium-dependent agonists inaugurated the current huge field of NO biology. It is now recognized that NO plays essential roles in many diverse physiological processes and in some pathophysiological events. Development of these concepts has been based largely on evidence obtained by limiting NO biosynthesis. This review is centred on the cardiovascular and particularly the renal functional and structural consequences of chronic pharmacological NO inhibition by L-arginine analogues. This study devoted special attention to the mechanisms of hypertension and organ injury that occur under these circumstances, while appreciating the inherent limitations surrounding interpretation of these data.

Comment

The current state of knowledge about this relatively novel model of experimental hypertension is discussed in this recent review. Without exception, the studies demonstrate sustained elevation of blood pressure, suggesting a role for NO, although not necessarily endothelium-derived NO, in blood pressure regulation.

The mechanism of hypertension in this model is probably more complex than originally thought. Guyton's hypothesis has it that sustained hypertension requires at least one of the following abnormalities: (1) increased cardiac output, (2) increased total peripheral resistance (TPR), or (3) impaired renal ability to excrete sodium |31|. Cardiac output appears to be reduced in this model; therefore, one or both of the other abnormalities must apply.

The withdrawal of the basal vasodilator tone of NO is important in raising TPR in the acute phase, and seems to persist into the chronic phase, resulting in unbalanced tonic action of endogenous vasoconstrictors, such as angiotensin II and prostanoids, although endothelin is thought to be less important. Indeed, the renin–angiotensin system (RAS) may even be stimulated by chronic NOS inhibition, perhaps as a consequence of renal structural injury |32, 33|. Stimulation of the sympathetic nervous system also appears to contribute to the increased TPR by inhibiting NOS in strategic areas of the central nervous system |34|. There is evidence that chronic NOS inhibition also causes an antinatriuresis in keeping with abnormality (3) of Guyton's hypothesis, which appears to be dose-dependent. At lower doses, TPR is unchanged, but a purely volume-dependent hypertension develops |32|. At higher doses, when NOS inhibition is complete, renal and systemic vasoconstriction predominate, and the animals develop a rapidly progressive and malignant hypertension, with vascular and parenchymal damage |33|.

By contrast with the renal parenchymal damage, which can be severe |33|, a peculiarity of this model of hypertension is the relative absence of vascular structural changes. Arnal *et al.* gave oral L-NAME to Wistar rats for 8 weeks and found no cardiac hypertrophy in the majority of animals |35|. They did find cardiac hypertrophy in some animals, but these were the animals with the highest blood pressure and RAS detected by increased plasma renin activity.

Conclusion

Since the advent of this model of experimental hypertension, it has become clear that NO is an important element in the maintenance of circulatory integrity, regulating such diverse functions as vascular tone, renal salt excretion and renin secretion. As all three NOS isoforms are inhibited, further investigation is needed to establish the relative importance of NO derived from the various isoforms in controlling renal and systemic haemodynamics in health and disease.

Vascular smooth muscle cell polyploidy and cardiomyocyte hypertrophy due to chronic NOS inhibition in vivo.
A M Devlin, M J Brosnan, D Graham, J J Morton, A R McPhasen, M McIntyre, *et al. Am J Physiol Heart Circ Physiol* 1998; **43**: H52–9.

BACKGROUND. The objective of this study was to assess the vascular and cardiac response to nitric oxide synthase (NOS) blockade in vivo. Wistar–Kyoto rats (WKY) were treated for 3 weeks with N^G-nitro-arginine methyl ester (L-NAME: 10 mg/kg day).

INTERPRETATION. These studies provide further insight to confirm that NO deficiency in vivo results in the development of vascular and cardiac hypertrophy.

Comment

In this study, Devlin *et al.* examined various changes in normotensive Wistar–Kyoto (WKY) rats made hypertensive with 3 weeks of L-NAME treatment. We studied several indices of vascular and cardiac hypertrophy, including:

- vascular smooth muscle cell polyploidy, using flow cytometry DNA analysis
- light microscopy of aortic wall
- heart/body weight ratio
- expression of skeletal α-actin within the ventricle

Main results. The L-NAME-induced hypertension was rapid in onset, with significant increases in systolic blood pressure (SBP) as early as 1 week after initiation of treatment. By 3 weeks, there was a significant increase in SBP (mmHg ± SEM) in the L-NAME-treated animals (172 ± 5.68, n=15) compared to untreated control animals (132 ± 4.00, n=16; $P<0.0001$). Table 8.7 details the measured indices of vascular and cardiac hypertrophy, which were all increased in the L-NAME-treated group. Note that the RAS was activated in the hypertensive animals (Table 8.7). Relaxation of aortic ring in vitro from the L-NAME-treated animals was attenuated compared to control animals, and this attenuation was reversed by L-arginine, the substrate for NOS.

Summary

Once again, this study demonstrates that vascular and cardiac hypertrophy can be a feature of this model of hypertension, but once again the RAS has been shown to be

Table 8.7 Comparison of indices of vascular and cardiac hypertrophy between L-NAME-treated hypertensive rats and untreated normotensive control rats

	Control (n)	L-NAME (n)	P
Systolic blood pressure (mmHg ± SEM)	132 ± 4.00 (16)	172 ± 5.68 (15)	<0.0001
VSMC polyploidy (% cells ± SEM in G_2+M)	16.6 ± 0.35 (16)	24.1 ± 1.1 (14)	<0.0001
Heart:body weight (mg/g ± SEM)	3.10 ± 0.06 (16)	4.20 ± 0.11 (15)	<0.0001
Ventricular skeletal α-actin mRNA (± SEM)*	0.173 ± 0.04	0.463 ± 0.07	0.03
Plasma renin activity (ng/ml/hr ± SEM)	12.2 ± 1.5 (8)	24.6 ± 4.6 (7)	<0.05
Angiotensin II (pg/ml ± SEM)	103 ± 9.3 (8)	292 ± 50 (7)	<0.01
ACE activity (nmol/ml/min ± SEM)	18.3 ± 1.2 (8)	16.7 ± 1.0 (7)	n.s.

VSMC = vascular smooth muscle cell.
ACE = angiotensin-converting enzyme; n.s. = not significant; SEM = standard error of the mean.
*mRNA expression as a ratio to the housekeeping gene, glyceraldehyde phosphate dehydrogenase.
Source: Devlin *et al.* (1998).

stimulated, as with the Arnal study |**35**|. Certainly, chronic NOS inhibition has been shown to produce glomerular damage |**36**|, and the subsequent stimulation of the RAS may be responsible for the vascular structural changes. This is confirmed by Takemoto *et al.*, who produced coronary vascular remodelling and myocardial hypertrophy in WKY after 4 and 8 weeks of NOS inhibition with L-NAME |**37**|. They showed that the cardiovascular structural changes could be prevented by co-administration of the angiotensin-converting enzyme inhibitor temocapril, but not with hydralazine, despite its producing a similar reduction in blood pressure. The different susceptibility of various strains of rat to NOS inhibitor-induced vascular changes may reflect altered sensitivity to renal damage and subsequent stimulation of the RAS, rather than altered sensitivity of heart and blood vessels *per se*. This altered sensitivity to renal damage may in turn reflect divergent genetic backgrounds.

Although local intrabrachial infusions of L-arginine analogues have been given to humans in many studies to investigate endothelial function, a systemic infusion of a pharmacological dose of a NOS inhibitor was given to humans for the first time by Haynes *et al.* |**38**|. A 5-minute infusion of L-NAME (3 mg/kg) in healthy volunteers produced a 10% increase in mean arterial pressure, a 19% decrease in heart rate and a 25% decrease in cardiac index, resulting in a 46% increase in calculated total peripheral resistance. Creatinine clearance was unchanged, but in contrast to the animal studies, they found a natriuresis with NOS inhibition, which they attributed to a pressure natriuresis.

An introduction to superoxide anion

While much attention has been focused on the role of NO in hypertension and cardiovascular disease, the role of superoxide (O_2^-) has also been examined in relation to endothelial dysfunction. Despite being essential for most forms of life, the high content of oxygen (O_2) in the atmosphere means that oxidation reactions are commonplace in our environment. Although our bodies use O_2 and oxidation reactions to good effect for generating energy and killing invaders, unwanted side-reactions are unavoidable. Therefore, to support aerobic metabolism, mechanisms had to evolve for the biological control of O_2. One such mechanism involves its complete reduction to water (Fig. 8.2), which produces the free radical O_2^- by the one electron reduction of molecular O_2 as the first intermediate in this pathway. The majority of O_2 is reduced by the cytochrome oxidase complex, which prevents release of the reactive intermediates. However, the evolution of a variety of superoxide dismutase (SOD) enzymes, catalase and peroxidase to remove the reactive intermediates suggests that a significant proportion of O_2 is reduced by this route. It has been estimated that a typical human cell metabolizes about 10^{12} molecules of O_2 per day and generates some 3×10^9 molecules of hydrogen peroxide (H_2O_2) per hour |**39**|. Although associated with so-called 'oxidative stress', O_2^- is an unusual species in that it can act as a reducing agent, donating its extra electron e.g. to form

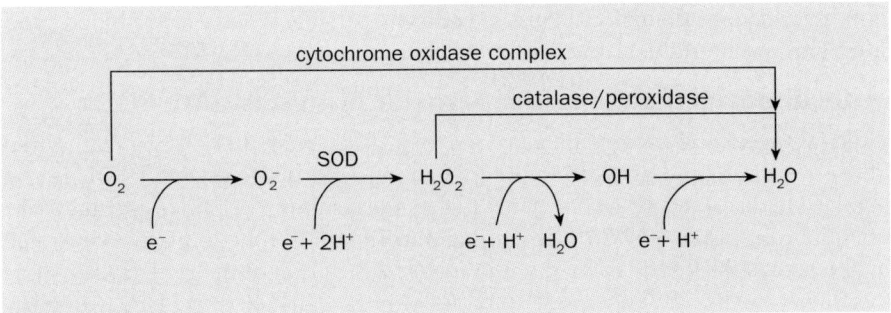

Fig. 8.2 Steps in the 4 electron (e⁻) reduction of molecular oxygen (O_2) to water (H_2O), via superoxide anion (O_2^-), hydrogen peroxide (H_2O_2) and hydroxyl radical (OH) intermediates. The majority of O_2 is reduced by the cytochrome oxidase complex, which prevents release of the reactive intermediates. However, the evolution of a variety of superoxide dismutase (SOD) enzymes, catalase and peroxidase, to remove the reactive intermediates, suggests that a significant proportion of O_2 is reduced by this route.

peroxynitrite ($ONOO^-$) with NO, or as an oxidizing agent, in which case it is reduced to H_2O_2. Under normal circumstances, the relatively high abundance of SOD enzyme ensures that the latter reaction occurs preferentially, even though the former reaction occurs more rapidly [40]. However, when NO is produced in large quantities, a significant amount of O_2^- reacts with NO to produce $ONOO^-$.

Superoxide dismutases

As described above, organisms that depend on oxidative metabolism have evolved a number of enzymes to reduce O_2^-, which is formed as an intermediate. One such family of enzymes are the superoxide dismutases, which catalyse the reaction of O_2^- with an electron and two protons to form H_2O_2 (Fig. 8.2). Three mammalian SODs have so far been identified; copper/zinc SOD (SOD1), manganese SOD (SOD2) and extracellular SOD (SOD3).

Cytosolic copper/zinc superoxide dismutase (Cu/Zn SOD)

This enzyme was the first member of the family to be discovered in mammals in 1969. The human gene for Cu/Zn SOD (*Sod1*) has been localized to chromosome 21. Therefore, patients with Down's syndrome (trisomy 21) have an extra copy of the gene, and have been shown to have Cu/Zn SOD activity 50% greater than the normal diploid population, in keeping with the gene dosage effect. This increased activity in Down's syndrome provides one piece of evidence for a role for O_2^- in hypertension. With a higher Cu/Zn SOD activity, Down's syndrome patients will have reduced O_2^- levels. If O_2^- excess is involved in the pathogenesis of hypertension, then one would expect Down's syndrome patients to have lower blood pressure. This was found to be the case in a well-controlled study by Morrison *et al.* [41].

Mitochondrial manganese superoxide dismutase (Mn SOD)

This was the second mammalian enzyme to be discovered in 1973. It is synthesized in the cytoplasm and directed to the mitochondria by a signal peptide, where it is involved in dismutating the O_2^- generated by the respiratory chain of enzymes. The essential role of Mn SOD in maintaining mitochondrial function is demonstrated by the neonatal lethality of mice with targeted disruption of the gene for Mn SOD (*Sod2*) [42]. Such *Sod2* 'knock-out' mice die within the first 10 days of life with dilated cardiomyopathy, which is in keeping with the fact that in the wild-type mice Mn SOD activity is greatest in the heart.

Extracellular copper/zinc superoxide dismutase (EC-SOD)

This is the third and currently the last mammalian SOD to be characterized. It was purified from human lung by Marklund in 1982. It is produced in fibroblasts and glial cells and secreted into the extracellular fluid, where it is the principal SOD. The enzyme is a glycoprotein, which binds sulphated polysaccharides, such as heparin and heparan sulphate. Therefore, EC-SOD will exist in the vasculature mainly bound to the surface of the endothelial cells and the extracellular matrix, both of which have an abundance of heparan sulphate, although some enzyme activity can be detected in the plasma. A genetic marker in the *Sod3* gene has been shown to reduce binding to endothelial cells, and increase serum EC-SOD levels [43]. It is not reported whether the carriers of this marker have altered blood pressure or cardiovascular risk.

Superoxide anion in hypertension

As mentioned previously, NO can be scavenged by O_2^- to form peroxynitrite ($ONOO^-$), effectively reducing the bioavailability of endothelium-derived NO. Therefore, circumstances which result in increased O_2^- can be harmful in several ways: first, by removing the beneficial effects of NO, and second, by the damaging effects of $ONOO^-$, which can be protonated to peroxynitrous acid, the cleavage products of which are among the most reactive oxygen species in the biological system. In addition, several studies have demonstrated that O_2^- can act as a vasoconstrictor [44, 45]. For all of these reasons, a role for O_2^- has been suggested in hypertension, and recently this has been extensively reviewed [46].

Superoxide anion in experimental hypertension

Since the landmark study on renovascular hypertension by Goldblatt *et al.* in 1934 [47], it has become clear that the renin–angiotensin system (RAS) plays a major role in hypertension. The mechanism of RAS-induced hypertension has generally been attributed to the vasoconstrictor effects of angiotensin II and the mineralocorticoid effects of aldosterone. However, recent work has revealed an additional potential mechanism. Angiotensin II has been shown to stimulate O_2^- generation by increasing the activity of the enzyme NAD(P)H cytochrome P-450 oxidoreductase, more commonly termed NAD(P)H oxidase, in aortas of rats made hypertensive by angiotensin II infusion |**48**|. This seems to be a fairly specific effect, as rats made hypertensive to a similar degree by infusion of noradrenaline showed no increase in NAD(P)H oxidase activity |**48**|. Blood pressure was reduced by 50 mmHg and vascular reactivity in response to ACh was restored by exogenous liposome-encapsulated SOD in the angiotensin II hypertensive rats, but not the noradrenaline hypertensive rats, which further implicates O_2^- in hypertension associated with high angiotensin II states |**49**|.

O_2^- has been implicated in other models of experimental hypertension. Grunfeld *et al.* demonstrated that, in aortas of the SHRSP model of genetic hypertension, excess O_2^- could exactly account for the reduced bioavailability of NO detected by their porphyrinic microsensor |**50**|. The following year, Tschudi *et al.* confirmed normal NO production, but increased decomposition by O_2^- in the mesenteric resistance vessels of SHRSP |**51**|. It has recently been confirmed that NO production is greater in SHRSP compared to the normotensive WKY strain |**52**|. Despite this greater production, it was demonstrated that NO bioavailability is reduced in the hypertensive strain. This suggests that NO may be scavenged by O_2^- in the hypertensive strain.

Superoxide anion production is increased in a model of genetic hypertension: role of the endothelium.
S Kerr, M J Brosnan, M McIntyre, J L Reid, A F Dominiczak, C A Hamilton. *Hypertension* 1999; **33**: 1353–8.

BACKGROUND. The hypothesis that the decreased NO availability observed in spontaneously hypertensive stroke-prone rats (SHRSP) is due to excess superoxide (O_2^-) was examined.

INTERPRETATION. These results show that O_2^- generation is increased in SHRSP and that the tissue and enzymatic sources of this excess O_2^- appear to be the endothelium and eNOS, respectively. The increase in O_2^- generation could explain the decreased availability of basal NO observed in this model of genetic hypertension.

Comment

In this study, O_2^- generation by aortic rings from SHRSP and WKY rats was quantified by lucigenin chemiluminescence. O_2^- generation was also quantified after removal of the endothelium; after inhibition of NOS with L-NAME; and after addition of tetrahydrobiopterin (BH_4), one of the cofactors essential for NOS function.

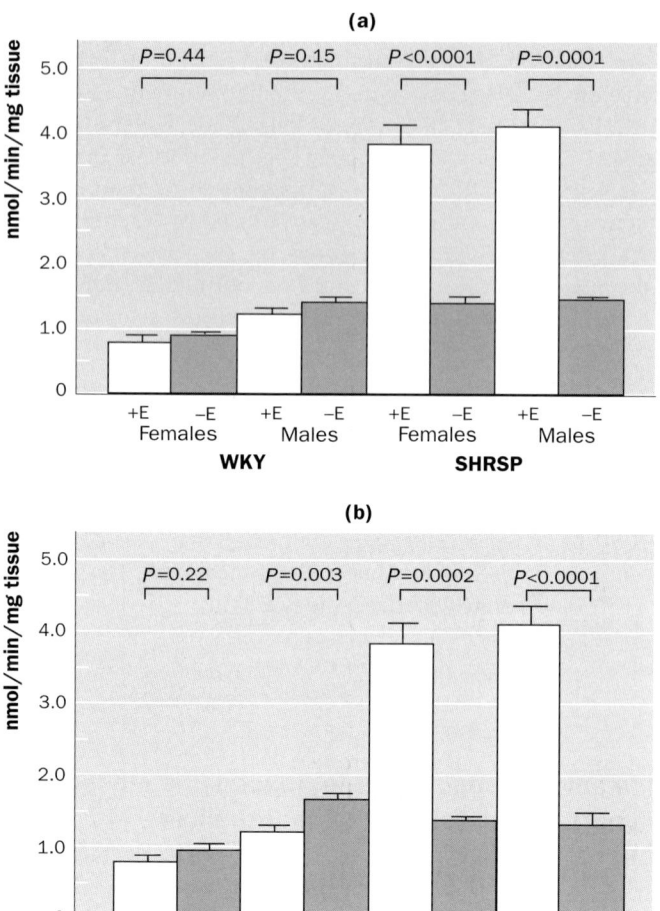

Fig. 8.3 (a) Effect of removal of the endothelium (E) on O_2^- generation in rings of aorta from male and female WKY and SHRSP. (b) Effect of inhibiting NOS with L-NAME (L-N) on O_2^- generation in rings of aorta from male and female WKY and SHRSP.

Main results. O_2^- generation (nmol/min/mg protein $\pm$ SEM) was significantly increased in aortas from SHRSP (3.96 ± 0.19, n=13) compared to WKY (1.02 ± 0.08, n=18, $P<0.0001$). As shown in Fig. 8.3, O_2^- generation in aortas from SHRSP was reduced to WKY levels by removal of the endothelium or inhibition of NOS by L-NAME. Incubation of aortas from SHRSP with BH_4 significantly reduced O_2^- generation from 4.04 ± 0.11 to 2.36 ± 0.40 nmol/min/mg protein

($P=0.0026$), but BH_4 incubation had no significant effect on O_2^- generation from aortas from WKY.

Summary

This study confirms that O_2^- generation is increased in aortas from SHRSP compared to WKY, and would at least partly explain the reduced NO availability in the hypertensive animals. The cellular and enzymatic sources of the O_2^- excess appear to be the endothelium and NOS, respectively.

O_2^- generation by NOS has been reported before. Purified rat brain NOS (NOS I) has been shown to produce O_2^- in a reaction which is inhibited by L-NAME, but not L-NMMA [53]. The reason why NOS changes from generating beneficial NO to generating harmful O_2^- remains unclear. Recent studies have implicated BH_4. Wever et al. [54] used purified NOS III to confirm that NOS III can indeed generate O_2^-. This O_2^- generation was not inhibited by L-arginine, but was dose-dependently inhibited by BH_4 [54]. Stroes et al. [55] demonstrated restoration of endothelial function in the forearm of hypercholesterolaemic humans by BH_4. It appears, therefore, that NOS is capable of generating both NO and O_2^-, and the relative proportion of each seems to be determined by the local concentration of BH_4.

Superoxide anion in human essential hypertension

The role of O_2^- in human essential hypertension is much less well studied. Certainly, endogenous O_2^- has been shown to affect tone in human vessels. Hamilton et al. determined NO and O_2^- levels in internal thoracic arteries (ITA) and saphenous veins (SV) in vitro, from patients undergoing coronary artery bypass grafting [56]. They found similar levels of carbachol-stimulated NO release in ITA and SV, but could detect virtually no basal release of NO in SV, despite easily detecting basal NO release in ITA. The NOS III enzyme was detected immunohistochemically in both vessels, suggesting that NO was being scavenged in SV. When the O_2^- chelator tiron was added to the organ bath, basal NO release increased to ITA levels. Interestingly, tiron also increased basal NO in ITA, albeit to a lesser degree, suggesting that O_2^- impairs NO vasodilator tone in human arteries, but more so in veins.

As with the rat enzyme, human NOS III has also been suggested as the source of O_2^- in cultured human umbilical vein endothelial cells stimulated with native low-density lipoprotein, as it can be inhibited by L-NAME [57]. However, there are no in vivo data implicating the endothelium as a source of O_2^- in human essential hypertension. Increased O_2^- generation, albeit by neutrophils, has been demonstrated in human essential hypertension [58]. Although the mechanism remains unclear, the effect can be reversed by β-adrenoceptor blockade with celiprolol [58]. This is in contrast to an earlier study by Seifert et al. [59], who found no difference in neutrophil superoxide-forming NAD(P)H oxidase in human essential hypertension. Red blood cell SOD activity was also found to be reduced in patients with essential hypertension compared to normotensive controls, but the groups were very poorly matched for age [60]. Although not directly measured in this study, the implication is that O_2^- would consequently be increased in the hypertensive group, perhaps contributing to the hypertension.

Polymorphism of the NADH/NAD(P)H oxidase *p22 phox* gene in patients with coronary artery disease.

N Inoue, S Kawashima, K Kanazawa, S Yamada, H Akita, M Yokoyama.
Circulation 1998; **97**: 135–7.

BACKGROUND. **Oxidative stress in the vasculature has been implicated in the pathogenesis of coronary artery disease (CAD). NADH/NAD(P)H oxidase is a key enzyme of superoxide production in the vasculature. *p22 phox*, an essential component of NADH/NA(P)DH oxidase, has four types of polymorphism. The C22 polymorphism changes histidine-72 to tyrosine, located in the potential heme-binding sites, whereas A640G polymorphism is located in the 3′ untranslated region.**

INTERPRETATION. The mutation of the potential heme-binding site of the *p22 phox* gene is a novel genetic marker that has a protective effect on coronary risk.

Comment

In contrast to the many reports relating to *Nos3* polymorphisms in hypertension, the only described polymorphism in any O_2^- related gene with regard to human cardiovascular disease involves the *p22 phox* gene, which encodes NAD(P)H oxidase. In this study, Inoue *et al.* describe a mutation, C242T, which changes histidine-72 to tyrosine in the potential haem-binding site of the enzyme. In addition they identified another polymorphism, A640G, in the 3′ untranslated region of the gene. They studied 201 CAD patients ($>75\%$ stenosis at coronary angiography) and 201 age- and sex-matched controls (without symptoms of CAD or peripheral vascular disease).

Main results. Although well matched for age and sex, the groups were poorly matched for other cardiovascular risk factors, e.g. smoking status ($P<0.001$) incidence of hypercholesterolaemia ($P<0.001$), incidence of diabetes ($P<0.001$) and incidence of hypertension ($P<0.001$) with each risk factor being more prevalent in the CAD group. The allele frequencies of the A640G polymorphism were not different between control and case patients. However, with regard to the C242T polymorphism, the frequency of the T allele was significantly increased in the control group (0.13) compared to cases (0.08, $P<0.02$). The odds ratio of the TC+TT versus the CC genotype between case patients and control subjects was 0.49 (95% confidence interval, CI 0.28–0.87). The association of the TC+TT genotype with CAD was significant and independent of other risk factors when subjected to logistic regression analysis ($P=0.15$).

Summary

This study provides some evidence for an association of the O_2^- generating system with CAD. Although the cases and controls are poorly matched for risk factors, the logistic regression analysis goes some way to validating the association. The fact that the mutation lies in the potential haem-binding site of the enzyme makes it a slightly more likely candidate; but, as with the *Nos3* polymorphisms described above, functional studies of the mutant enzyme would be necessary to confirm that it represents a genetic predisposition to cardiovascular disease. Mutations in the *Sod2* gene have been reported in various neurodegenerative diseases, but no *Sod* gene mutations have been thus far linked to hypertension or cardiovascular disease.

Conclusions

There remains little doubt that NO is an important molecule in cardiovascular physiology. However, through its interaction with NO, O_2^- is now emerging as a molecule of equal, if not potentially greater, importance in cardiovascular pathology, and perhaps even physiology. It is now becoming clear that the balance between these two radicals is more important than are the absolute levels of either alone. Pharmacological intervention to tip this balance in favour of NO may be useful in the prevention and treatment of a host of diseases common in the western world, including hypertension, diabetes and atherosclerotic cardiovascular disease.

References

1. Furchgott RF, Zawadski JV. The obligatory role of endothelial cells in the relaxation of arterial smooth muscle by acetylcholine. *Nature* 1980; **228**: 373–6.
2. Palmer RMJ, Ferrige AG, Moncada S. Nitric oxide release accounts for the biological activity of endothelium-derived relaxing factor. *Nature* 1987; **327**: 524–6.
3. Palmer RMJ, Ashton DS, Moncada S. Vascular endothelial cells synthesize nitric oxide from L-arginine. *Nature* 1988; **333**: 664–6.
4. Hecker M, Sessa WC, Harris HJ, Anggard EE, Vane JR. The metabolism of L-arginine and its significance for the biosynthesis of endothelium-derived relaxing factor: cultured endothelial cells recycle L-citrulline to L-arginine. *Proc Nat Acad Sci USA* 1990; **87**: 8612–6.
5. Wu G, Meininger CJ. Regulation of L-arginine synthesis from L-citrulline by L-glutamine in endothelial cells. *Am J Physiol Heart Circ Physiol* 1993; **265**: H1965–71.
6. Shepherd JT. Increased systemic vascular resistance and primary hypertension: the expanding complexity. *J Hypertens* 1990; **8**(Suppl 7): S15–S27.
7. Folkow B. Physiological aspects of primary hypertension. *Physiol Rev* 1982; **62**: 347–504.
8. Vallance P, Collier J, Moncada S. Effects of endothelium-derived nitric oxide on peripheral arteriolar tone in man. *Lancet* 1989; **2**: 997–1000.
9. Angus JA, Dyke AC, Jennings GL, Korner PI, Sudhir K, Ward JE, *et al*. Release of

endothelium-derived relaxing factor from resistance arteries in hypertension. *Kidney Int Suppl* 1992; **37**: S73–8.

10. Salom MG, Lahera V, Miranda-Guardiola F, Romero JC. Blockade of pressure natriuresis induced by inhibition of renal synthesis of nitric oxide in dogs. *Am J Physiol —Renal Fluid and Electrolyte Physiology* 1992; **262**: F718–22.

11. Dominiczak AF, Bohr DF. Nitric oxide and its putative role in hypertension. *Hypertension* 1995; **25**: 1202–11.

12. Chen PY, Sanders PW. L-arginine abrogates salt-sensitive hypertension in Dahl/Rapp rats. *J Clin Invest* 1991; **88**: 1559–67.

13. Huang PL, Huang Z, Mashimo H, Bloch KD, Moskowitz MA, Bevan JA, *et al.* Hypertension in mice lacking the gene for endothelial nitric oxide synthase. *Nature* 1995; **377**: 239–42.

14. Shesely EG, Maeda N, Kim HS, Desai KM, Krege JH, Laubach VE, *et al.* Elevated blood pressures in mice lacking endothelial nitric oxide synthase. *Proc Nat Acad Sci USA* 1996; **93**: 13176–81.

15. Deng AY, Rapp JP. Locus for the inducible, but not a constitutive, nitric oxide synthase cosegregates with blood pressure in the Dahl salt-sensitive rat. *J Clin Invest* 1995; **95**: 2170–7.

16. Dukhanina OI, Dene H, Deng AY, Choi CR, Hoebee B, Rapp JP. Linkage map and congenic strains to localize blood pressure QTL on rat chromosome 10. *Mamm Genome* 1997; **8**: 229–35.

17. Panza JA, Quyyumi AA, Brush JE, Epstein SE. Abnormal endothelium-dependent vascular relaxation in patients with essential hypertension. *N Engl J Med* 1990; **323**: 22–7.

18. Taddei S, Virdis A, Mattei P, Salvetti A. Vasodilatation to acetylcholine in primary and secondary forms of human hypertension. *Hypertension* 1993; **21**: 929–33.

19. Linder L, Kiowski W, Buhler FR, Luscher TF. Indirect evidence for release of endothelium-derived relaxing factor in human forearm circulation *in vivo.* Blunted response in hypertension. *Circulation* 1990; **81**: 1762–7.

20. Cockcroft JR, Chowienczyk PJ, Benjamin N, Ritter JM. Preserved endothelium-dependent vasodilatation in patients with essential hypertension. *N Engl J Med* 1994; **330**: 1036–40.

21. Calver A, Collier J, Moncada S, Vallance P. Effect of local intra-arterial N(G)-monomethyl-L-arginine in patients with hypertension: the nitric oxide dilator mechanism appears abnormal. *J Hypertens* 1992; **10**: 1025–31.

22. Chowienczyk PJ, Cockcroft JR, Ritter JM. Blood flow responses to intra-arterial acetylcholine in man: effects of basal flow and conduit vessel length. *Clin Sci* 1994; **87**: 45–51.

23. Laurent S, Lacolley P, Brunel P, Laloux B, Pannier B, Safar M. Flow-dependent vasodilation of brachial artery in essential hypertension. *Am J Physiol* 1990; **258**: H1004–11.

24. Wang XL, Sim AS, Badenhop RF, McCredie RM, Wilcken DEL. A smoking-dependent risk of coronary artery disease associated with a polymorphism of the endothelial nitric oxide synthase gene. *Nat Med* 1996; **2**: 41–5.

25. Hibi K, Ishigami T, Tamura K, Mizushima S, Nyui N, Fujita T, *et al.* Endothelial nitric oxide synthase gene polymorphism and acute myocardial infarction. *Hypertension* 1998; **32**: 521–6.

26. Bonnardeaux A, Nadaud S, Charru A, Jeunemaitre X, Corvol P, Soubrier F. Lack of

evidence for linkage of the endothelial cell nitric oxide synthase gene to essential hypertension. *Circulation* 1995; **91**: 96–102.

27. Friend LR, Morris BJ, Gaffney PT, Griffiths LR. Examination of the role of nitric oxide synthase and renal kallikrein as candidate genes for essential hypertension. *Clin Exp Pharmacol Physiol* 1996; **23**: 564–6.

28. Hunt SC, Williams CS, Sharma AM, Inoue I, Williams RR, Lalouel JM. Lack of linkage between the endothelial nitric oxide synthase gene and hypertension. *J Hum Hypertens* 1996; **10**: 27–30.

29. Taddei S, Virdis A, Mattei P, Ghiadoni L, Sudano I, Salvetti A. Defective L-arginine-nitric oxide pathways in offspring of essential hypertensive patients. *Circulation* 1996; **94**: 1298–303.

30. Jilma B, Kastner J, Mensik C, Vondrovec B, Hildebrandt J, Krejcy K, *et al.* Sex differences in concentrations of exhaled nitric oxide and plasma nitrate. *Life Sci* 1996; **58**: 469–76.

31. Guyton AC. Long-term arterial pressure control: an analysis from animal experiments and computer and graphic models. *Am J Physiol* 1990; **259**: R865–77.

32. Yamada SS, Sassaki AL, Fujihara CK, de Malheiros DMAC, Nucci G, Zatz R. Effect of salt intake and inhibitor dose on arterial hypertension and renal injury induced by chronic nitric oxide blockade. *Hypertension* 1996; **27**: 1165–72.

33. Ribeiro MO, Antudes E, de-Nucci G, Lovisolo SM, Zata R. Chronic inhibition of nitric oxide synthase. A new model of arterial hypertension. *Hypertension* 1992; **20**: 298–303.

34. Cunha RS, Cabral AM, Vasquez EC. Evidence that the autonomic nervous system plays a major role in the L-NAME-induced hypertension in conscious rats. *Am J Hypertens* 1993; **6**: 806–9.

35. Arnal JF, El Amrani AI, Chatellier G, Menard J, Michel JB. Cardiac weight in hypertension induced by nitric oxide synthase blockade. *Hypertension* 1993; **22**: 380–7.

36. Baylis C, Mitruka B, Deng A. Chronic blockade of nitric oxide synthesis in the rat produces systemic hypertension and glomerular damage. *J Clin Invest* 1992; **90**: 278–81.

37. Takemoto M, Egashira K, Usui M, Numaguchi K, Tomita H, Tsutsui H, *et al.* Important role of tissue angiotensin-converting enzyme activity in the pathogenesis of coronary vascular and myocardial structural changes induced by long-term blockade of nitric oxide synthesis in rats. *J Clin Invest* 1997; **99**: 278–87.

38. Haynes WG, Noon JP, Walker BR, Webb DJ. Inhibition of nitric oxide synthesis increases blood pressure in healthy humans. *J Hypertens* 1993; **11**: 1375–80.

39. Newcomb TG, Loeb LA. Oxidative DNA damage and mutagenesis. In: Nickoloff J, Hoekstra M (eds): *DNA Damage and Repair.* Totowa, NJ: Humana Press, 1998, pp. 65–84.

40. Beckman JS, Chen J, Ischiropoulos H, Crow JP. Oxidative chemistry of peroxynitrite. In: Packer L (ed.): *Methods of Enzymology.* San Diego, CA: Academic Press Inc., 1994, pp. 229–40.

41. Morrison RA, McGrath A, Davidson G, Brown JJ, Murray GD, Lever AF. Low blood pressure in Down's syndrome. A link with Alzheimer's disease? *Hypertension* 1996; **28**: 569–75.

42. Li Y, Huang TT, Carlson EJ, Melov S, Ursell PC, Olson JL, *et al.* Dilated cardiomyopathy and neonatal lethality in mutant mice lacking manganese superoxide dismutase. *Nat Genet* 1995; **11**: 376–81.

43. Yamada H, Yamada Y, Adachi T, Goto H, Ogasawara N, Futenma A, *et al.* Polymorphism

of extracellular superoxide dismutase (EC-SOD) gene: relation to the mutation responsible for high EC-SOD level in serum. *Jpn J Hum Genet* 1997; **42**: 353–6

44. Auch-Schwelk W, Katusic ZS, Vanhoutte PM. Contractions to oxygen-derived free radicals are augmented in aorta of the spontaneously hypertensive rat. *Hypertension* 1989; **13**: 859–64.

45. Cosentino F, Sill JC, Katusic ZS. Role of superoxide anions in the mediation of endothelium-dependent contractions. *Hypertension* 1994; **23**: 229–35.

46. McIntyre M, Bohr DF, Dominiczak AF. Endothelial dysfunction in hypertension: the role of superoxide anion. *Hypertension* 1999; **34**: 539–45.

47. Goldblatt H, Lynch J, Hanzal RF, Summerville WW. Studies on experimental hypertension I: the production of persistent elevation of systolic blood pressure by means of renal ischaemia. *J Exp Med* 1934; **59**: 347–79.

48. Rajagopalan S, Kurz S, Munzel T, Tarpey M, Freeman BA, Griendling KK, *et al.* Angiotensin II-mediated hypertension in the rat increases vascular superoxide production via membrane NADH/NADPH oxidase activation. Contribution to alterations of vasomotor tone. *J Clin Invest* 1996; **97**: 1916–23.

49. Laursen JB, Rajagopalan S, Galis Z, Tarpey M, Freeman BA, Harrison DG. Role of superoxide in angiotensin II-induced but not catecholamine-induced hypertension. *Circulation* 1997; **95**: 588–93.

50. Grunfeld S, Hamilton CA, Mesaros S, McClain SW, Dominiczak AF, Bohr DF, *et al.* Role of superoxide in the depressed nitric oxide production by the endothelium of genetically hypertensive rats. *Hypertension* 1995; **26**: 854–7.

51. Tschudi MR, Mesaros S, Luscher TF, Malinski T. Direct in situ measurement of nitric oxide in mesenteric resistance arteries: increased decomposition by superoxide in hypertension. *Hypertension* 1996; **27**: 32–5.

52. McIntyre M, Hamilton CA, Rees DD, Reid JL, Dominiczak AF. Sex differences in the abundance of endothelial nitric oxide in a model of genetic hypertension. *Hypertension* 1997; **30**: 1517–24.

53. Pou S, Pou WS, Bredt DS, Snyder SH, Rosen GM. Generation of superoxide by purified brain nitric oxide synthase. *J Biol Chem* 1992; **267**: 24173–6.

54. Wever RMF, van Dam T, van Rijn HJ, de Groot F, Rabelink TJ. Tetrahydrobiopterin regulates superoxide and nitric oxide generation by recombinant endothelial nitric oxide synthase. *Biochem Biophys Res Commun* 1997; **237**: 340–4.

55. Stroes E, Kastelein J, Cosentino F, Erkelens W, Wever R, Koomans H, *et al.* Tetrahydrobiopterin restores endothelial function in hypercholesterolemia. *J Clin Invest* 1997; **99**: 41–6.

56. Hamilton CA, Berg G, McIntyre M, McPhaden AR, Reid JL, Dominiczak AF. Effects of nitric oxide and superoxide on relaxation in human artery and vein. *Atherosclerosis* 1997; **133**: 77–86.

57. Pritchard Jr KA, Groszek L, Smalley DM, Sessa WC, Wu M, Villalon P, *et al.* Native low-density lipoprotein increases endothelial cell nitric oxide synthase generation of superoxide anion. *Circ Res* 1995; **77**: 510–18.

58. Mehta JL, Lopez LM, Chen L, Cox OE. Alterations in nitric oxide synthase activity, superoxide anion generation, and platelet aggregation in systemic hypertension, and effects of celiprolol. *Am J Cardiol* 1994; **74**: 901–5.

59. Seifert R, Hilgenstock G, Fassbender M, Distler A. Regulation of the superoxide-forming NADPH oxidase of human neutrophils is not altered in essential hypertension. *J Hypertens* 1991; **9**: 147–53.

60. Jun T, KeYan F, Catalano M. Increased superoxide anion production in humans: a possible mechanism for the pathogenesis of hypertension. *J Hum Hypertens* 1996; **10**: 305–9.

9

Mineralocorticoid hypertension: from recent research to clinical developments

Introduction

High blood pressure associated with excessive renal sodium reabsorption in the distal renal tubule, expansion of the extracellular fluid compartment and increased body sodium content, leading to suppression of synthesis and release of renin, is defined as mineralocorticoid hypertension (for a review, see Stewart 1999 [1]). Mineralocorticoid hypertension results from excessive activation of the epithelial sodium channel, which is normally regulated by the mineralocorticoid receptor. Recently, detailed understanding of the various biochemical and molecular mechanisms that result in a common clinical phenotype has shed light on the basic mechanisms involved in blood pressure and volume homeostasis. In turn, this has identified important candidate mechanisms that might contribute to the development of essential hypertension. In this regard, it is important to note that the majority of studies on the genetic basis of human essential hypertension have focused on candidate genes encoding components of the renin–angiotensin–aldosterone system or on genes involved in renal sodium retention. For example, some, but not all, studies have supported the involvement of the angiotensinogen locus in human essential hypertension [2–4]. In addition, the gene encoding human aldosterone synthase (*CYP11B2*) has been reported, in several studies in the last 12 months, to be associated with high blood pressure and increased urinary aldosterone excretion.

Evaluation of the angiotensin locus in human essential hypertension.

E Brand, N Chatelain, B Keavney, M Caulfield, L Citterio, J M C Connell, *et al. Hypertension* 1998; **31**: 725–9.

BACKGROUND. Different family and case–control studies support genetic linkage and association at the human angiotensinogen (AGT) locus with essential hypertension. To extend these previous observations, a European collaborative study of nine centres was set up to create a large resource of affected sibling pairs.

METHODS AND RESULTS. The AGT locus was studied using a highly polymorphic dinucleotide repeat in the 3'-flanking region of the gene in 350 European families, comprising 630 affected sibling pairs. Statistical analyses using two different methods did not show any evidence for linkage either in the whole panel or in family subsets selected for severity or early onset of disease.

INTERPRETATION. Although several arguments from association studies suggest a role of the AGT gene in essential hypertension, this large family study did not replicate the initial linkage reported in smaller studies. Our results highlight the difficulty of identifying susceptibility genes by linkage analysis in complex diseases.

Comment

The role of the AGT locus in hypertension has been the subject of a number of studies over the last year. In this investigation, a large sibling pair collection from across Europe was investigated and showed no evidence for linkage of the AGT locus with hypertension. This study suggests that previous investigations may have shown false-positive results due to small numbers, and illustrates the importance of performing appropriately powered studies in the investigation of the genetic basis of hypertension.

Structural analysis and evaluation of the aldosterone synthase gene in hypertension.

E Brand, N Chatelain, P Mulatero, I Fery, K Curnew, X Jeunemaitre, *et al.*
Hypertension 1998; **32**: 198–204.

BACKGROUND. Anomalies in either of the tightly linked genes encoding the enzymes *CYP11B1* (11 beta-hydroxylase) or *CYP11B2* (aldosterone synthase) can lead to important changes in arterial pressure and are responsible for several monogenically inherited forms of hypertension. Mutations in these genes or their regulatory regions could thus contribute to genetic variation in susceptibility to essential hypertension. To test this hypothesis, the authors performed two complementary studies of the *CYP11B1/CYP11B2* locus in essential hypertension.

METHODS AND RESULTS. After characterizing a DNA contig containing the *CYP11B1* gene and mapping the gene in the Centre d'Etudes du Polymorphisme Humain reference panel of families, a linkage study was performed with 292 hypertensive sibling pairs and a highly informative microsatellite marker near *CYP11B1*. Also analysed were the association of two frequent bi-allelic polymorphisms of the *CYP11B2* gene, one in the promoter at position −344 (−344C/T) and the other a common gene conversion in intron 2, with hypertension in 380 hypertensive patients and 293 normotensive individuals. Statistical analyses did not show significant linkage of the *CYP11B1* microsatellite marker to hypertension.

INTERPRETATION. No positive association with hypertension was found with the gene conversion in intron 2, but a positive association with hypertension was found with the

–344T allele. The hypertensive and normotensive samples differed significantly in both genotype (P=0.023) and allele frequencies (P=0.010). Our data suggest a modest contribution of the *CYP11B2* gene to essential hypertension.

Aldosterone excretion rate and blood pressure in essential hypertension are related to polymorphic differences in the aldosterone synthase gene *(CYP11B2)*.

E Davies, C D Holloway, M C Ingram, G C Inglis, E C Friel, C Morrison, *et al.*
Hypertension 1999; **33**: 703–7.

BACKGROUND. **Significant correlation of body sodium and potassium with blood pressure (BP) may suggest a role for aldosterone in essential hypertension. In patients with this disease, the ratio of plasma renin to plasma aldosterone may be lower than in control subjects, and plasma aldosterone levels may be more sensitive to angiotensin II infusion. Because essential hypertension is partly genetic, it is possible that altered control of aldosterone synthase gene expression or translation may be responsible. We compared the frequency of two linked polymorphisms, one in the steroidogenic factor-1 (SF-1) binding site and the other an intronic conversion (IC), in groups of hypertensive and normotensive subjects. In a larger population, the relationship of aldosterone excretion rate to these polymorphisms was also evaluated.**

METHODS AND RESULTS. **In 138 hypertensive subjects, there was a highly significant excess of TT homozygosity (SF-1) over CC homozygosity compared with a group of individually matched normotensive control subjects. The T allele was significantly more frequent than the C allele in the hypertensive group compared with the control group. Similarly, there was a highly significant relative excess of the conversion allele over the 'wild-type' allele and of conversion homozygosity over wild-type homozygosity in the hypertensive group compared with the control group. In 486 subjects sampled from the North Glasgow Monitoring of Trends and Determinants in Cardiovascular Disease (MONICA) population, SF-1 and IC genotypes were compared with tetrahydroaldosterone excretion rate. Subjects with the SF-1 genotypes TT or TC had significantly higher excretion rates than those with the CC genotype. The T allele was associated with higher excretion rates than the C allele. However, no significant differences were found in excretion rate between subjects of different IC genotype.**

INTERPRETATION. Urinary aldosterone excretion rate may be a useful intermediate phenotype linking these genotypes to raised BP. However, no causal relationship has yet been established, and it is possible that the polymorphisms may be in linkage with other causative mutations.

Comment

These two studies have examined the association of a polymorphism associated with the gene encoding aldosterone synthase (see Fig. 9.1) with hypertension. In both studies, a case–control approach showed a positive finding with the same polymorphism and essential hypertension. In the first study (Brand *et al.*), a separate

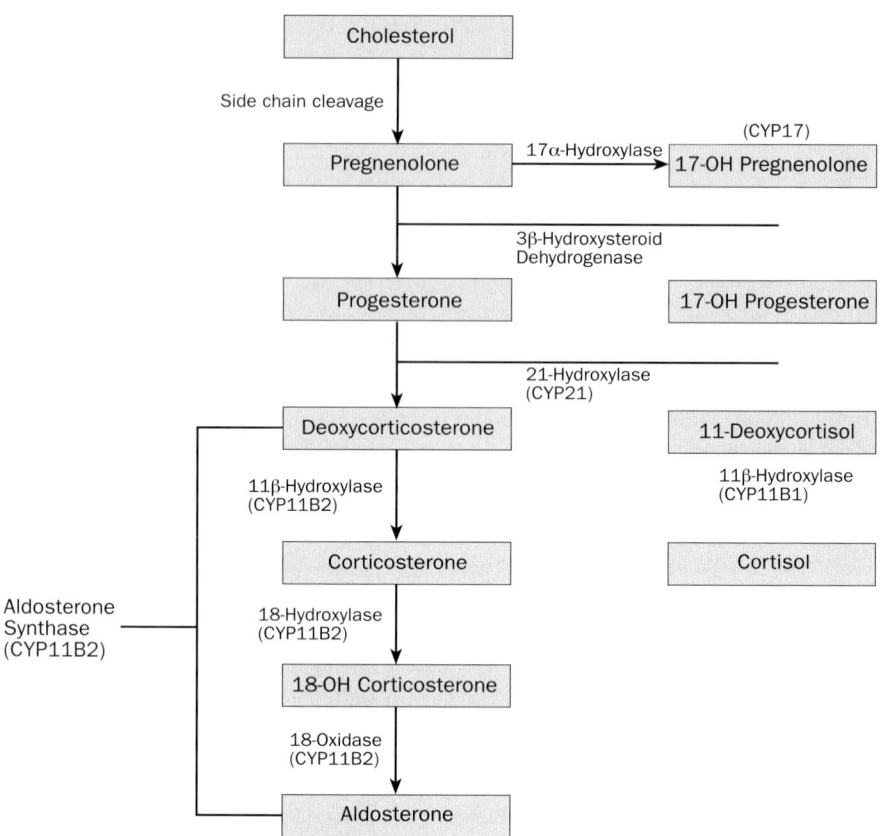

Fig. 9.1 The conversions carried out by aldosterone synthase (zona glomerulosa) and 11β-hydroxylase (zona fasciculata) are shown.

linkage study using hypertensive sibling pairs failed to show any association of a microsatellite marker around this locus with hypertension. However, linkage studies of this type may be less powerful than case–control analyses, and the positive findings with the polymorphism in the 5-promoter region of the aldosterone synthase gene do suggest that this is a real effect. Furthermore, in the second paper, this genetic variant was associated with increased aldosterone metabolite levels in urine. Thus there is a plausible physiological explanation (increased aldosterone production) for the association between this genetic change and hypertension.

Primary aldosteronism (PA) is the most common form of mineralocorticoid excess. By definition, the syndrome occurs as a result of excessive and inappropriate aldosterone production. Solitary benign adenomas of the adrenal cortex (Conn's adenomas) account for 70% of patients with PA, while the majority of the remainder have bilateral adrenal hyperplasia (described in greater detail below). In a very small number of patients, an autosomal dominant form of aldosterone excess (glucocorticoid remediable aldosteronism: GRA) is present. Again, this is described in detail below. Other forms of mineralocorticoid hypertension include constitutive activation of the epithelial sodium channel (Liddle's syndrome) and altered corticosteroid metabolism, in which cortisol acts as a mineralocorticoid hormone (syndrome of apparent mineralocorticoid excess). Again, these are discussed in greater detail below.

Normal physiology of the renin–angiotensin–aldosterone system

In order to understand recent developments in mineralocorticoid hypertension it is necessary to review, briefly, the physiological regulation of the renin–angiotensin–aldosterone system. Aldosterone is produced in the zona glomerulosa cells of the adrenal cortex from cholesterol, in a series of biochemical reactions that involve sequential hydroxylation and dehydrogenation steps. These are summarized in Fig. 9.1. The unique components of the pathway in aldosterone formation are in the 18-hydroxylation of corticosterone followed by a dehydration to yield aldosterone. These steps are catalysed by the enzyme, aldosterone synthase. Expression of this enzyme is regulated by angiotensin II and extracellular potassium concentration [4].

Aldosterone secretion is normally regulated by changes in body sodium status through the activity of the renin–angiotensin system (for a review, see Fraser 1988 [5]). Loss of sodium (or volume depletion) stimulates the system; this results in synthesis and release of renin by the juxta-glomerular apparatus of the kidney. In turn, renin, through generation of angiotensin I and its subsequent conversion to angiotensin II determines aldosterone release. Potassium also stimulates aldosterone secretion in an interactive way with angiotensin II. Thus the sensitivity of aldosterone to angiotensin II stimulation is determined by prevailing potassium levels. The pituitary hormone ACTH acutely stimulates aldosterone secretion from the adrenal cortex, but after chronic administration, aldosterone synthesis and release is suppressed.

The adrenal cortex produces relatively small amounts of aldosterone (up to 150 μg daily), and this is very much less than the amount of cortisol secreted (over 100-fold less). A paradox that remained ill understood for many years was the fact that cortisol and aldosterone showed similar binding affinity for the mineralocorticoid receptor in vitro. This led to a conceptual difficulty in identifying a means by which aldosterone could act as a specific mineralocorticoid hormone in the presence of much higher cortisol concentration. However, it is now clear that the mineralocorticoid receptor is protected from activation by cortisol by the enzyme 11β-hydroxysteroid dehydrogenase (type 2), which converts cortisol to the inactive metabolite cortisone, thus allowing aldosterone to occupy the receptor [6]. In circumstances where this enzyme is inhibited pharmacologically or is inactive owing to genetic mutations, cortisol acts as a mineralocorticoid (syndrome of apparent mineralocorticoid excess) |7| and this is reviewed below.

Mineralocorticoid receptors are present in the distal renal tubule, vascular smooth muscle cells, heart, distal colon, salivary gland and central nervous system. In the kidney, occupation of the receptor leads to increased activity of the epithelial sodium channel on the luminal membrane. This heterotrimeric protein, composed of three subunits (α, β and γ), transports sodium from the lumen of the tubule into the cell |8|.

The exchanger is coupled to an intracellular protein (Nedd4), whose function appears to be to terminate activity of the exchanger. Mineralocorticoid receptor occupancy also increases synthesis of the energy-dependent sodium–potassium transporter, so that the net effect of excess aldosterone action in the kidney is to increase transport of sodium from the lumen of the renal tubule into the bloodstream in exchange for potassium and hydrogen.

The role of the mineralocorticoid receptor in other tissues in relation to cardiovascular regulation is less clear. Nonetheless, recent evidence shows that mineralocorticoid action on the heart increases cardiac fibrosis |9| and that this can be blocked by specific aldosterone antagonists |10|. In blood vessels, aldosterone causes increased catecholamine and angiotensin-II-induced vasoconstriction. Finally, activation of mineralocorticoid receptors in the central nervous system has a direct effect to raise BP through activation of central sympathetic outflow |11|. In addition, these receptors regulate sodium and water homeostasis by modifying ingestive behaviour.

Clinical forms of mineralocorticoid hypertension

Liddle's syndrome

This rare form of hypertension was first identified in 1963 by Liddle, who described a family with high BP and low renin but low, rather than high, aldosterone levels |12|. Although Liddle recognized that the defect lay in the renal tubule, progress in identifying the cause of the hypertension was not made until cloning of the mineralocorticoid-dependent epithelial sodium channels in the renal tubule was achieved. In all cases of Liddle's syndrome thus described, activating mutations affecting either the β or γ subunits are present |8, 13|. (These subunits are encoded by two genes on chromosome 16 in man.) In each instance, the mutations lead to loss of the intracellular cytoplasmic tail of the subunit, which is thought to act as an anchor site for the Nedd4 protein described above. Given that interaction of the subunits with Nedd4 represents a likely mechanism for channel inactivation, the mutations result in constitutive overactivity of the sodium channel.

Defective regulation of the epithelial Na$^+$ channel by Nedd4 in Liddle's syndrome.

H Abriel, J Loffig, J F Rebhun, J H Pratt, L Schild, J D Horisberger, *et al.*
J Clin Invest 1999; **103**: 667–73.

BACKGROUND. Liddle's syndrome is an inherited form of hypertension linked to mutations in the epithelial sodium channel (ESC). ENaC is composed of three subunits (α, β, γ), each containing a COOH-terminal PY motif (xPPxY). Mutations causing Liddle's syndrome alter or delete the PY motifs of β- or γ-ENaC. The authors recently demonstrated that the ubiquitin–protein ligase Nedd4 binds these PY motifs, and that ENaC is regulated by ubiquitination.

METHODS AND RESULTS. This study investigates, using the *Xenopus* oocyte system, whether Nedd4 affects ENaC function. Overexpression of wild-type Nedd4, together with ENaC, inhibited channel activity, whereas a catalytically inactive Nedd4 stimulated it, probably by acting as a competitive antagonist to endogenous Nedd4. These effects were dependent on the PY motifs, because no Nedd4-mediated changes in channel activity were observed in ENaC lacking them. The effect of Nedd4 on ENaC missing only one PY motif (of β-ENaC), as originally described in patients with Liddle's syndrome, was intermediate. Changes were due entirely to alterations in ENaC numbers at the plasma membrane, as determined by surface binding and immunofluorescence.

INTERPRETATION. These results demonstrate that Nedd4 is a negative regulator of ESC, and suggest that the loss of Nedd4 binding sites in ENaC observed in Liddle's syndrome may explain the increase in channel number at the cell surface, increased sodium reabsorption by the distal nephron, and hence the hypertension.

Comment

Liddle's syndrome is associated with a mutation in the ESC—this mutation causes loss of a cytoplasmic tail in the protein of the channel. In this paper, Abriel and colleagues demonstrate that an intracellular protein binds to the cytoplasmic tail of the channel to regulate its activity. Thus the mutation in Liddle's syndrome that leads to loss of this cytoplasmic tail results in failure of the intracellular protein (Nedd4) to bind. In turn, this results in constitutive overactivity of the channel. There is, therefore, a clear biological mechanism which accounts for the increased sodium channel activity in Liddle's syndrome, and the relationship between genetic variation, protein structural change and ultimate biological functional outcome is clear.

Liddle's syndrome responds clinically to treatment with amiloride, which specifically blocks the ESC. As aldosterone levels are not high, the aldosterone receptor antagonist, spironolactone, is ineffective in this circumstance.

Although it is rare, one important feature of Liddle's syndrome is the possible candidate role it highlights for the ESC in hypertensive subjects. Baker and colleagues have described an association between a mutation in the ESC and hypertension in Afro-Caribbean subjects. Although other reports have not yet confirmed this observation, excessive renal tubular sodium reabsorption through this means provides an attractive pathophysiological mechanism for other more common types of hypertension.

Association of hypertension with T594M mutation in β subunit of epithelial sodium channels in black people resident in London.

E H Baker, Y B Dong, G A Sagnella, M Rothwell, A K Onipinla, N D Markandu, *et al. Lancet* 1998; **351**: 1388–92.

BACKGROUND. Liddle's syndrome is a rare inherited form of hypertension in which mutations of the epithelial sodium channel (ESC) result in increased renal sodium reabsorption. Essential hypertension in black patients also shows clinical features of sodium retention, so we screened black people for the T594M mutation, the most commonly identified sodium-channel mutation.

METHODS AND RESULTS. In a case–control study, 206 hypertensive (mean age 48.0 [SD 11.8] years, men:women 80:126) and 142 normotensive (48.7 [7.4] years; 61:81) black people who lived in London, UK, were screened for T594M. Part of the last exon of the ESC beta-subunit from genomic DNA was amplified by polymerase chain reaction (PCR). The T594M variant was detected by single-strand conformational polymorphism analysis of PCR products and confirmed by DNA sequencing. *Findings:* 17 (8.3%) of 206 hypertensive participants compared with three (2.1%) of 142 normotensive participants possessed the T594M variant (odds ratio [OR]=4.17 [95% confidence interval, CI 1.12–18.25], *P*=0.029). A high proportion of participants with the T594M variant were women (15 of 17 hypertensive participants and all three normotensive participants), whereas women constituted a lower proportion of the individuals screened (61.2% hypertensive, 57.7% normotensive). However, the association between the T594M variant and hypertension persisted after adjustment for sex and Body-Mass Index (Mantel-Haenszel OR=5.52 [1.40–30.61], *P*=0.012). Plasma renin activity was significantly lower in 13 hypertensive participants with the T594M variant (median=0.19 ng/ml/h) than in 39 untreated hypertensive individuals without the variant (median=0.45 ng/ml/h), *P*=0.009).

INTERPRETATION. Among black London people the T594M sodium-channel beta-subunit mutation occurs more frequently in people with hypertension than those without. The T594M variant may increase sodium-channel activity, and could raise BP in affected people by increasing renal tubular sodium reabsorption. These findings suggest that the T594M mutation could be the most common secondary cause of essential hypertension in black people identified to date.

Comment

In this case–control study of black people in London, the frequency of a polymorphism (T594M) in the codon region of the gene for the β-subunit of the ESC was examined. This genetic variation changes a threonine for a methionine residue.

Activating mutations of this gene cause the rare monogenic form of hypertension, Liddle's syndrome.

The mutant allele was present more frequently in hypertensive subjects (8.3%) than normotensives (2.1%). There was a slightly lower plasma renin activity in the hypertensives with the mutation than in those with only the wild-type allele. The hypertensive group is well matched with the controls, apart from weight—the hypertensives were significantly heavier.

Case–control studies are open to criticism, as it can be difficult to ensure that the two groups are derived from the same population. Thus differences in the distribution of a genetic marker between cases and controls might represent heterogeneity of population, rather than a true association with disease. In this study the matching seems to be carefully performed. For case–control association studies, a positive association suggests that the causal gene is very close (in genetic terms) to the marker studied, owing to the large number of genetic recombinations that occur in a sample derived from a free-breeding population. Thus this result suggests that the β-subunit of the ESC is an important candidate gene for hypertension. In genetic studies, it is important to establish a plausible biological link between genotype and ultimate phenotype (high BP in this instance). In this paper, there was a small reduction in plasma renin activity in subjects bearing the mutant allele, suggesting that this was associated with excessive renal sodium retention. However, it should be noted that numbers were small, and no difference was seen in normotensive patients.

Finally, despite the positive nature of this study, only a minority of hypertensive subjects carried the mutant allele, and its contribution to essential hypertension must be small. The importance of this study lies in the link that it provides between a monogenic disorder—Liddle's syndrome—and a common clinical phenotype—essential hypertension, with a plausible biochemical intermediate phenotype (low renin activity).

Syndrome of apparent mineralocorticoid excess

As was detailed above, cortisol can, potentially, act as a mineralocorticoid receptor agonist. Indeed, when present in very high concentrations, cortisol displays classical mineralocorticoid effects: when healthy volunteers are given high doses of hydrocortisone, they retain sodium avidly, lose potassium and become hypertensive [14]. Similarly, subjects with ectopic ACTH syndrome show classical features of mineralocorticoid hypertension, with profound hypokalaemia. Under more usual physiological circumstances, however, the mineralocorticoid receptor is protected from the effects of cortisol by the type 2 11β-hydroxysteroid dehydrogenase enzyme, which converts cortisol to cortisone [14]. The type 2 enzyme is found in the kidney, large bowel and salivary gland; it is also present in placenta, brain and vascular endothelium (for a review, see Albiston et al. [15]).

The syndrome in which cortisol can act as a mineralocorticoid owing to inactivation of this enzyme was first described in children in 1979 [16]. However, the role of 11β-hydroxysteroid dehydrogenase in this syndrome was not appreciated until

1988, when Stewart and colleagues described abnormalities in cortisol to cortisone conversion in an adult with severe hypertension |7|. Since then, a number of kindreds showing autosomal-recessive inheritance of this defect have been described. In most instances, heterozygote subjects are apparently normal. The syndrome responds to inhibition of cortisol production by dexamethasone; alternatively, spironolactone or amiloride can be effective.

As with other rare monogenic forms of hypertension, the syndrome of apparent mineralocorticoid excess offers a potential candidate mechanism that may be involved in essential hypertension. Given that heterozygote subjects (with loss of one allele encoding 11β-hydroxysteroid dehydrogenase) have no phenotypic abnormality, it seems unlikely that minor mutations at this locus will have major consequences for cortisol metabolism and, hence, the development of hypertension. Nonetheless, there have been reports of associations between polymorphisms at the 11β-HSD2 locus and hypertension in subjects with sodium sensitivity, and more detailed investigation of this is necessary |**17**|. An alternative mechanism by which this system may be involved in hypertension may be in the presence of inhibitors of 11β-hydroxysteroid dehydrogenase function. Thus the active derivative of liquorice, glycyrrhetinic acid, causes hypertension and sodium retention through inhibition of 11β-hydroxysteroid dehydrogenase type 2 activity |**18**|.

Impact of dietary Na⁺ on glycyrrhetinic acid-like factors (kidney 11β-HSD2-GALFS) in human essential hypertension.

D J Morris, Y H Lo, W R Litchfield, G H Williams. *Hypertension* 1998; **31**: 469–72.

BACKGROUND. Previous studies by these authors have shown that human urine contains glycyrrhetinic acid-like factors (GALFs) that possess inhibitory activity against kidney 11β-hydroxysteroid dehydrogenase isoform 2 (HSD2). The present studies were undertaken to determine the impact of dietary sodium intake on the levels of kidney 11β-(HSD2)-GALFs.

METHODS AND RESULTS. The excretion of kidney 11β-(HSD2)-GALFs in 24-hour urine samples of 30 unmedicated subjects (10 normotensive and 10 high/normal-renin and 10 low-renin essential hypertensive subjects) on both 200- and 10-mmol sodium diets was studied. No differences in the urinary levels of kidney 11β-(HSD2)-GALFs were observed among the three groups on the high-sodium diet. However, with a low-sodium diet, the levels of kidney 11β-(HSD2)-GALFs were significantly increased in hypertensive subjects but not in normal subjects. Levels increased from 8.3 ± 1.4 to 17.3 ± 2.9 and 6.7 ± 1.3 to 10.6 ± 1.4 carbenoxolone sodium units/d in high/normal-renin ($P=0.01$) and low-renin hypertensive subjects ($P=0.07$), respectively; normal subjects changed from 8.0 ± 1.9 to 10.6 ± 2.4.

INTERPRETATION. The levels of kidney 11β-(HSD2)-GALFs were significantly higher in the high/normal-renin hypertensive subjects than in either the control normotensive subjects or the low-renin hypertensive subjects when challenged with the low-sodium diet

($P<$0.05 by Wilcoxon rank-sum test). The greater response of the high/normal-renin essential hypertensive subjects indicated that they may utilize kidney 11β-(HSD2)-GALFs when challenged with a low-sodium diet, whereas the low-renin essential hypertensive subjects do not.

Comment

Studies showing an association between 11β-hydroxysteroid dehydrogenase activity, altered sodium balance and hypertension have largely focused on the rare genetic syndromes that lead to loss of 11β-HSD2 activity (syndrome of apparent mineralo-corticoid excess). However, this paper suggests that in essential hypertension, inhibitors of the enzyme may also give rise to reduced function. In turn, this would result in decreased cortisol to cortisone conversion, and excessive binding of corti-sol to the mineralocorticoid receptor. In the paper of Morris *et al.*, a bio-assay was used to examine the presence of inhibitors of the enzyme in the urine of patients with hypertension in comparison to normal controls. The study was carried out during high- and low-sodium intakes, and hypertensive subjects were divided into those with high- or low-renin activity. The main finding of the study was that patients with high renin activity showed a significantly greater increase in the in-hibitor of the enzyme when changing from a low to a high salt intake in comparison to low-renin patients or control subjects. As the increase in enzyme inhibitor activi-ty during low-sodium intake might be regarded as an appropriate homeostatic re-sponse to allow increased cortisol availability to the mineralocorticoid receptor, the significance of the greater increase in high-renin hypertensive patients is uncertain. Nonetheless, the paper does identify an interesting biological mechanism that may help regulate renal sodium retention during altered salt intake, and provides another potential biological function that may, when functioning abnormally, contribute to development of volume-dependent hypertension.

It is possible that endogenous inhibitors of this enzyme exist—there are recent reports of increased concentration of these type of inhibitors in hypertensive sub-jects |**24**|. Again, more detailed studies of this phenomenon in larger groups of patients with hypertension are required.

Other non-aldosterone-dependent forms of mineralocorticoid hypertension

Rarely, other steroid hormones can cause mineralocorticoid hypertension. Of these, the commonest is deoxycorticosterone, which is a precursor steroid pro-duced by the adrenal cortex (see Fig. 9.1). Some subjects with adrenal carcinomas produce deoxycorticosterone to excess. Although the hormone has weaker affinity for the mineralocorticoid receptor than aldosterone, deoxycorticosterone can cause hypertension with suppression of renin. The other situations in which deoxy-corticosterone is present in excess are the syndromes of 11β-hydroxylase deficiency and 17α-hydroxylase deficiency. These conditions are, however, excessively rare, and the reader is referred to a review for a more detailed description |**5**|.

11β-hydroxylase deficiency does, however, illustrate one important feature which is relevant to essential hypertension. The enzyme is the key control step in the zona fasciculata, which converts deoxycortisol to cortisol, and deoxycorticosterone to corticosterone (see Fig. 9.1). In the rare autosomal recessive condition of enzyme deficiency, complete lack of this activity leads to major build-up of deoxycorticosterone. Deficiency of cortisol leads to excessive ACTH stimulation of the gland, and the syndrome responds to treatment with dexamethasone. As with the other rare forms of hypertension, however, it is clear that lesser abnormalities might lead to mild forms of deoxycorticosterone excess, which could contribute to the development of more common forms of hypertension. At present, few studies have examined this in great detail. There are, however, reports of increased deoxycorticosterone levels in the plasma of patients with hypertension, both in the basal situation and after ACTH stimulation |19|. Thus this rare circumstance again illustrates a potential candidate mechanism by which high BP might occur through a mineralocorticoid-dependent mechanism.

Mineralocorticoid hypertension due to aldosterone excess

Primary aldosteronism

Glucocorticoid remediable aldosteronism (GRA)

GRA is a rare, autosomal dominantly inherited form of primary aldosteronism (PA). It occurs as a result of the presence of a chimeric gene, comprising the 5′ regions from 11β-hydroxylase (*CYP11B1*), which contain the ACTH-responsive elements, attached to the 3′ coding regions of aldosterone synthase (*CYP11B2*) |20|. This gene, whose expression is regulated by ACTH, leads to production of aldosterone synthase in the zona fasciculata. The chimeric gene occurs as a result of unequal recombination between *CYP11B1* and *CYP11B2* during meiosis. Subjects with GRA have aldosterone excess, with variable severity of hypertension, often from a young age. Aldosterone excess (and BP) respond to administration of an aldosterone receptor antagonist, such as spironolactone, or treatment with amiloride. Aldosterone production can also be suppressed with a glucocorticoid such as dexamethasone, and this provides an alternative form of treatment.

Intracranial aneurysm and hemorrhagic stroke in glucocorticoid remediable aldosterone.
W R Litchfield, B F Anderson, R J Weiss, R P Lifton, R G Dluhy.
Hypertension 1998; **31**: 445–50.

BACKGROUND. **There are anecdotal reports of early cerebrovascular complications occurring in patients with GRA. The issue has never been systematically evaluated.**

This study retrospectively reviewed the International Registry for GRA to see if there was an association between cerebrovascular complications and GRA.

METHODS AND RESULTS. The authors searched the records of 376 patients from 27 genetically proven GRA pedigrees for premature death or cerebrovascular complications. Each case was subsequently verified through the referring physician or autopsy reports. The number of complications occurring in patients with proven GRA was compared to GRA-negative subjects from the same pedigrees. There were 18 cerebrovascular events in 15 patients with proven GRA (n=167) and none in the GRA-negative group (n=194; $P<0.001$). There were an additional 15 events in 15 subjects that were suspected of having GRA based on clinical history. Seventy per cent of events were hemorrhagic strokes; the overall case fatality rate was 61%. The mean (± SD) age at the time of the initial event was 31.7 ± 11.3 years. In total, 48% of all GRA pedigrees and 18% of all GRA patients had cerebrovascular complications, which is similar to the frequency of aneurysm in adult polycystic kidney disease. GRA is associated with high morbidity and mortality from early onset of hemorrhagic stroke and ruptured intracranial aneurysms.

INTERPRETATION. Screening for intracranial aneurysm with magnetic resonance angiography is advised for patients with genetically proven GRA.

Comment

Glucocorticoid remediable aldosteronism is a rare genetic cause of hypertension caused by excessive aldosterone production from the adrenal gland. In this paper, the authors report an apparent high rate of cerebrovascular events in patients with GRA (of these, most were due to cerebral haemorrhages due to intracranial aneurysm), and recommend that patients with proven GRA be prospectively screened for the presence of aneurysms.

While the finding is of interest, the patient population studied here is highly selected and may be subject to reporting bias. Thus detailed investigation to look for a cause of hypertension may be more likely in families that present with severe early-onset disease associated with cerebral haemorrhage. In order to be certain that there was a true increased risk of intracranial aneurysm associated with GRA, a more thorough screening programme would be necessary, comparing family members with or without the genetic defect. Nonetheless, it is certainly prudent to ensure that patients with GRA have optimal BP control.

GRA can be readily diagnosed by genetic means (either by a Southern blotting technique to identify a unique restriction fragment or by a recently reported reliable polymerase chain reaction method that provides a simple and rapid means of screening families at risk).

Rapid diagnosis and identification of cross-over sites in patients with glucocorticoid remediable aldosterone.

A A MacConnachie, K F Kelly, A McNamara, S Loughlin, I J Gates, G C Inglis, et al. J Clin Endocrinol Metab 1998; **83**: 4328–31.

BACKGROUND. Glucocorticoid remediable aldosteronism (GRA) is an autosomal dominant cause of PA and high blood pressure resulting from a chimeric 11 beta-hydroxylase/aldosterone synthase gene. Abnormal expression of aldosterone synthase causes PA, which can be inhibited by glucocorticoids. Diagnosis of GRA has depended on the identification of a restriction enzyme product in genomic DNA of affected individuals. Recently, a two-tube-long polymerase chain reaction (PCR) method was described that allowed diagnosis of GRA in a kindred group in Australia. A similar long PCR method confirmed the diagnosis of GRA in members of five northeastern Scotland families previously identified by Southern blotting, and detected affected members of five GRA families previously identified in Glasgow. A multiplex PCR protocol is described here that allows the control aldosterone synthase amplification and chimeric gene amplification to be carried out in the same tube.

METHODS AND RESULTS. We describe the regions of cross-over in each of 10 kindreds identified in Scotland. To identify cross-over regions in each of the kindreds, the chimeric long PCR product was cloned and sequenced.

INTERPRETATION. Five cross-over sites were identified ranging from intron 2 to exon 4, indicating the reliability of the method in identifying chimeric genes resulting from different sites of cross-over.

Comment

The diagnosis of GRA has hitherto relied on demonstration of primary aldosterone excess by biochemical means, followed by a demonstration that aldosterone can be effectively suppressed by administration of a glucocorticoid. This test can give rise to false-positive results. Following the identification of the genetic cause of the disorder by Lifton, diagnosis can be made using Southern blotting, but this is a time-consuming procedure. The above paper reports a rapid and reliable long PCR-based technique which allows the diagnosis of GRA to be made in a single step. No cases of GRA were missed using this technique. In the future, diagnosis of GRA (once suspected) may be best made using a molecular approach such as this rather than cumbersome biochemical methods.

Common forms of primary aldosteronism

Following the first description by Conn in 1955 |**21**|, the frequency of PA due to adrenal adenoma was thought to be low. However, more recent screening tests have been used to investigate large populations of hypertensive patients, and these have reported high prevalence of PA |**22, 23**|. Most of these studies have used tests based on measurement of the ratio of aldosterone to renin (discussed in greater detail below). These investigations have suggested that PA may occur in up to 15% of the hypertensive population: this includes a recent study from Dundee, where patients in General Practice Hypertension Clinics were studied |**24**|. However, several of these screening investigations based on the aldosterone:renin ratio are heavily influenced by the denominator in the equation. Thus very minor changes in renin activity will result in an abnormal ratio. It is unclear, from these studies, how many patients would be reliably diagnosed as having PA if the ratio were only so interpreted along with a corresponding requirement for the aldosterone level, itself, to be frankly elevated. It is noteworthy that in a recent large series (3900 subjects) who were very thoroughly screened for PA with measurements that included urinary aldosterone excretion as well as plasma measurements, a prevalence of 6.5% was reported—in only half of these subjects were adrenal adenomas identified |**25**|. This figure is consistent with other large series. Again, in a recent paper reported from Italy within the last year, a figure of 3.6% was reported for the prevalence of aldosterone-producing adenomas using sophisticated statistical modelling techniques |**26**|, although these are likely to be useful in clinical practice |**27**|.

Screening for primary aldosteronism with a logistic multivariate discriminant analysis.

G R Rossi, E Rossi, E Pavan, N Rosati, R Zecchel, A Semplicini, *et al. Clin Endocrinol* 1998; **49**: 713–23.

BACKGROUND. Primary aldosteronism (PA) is the most common endocrine cause of curable hypertension, but no single test unequivocally identifies it. Accordingly, the authors investigated the usefulness of a logistic multivariate discriminant analysis (MDA) approach for PA screening,

METHODS AND RESULTS. Generation of a logistic MDA function based on retrospective analysis of biochemical tests in a large cohort of referred patients with or without confirmed Conn's adenoma (CA) was followed by prospective validation of the model. The authors investigated 574 selected hypertensives: 206 (32 with and 174 without CA) retrospectively, 48 (with a 13% prevalence of CA) prospectively for the validation of the model, and 320 referred hypertensives (with a 3.4% prevalence of CA) similarly evaluated. Patients were referred to a specialized centre for hypertension (4th Clinica Medica–University of Padua) and to the Department of Internal Medicine of a regional hospital (Reggio Emilia),

Measurements: in all patients we measured several demographic and biochemical variables and performed a captopril test. A stepwise analysis of variance, based on a model fitted with several different variables, identified baseline (sALDO) and captopril-suppressed plasma aldosterone (cALDO), supine plasma renin activity (sPRA) and potassium as the most informative. Therefore, two models of logistic MDA with sPRA, potassium, and either sALDO (model A) or cALDO (model B) were developed and used. Receiver–operator curve analysis was also performed to assess the optimal cut-off values.

The model B MDA provided the best performance, and identified CA with 100% sensitivity and 81% accuracy. When used prospectively it showed 100% sensitivity, both in the Padua (88% accuracy) and in the Reggio Emilia series (90% accuracy). However, at both institutions most patients with idiopathic hyperaldosteronism (IHA) were also detected.

INTERPRETATION. Thus, although developed from patients with confirmed CA, a strategy based on MDA can be used prospectively for accurate screening for PA. Furthermore, it was proven to be accurate and applicable to patients tested with similar modalities at a different institution. Although this approach did not provide a clear-cut discrimination of CA from IHA, it may avoid unnecessary and costly further testing in patients with a low probability of PA.

Comment

This paper addresses the prevalence of PA in a hypertensive population and assesses the best methods of screening for the disorder. The first paper sets the scene for the second, and represents a very large (3900 subjects) screen of hypertensive patients for PA in a prospective manner. Measurements were made of renin in plasma, and of urinary aldosterone (and its major metabolites): 257 cases of PA were detected (6.6%), of whom 146 (3.9% of total) had adenomas.

In the second paper, an Italian group first examined retrospectively a population with high prevalence of aldosterone-producing adenomas (32 of 206) using mathematical modelling techniques to identify the best screening and diagnostic methods. They then used this to study, prospectively, an unselected hypertensive population to assess the utility of the methodology. They identified that a combination of supine plasma renin, serum potassium and aldosterone measurement after administration of captopril provided the best combination of tests, with a positive predictive value, in the retrospective study, of 40%. In the more realistic prospective study the accuracy of the tests was 90%, and the positive predictive value 26%. The prevalence of adenomas in this latter population was 3.6%, a value remarkably similar to that identified in the exhaustive screen of 3900 subjects detailed above.

The prevalence of primary aldosteronism

Debate continues on the true prevalence of PA. The very large German series gives an estimated figure of around 6.6%, which is less than several smaller studies that have relied solely on a ratio of aldosterone:renin. The prevalence of aldosterone-producing adenomas in the series was 3.9%. It is of interest that the Italian paper, which used sophisticated modelling techniques to assess the best combination of tests, reported a very similar value in a prospective study on unselected hypertensives. Thus it seems likely that the true prevalence of PA is around 6–8%, with more than 50% of these subjects harbouring an adenoma.

The Rossi paper identifies the importance of tests with high positive predictive value. In unselected hypertensives, their 'best' combination of tests gave a positive predictive value of 26%. In other words, patients picked up on screening had a 1 in 4 chance of being 'true' positives and having an aldosterone-producing adenoma. This rigorous type of approach to the assessment of screening tests is important—particularly if the condition is relatively uncommon, as in this instance. While it is unlikely that few centres will wish to establish complex multivariate models to verify screening procedures, simple combinations of tests may limit the number of patients subjected unnecessarily to an expensive investigation.

There are reports that some patients with PA due either to adenoma or bilateral adrenal hyperplasia can have a familial form of the disorder (referred to as Familial Hyperaldosteronism Type 2) inherited in an autosomal-dominant manner [28]. The molecular cause of this is uncertain: PA is reported in association with multiple endocrine neoplasia Type 1, but this appears not to be the cause of the distinct form described above.

Adrenal pathology in primary aldosteronism

Aldosterone-producing tumours (Conn's adenomas) are benign. The tumour size is generally of 1–2 cm, and when its surface is cut, the tumour has a bright yellow appearance. The histological appearance shows the presence of zona fasciculata- and zona glomerulosa-type cells—there may be a relationship between the histological appearance of the tumour and the degree of responsiveness of aldosterone to angiotensin II in patients with PA, although this has little practical value.

There are few consistent reports of pathological findings in patients with non-tumorous bilateral adrenal hyperplasia. In some instances, diffuse hyperplasia of the zona glomerulosa has been described, and there are descriptions of multiple nodules being present within the gland. However, similar appearances are reported in post-mortem findings in patients with essential hypertension, and this raises the possibility that there may be no clear demarcation between patients with low renin essential hypertension and patients with bilateral adrenal hyperplasia with modest aldosterone excess [29]. Thus in both circumstances, renal levels are suppressed, aldosterone levels are inappropriate for the level of renin, and there may be patho-logical findings on examination of the adrenal gland. This, in turn, raises the question of the underlying cause of essential hypertension, and suggests that subtle changes in regulation of the renin–angiotensin–aldosterone system may take place in a substantial proportion of patients with this disorder.

Causes and consequences of high blood pressure in primary aldosteronism

Aldosterone excess, in the acute phase, causes renal sodium and water retention and consequent volume expansion. This causes an increase in cardiac output. However, patients with chronic PA do not show sustained increase in cardiac output, and high BP is likely to be maintained by other mechanisms. In this regard, the presence of aldosterone receptors in vascular smooth muscle cells and the central nervous system may be of relevance. As was mentioned above, aldosterone promotes vasoconstriction in response to other agonists and has central effects to raise BP. Thus the maintenance of high BP in PA is likely to be complex.

Primary aldosteronism was previously thought to be a relatively benign form of hypertension. However, it is clear that high BP in this disorder can be severe and resistant to therapy. Indeed, patients with malignant hypertension due to PA are well described |30|. In addition, aldosterone excess has distinct effects on cardiovascular structure and function. Thus in experimental models, aldosterone has recently been reported to cause severe changes in cardiac collagen content and cardiac histological appearance |9|. It is of relevance that these changes are greatly exacerbated by a high sodium intake, and can be prevented by use of aldosterone receptor blockers |10|. In human subjects, studies of cardiac histological changes are not available. However, patients with PA are reported to have more severe left ventricular hypertrophy than those with corresponding levels of BP due to essential hypertension |31|. Additionally, abnormal left ventricular motion is described, including abnormal diastolic relaxation.

The effects of aldosterone on renal structure in man are not well reported. However, there is evidence from other forms of renal disease that aldosterone can be an important component in determining the rate of progression |32|. Furthermore, in animal studies, aldosterone excess causes very significant renal damage and, in addition, is a potent risk factor for development of stroke. As with cardiac changes, these abnormalities can be reversed by aldosterone receptor antagonism.

Role of aldosterone in renal vascular injury in stroke-prone hypertensive rats.
R Rocha, P N Chander, A Zuckerman, C T Stier. *Hypertension* 1999; **33**: 1–6.

BACKGROUND. Stroke-prone spontaneously hypertensive rats (SHRSP) on 1% NaCl drinking solution and Stroke-Prone Rodent Diet develop severe hypertension and glomerular and vascular lesions characteristic of thrombotic microangiopathy seen in malignant nephrosclerosis. The authors recently reported that spironolactone, a mineralocorticoid receptor antagonist, markedly reduced proteinuria and malignant nephrosclerotic lesions in these animals. This observation, together with our previous findings that angiotensin-converting enzyme inhibitors prevent the development of vascular damage, suggests that mineralocorticoids, as part of the renin–angiotensin–aldosterone system, play a pathophysiological role in this model. The present study examined whether chronic (2-week) infusion of aldosterone can reverse the renal vascular protective effects of captopril in SHRSP.

METHODS AND RESULTS. SHRSP received vehicle (n=8); captopril alone (50 mg/kg/day, orally) (n=10); aldosterone infusion alone (40 µg/kg/day, SC) (n=7); or captopril and aldosterone at 20 (n=6) or 40 (n=7) µg/kg/day. Systolic BP was markedly elevated in all groups. Vehicle- and aldosterone-infused SHRSP developed severe proteinuria and comparable degrees of renal injury (21 ± 3% and 29 ± 3%, respectively), manifested as thrombotic and proliferative lesions in the arterioles and glomeruli. Captopril treatment reduced plasma aldosterone levels concomitantly with marked reductions in proteinuria and the absence of histologic lesions of malignant nephrosclerosis. Aldosterone substitution at 20 or 40 µg/kg/day in captopril-treated SHRSP resulted in the development of severe renal lesions (16 ± 3% and 21 ± 2%, respectively) and proteinuria comparable with that observed in SHRSP given either aldosterone or vehicle alone. These findings support a major role for aldosterone in the development of malignant nephrosclerosis in saline-drinking SHRSP, independent of the effects of BP.

Mineralocorticoid blockade reduced vascular injury in stroke-prone hypertensive rats.

R Rocha, P N Chander, K Khanna, A Zuckerman, C T Stier. *Hypertension* 1998; **31**: 451–8.

BACKGROUND. Chronic treatment of saline-drinking stroke-prone spontaneously hypertensive rats (SHRSP) with agents that interfere with the formation or actions of angiotensin II (Ang II) prevents the development of stroke and renal vascular damage. Ang II, in addition to its direct vascular effects, stimulates the synthesis and release of aldosterone.

METHODS AND RESULTS. To assess the role of aldosterone in the development of pathological changes in these rats, we implanted time-release pellets containing 200 mg of the mineralocorticoid receptor antagonist, spironolactone, into 14 SHRSP at 7.5 weeks of age. Eight SHRSP littermates received placebo pellets. Over the period of study (3 to 4 weeks), systolic BP was not different between the groups. Spironolactone did not enhance water and electrolyte excretion. All placebo-treated SHRSP developed marked proteinuria (150 ± 6 mg/d), whereas in spironolactone-treated SHRSP, urinary protein excretion (UPE) averaged 39 ± 9 mg/d (*P*<0.0001). In a second study to assess effects on survival, six SHRSP received spironolactone (10 mg/kg/d) and six received vehicle. All but one of the control rats displayed signs of stroke and died by 16 weeks of age, while the spironolactone- treated SHRSP remained asymptomatic through 19 weeks of age (*P*<0.03). At 16 weeks of age, spironolactone-treated SHRSP were severely hypertensive (247 ± 3 mmHg), yet UPE remained at baseline levels. In contrast, preterminal UPE averaged 136 ± 13 mg/d in control rats (*P*<0.0001). In both studies, histopathological examination revealed a

marked protective effect of spironolactone against the development of malignant nephrosclerotic and cerebrovascular lesions.

INTERPRETATION. These observations indicate a vascular and end organ-protective effect of spironolactone in the absence of lowered BP in saline-drinking SHRSP, and are consistent with a major role for mineralocorticoids as hormonal mediators of vascular injury.

Comment

These two papers from the same group provide important information about the tissue effects of aldosterone excess. In the first paper, SHRSP rats were given either spironolactone (a specific aldosterone receptor antagonist) or placebo. The drug had no effect on BP, though it must be noted that this was not recorded over the 24-hour period. Nonetheless, spironolactone-treated rats did not develop proteinuria, and had significantly less histological damage in renal glomeruli, blood vessels and cerebral blood vessels. Importantly, a marked benefit in survival was seen in the spironolactone-treated group (none of which developed strokes) in comparison with the placebo group (all of which died).

In the second paper, SHRSP were treated with captopril, or with this drug and aldosterone, for 2 weeks. Captopril reduced aldosterone levels very significantly when compared with rats given captopril and aldosterone. No significant difference in BP was seen among the groups. However, while captopril caused a marked fall in urine protein excretion, and histological evidence of renal and vascular injury, this was not prevented in animals given captopril and aldosterone.

In summary, evidence in the last year has accumulated that aldosterone is a hormone with potentially very deleterious effects on cardiac, renal and cerebro-vascular structure and function. This emphasizes the notion that PA is a subtype of hypertension that is not only treatable, but can, if not identified, pose particular risks to cardiovascular structure and function.

Diagnosis of primary aldosteronism

The diagnosis of PA is a two-step procedure. Firstly, aldosterone excess needs to be identified; thereafter, the cause needs to be studied. If PA affects up to 5% of hypertensive patients, half of whom may have an adenoma, it is worth considering which screening tests are appropriate or necessary in hypertensive populations.

Screening for primary aldosteronism

If the frequency of PA is as high as 15%, then screening programmes to detect the disorder would be reasonable in hypertensive clinics. However, this may be less persuasive an argument if the true prevalence is closer to 5%. Under these circumstances, looking for PA in subgroups of patients at particular risk would be a reasonable approach. For example, screening should be carried out in patients who are shown to be resistant to conventional antihypertensive drugs (in practice, those whose BP is not well controlled on two agents), patients who have a positive family history of PA and patients who are hypokalaemic. In this regard, however, it is noteworthy that frank hypokalaemia is now recognized to be presented in less than 50% of patients with PA, and is not a reliable marker for the disorder |33|.

As was detailed above, simultaneous measurement of aldosterone and renin is the single best screening test for the disorder. It should be borne in mind, however, that plasma-renin activity measurements tend to be lower with age, particularly in patients with low-renin hypertension. As the denominator of the aldosterone:renin ratio, low plasma-renin activity measurements (in other words, values less than 1) can have a profound effect on the ratio, and lead to high levels of false-positive results. It is necessary, therefore, to set a fairly high cut-off for an aldosterone:renin ratio if large numbers of patients are not to be unnecessarily investigated. Under these circumstances, it would be pragmatic either simultaneously to use a threshold measurement of aldosterone, below which further investigations would not be appropriate, or to set a high threshold for the ratio. Given that aldosterone and renin assays vary from laboratory to laboratory, measurements and ranges need to be determined locally.

One advantage of the use of the aldosterone:renin ratio is the relatively robust nature of the measurement in relation to sodium intake and concurrent drug therapy. The majority of agents used to treat hypertension causes parallel changes in both aldosterone and renin. For this reason, few agents have a major distorting effect on the ratio, which facilitates its utility as a screening test. It is, of course, important to note that this is not the case when more detailed investigations are being carried out, where numerous drugs do suppress renin levels in patients with PA. In contrast, few agents can stimulate renin in patients with genuine aldosterone excess and a high renin measurement generally excludes PA.

When an abnormal aldosterone:renin ratio is present, the diagnosis of PA should be confirmed by other means. It is in those circumstances that patients should be asked to discontinue concurrent drug therapy, probably with the exception of α-blocking drugs.

Confirmatory tests for primary aldosteronism

Confirmation of the diagnosis should be made by careful measurements of aldosterone and renin—it is now accepted that a measurement made after recumbency (at least 30 minutes) or overnight rest while a patient is taking a normal sodium and potassium diet is appropriate. In normal subjects, renin and aldosterone rise after ambulation, while in patients with Conn's adenomas this is not normally the case: indeed, aldosterone levels generally fall, owing to an underlying ACTH-dependent diurnal rhythm. Thus a measurement of aldosterone and renin after 2 hours' ambulation is generally performed. Simultaneous measurement of cortisol allows one to make an indirect assessment of the concurrent effect of ACTH on aldosterone. When renin is low and aldosterone is high after recumbency, and where values are either unchanged or lower after 2 hours' ambulation, the diagnosis of PA is virtually certain, and the most likely cause is an aldosterone-producing adenoma.

Patients with bilateral adrenal hyperplasia (and a small subgroup of patients with aldosterone-producing adenomas) show responses of aldosterone to angiotensin II. In those circumstances, aldosterone can show a small rise after ambulation. However, this test, on its own, is not a sufficiently sensitive means of distinguishing between the presence or absence of a primary aldosterone-producing adenoma.

Measurement of urinary aldosterone excretion over a 24-hour period (either free aldosterone or aldosterone metabolite excretion) can be carried out. However, these measurements entail the need to make a 24-hour urine collection. Further tests to confirm the presence of PA are described below: in practice, a number of these are of little further value over the simple, carefully performed, baseline measurements of renin and aldosterone described above.

Saline infusion

The simplest test described is the infusion of normal saline (1.25 l over a 2-hour period). In normal subjects, plasma aldosterone levels are suppressed by this, while in patients with PA, levels remain elevated (> 240 pmol/l) |34|.

Fludrocortisone suppression test

Administration of fludrocortisone (0.5 mg 4 times daily for 2 days) should invariably suppress aldosterone in normal subjects. In patients with PA, levels remain elevated. Although this is regarded as a definitive test, it may entail admission of patients to hospital, and carries with it a substantial risk of provoking severe hypokalaemia |35|.

Captopril test

This test involves administation of captopril (25 mg) with measurements of renin and aldosterone before and 2 hours after drug therapy is described. In normal subjects, this will suppress aldosterone levels, while in patients with Conn's adenomas, this is not the case. However, as noted above, aldosterone levels tend to fall during the day in patients with Conn's adenomas, and the captopril test has not been routinely assessed in a large number of patients, so that its true value remains uncertain.

In summary, confirmation of PA may best be made by careful measurements of aldosterone and renin in patients taking a normal dietary sodium intake and in whom drug therapy has been withdrawn.

Differential diagnosis of primary aldosteronism

In practice, the key differential diagnosis is to decide whether or not a patient has a single aldosterone-producing adenoma that might be removed surgically. It is, of course, worth considering whether patients might have rare inherited forms of PA such as GRA; positive family history and young age of onset would provide useful clues in this regard that should lead to the use of a genetic screening test.

Although aldosterone levels may be, on average, higher in patients with adenomas and in bilateral hyperplasia, this would be insufficient on its own to distinguish the two disorders. Other biochemical measurements, such as levels of 18-hydroxy-corticosterone and 18-hydroxycortisol are described as differentiating the two conditions [1], but these are not routinely performed. Similarly, although the dynamic tests described above may provide diagnostic pointers (with the notion that patients with aldosterone-producing adenomas do not show a rise in aldosterone on ambulation), this is not invariable, and should not be, on its own, relied on as a means of distinguishing between the two. For this reason, the simplest and best means of diagnosing a single aldosterone-producing adenoma is to image the adrenal glands and, if necessary, sample aldosterone levels in adrenal veins.

Definitive procedures to identify the presence of an adrenal adenoma

Imaging of the adrenal glands can be carried out by either computed tomography (CT) or magnetic resonance imaging (MRI) scanning. Both techniques are useful in identification of adrenal adenomas, although it should be noted that small lesions (in practice, < 1 cm) may be below the limit of accurate resolution of either technique. For this reason, a negative adrenal scan does not exclude the presence of a small tumour.

In some patients with bilateral hyperplasia, CT scanning may show enlargement of the glands, with small nodules. However, it is also important to note that the presence of non-functional nodules within the adrenal is common. For this reason, it is not absolutely certain that patients with a demonstrable small lesion on CT scanning do, indeed, have PA as a result. It is suggested, therefore, that adrenal vein sampling should be carried out in situations of doubt, or where CT scanning is unhelpful. In these circumstances, simultaneous measurement of cortisol and aldosterone concentrations in both adrenal veins is appropriate. Cortisol measurements are necessary to confirm the technical success of the procedure. A successful demonstration of a unilateral lesion is helpful in identifying patients who are best treated surgically.

Surgical treatment

Surgical removal of an aldosterone-producing adenoma is normally the most appropriate treatment for patients with a unilateral lesion. However, before surgery is carried out, patients should be rendered normotensive by appropriate medical treatment. This is important, as use of an aldosterone receptor blocker or amiloride will also correct the major deficit in body potassium that would otherwise be present.

Recent surgical studies have demonstrated that laparoscopic adrenalectomy is a safe procedure that can reliably cure patients with PA |35|: the technique carries with it a low morbidity and entails a very short hospital stay for patients. Removal of Conn's adenomas cures hypertension in approximately two-thirds of patients and improves blood pressure control in the remainder.

Medical therapy

Medical therapy is appropriate for patients with bilateral adrenal hyperlasia, and in those patients with PA due to an adenoma where surgery is contraindicated. In those subjects, use of a mineralocorticoid receptor antagonist or amiloride is appropriate.

Spironolactone has been the most widely used mineralocorticoid receptor-blocking drug. It may need to be given in relatively high dose in patients with PA (up to 400 mg/day), and this may cause significant side-effects, particularly in male patients. These include gynaecomastia, diminished libido, impotence and dyspepsia. The newly developed receptor antagonist, eplerenone, is reportedly free of these side-effects, although large-scale studies demonstrating its use in PA are still awaited. An alternative to spironolactone is amiloride, which blocks the epithelial sodium channel. This effectively lowers blood pressure in PA; but, as with spironolactone, may need to be given in high doses (up to 60 mg/day).

In any medically treated patient it is important to monitor plasma potassium concentration. Plasma renin measurements may give some guide to the effectiveness of aldosterone blockade; where renin levels remain low, it is unlikely that effective aldosterone antagonism is being provided.

Summary

In the last few years, PA has been recognized as the most common cause of secondary hypertension. Recent screening studies have suggested that the prevalence may be as high as 15% in selected patient groups. Effective screening tests, using aldosterone:renin ratios, have now been described, and recent advances in therapy (laparoscopic surgery) and new drugs (novel aldosterone receptor antagonists) have provided alternative treatment options. In the context of essential hypertension, a better understanding of the physiology of regulation of the renin–angiotensin–aldosterone system and of the rare monogenic disorders that can cause mineralocorticoid hypertension have identified key mechanisms that may be relevant in the pathophysiology of common forms of hypertension and may, in the future, identify novel therapeutic targets.

References

1. Stewart PM. Mineralocorticoid hypertension. *Lancet* 1999; **353**: 1341–47.

2. Jeanemaitre X, Soubrier F, Kotelertster YV, Lifton RP, Williams CS, Charru A. Molecular basis of human hypertension: role of angiotensinogen. *Cell* 1992; **71**: 169–80.

3. Caulfield M, Lavender P, Newal-Price J, Farral M, Kamdar S, Daniel H. Linkage of the angiotensinogen gene locus to essential hypertension in African Caribbeans. *J Clin Invest* 1995; **96**: 687–92.

4. Mournet E, Dupont B, Bitek A, White PC. Characterization of two genes encoding human steroid 11β-hydroxylase (P-450 11β). *J Biol Chem* 1989; **264**: 20961–7.

5. Fraser R. Inborn errors of corticosteroid biosynthesis and metabolism: their effects on electrolyte metabolism. In: Robertson JIS (ed.): *Handbook of Hypertension*. Vol. 15: Clinical Hypertension. Amsterdam: Elsevier, 1988: 420–60.

6. Funder JW, Pearce PT, Smith R, Smith AL. Mineralocorticoid action: target tissue specificity is enzyme, not receptor, mediated. *Science* 1988; **242**: 583–5.

7. Edwards CRW, Stewart PM, Burt D, Brett L, McIntyre MA, Jutanto WS, *et al*. Localisation of 11β-hydroxysteroid dehydrogenase-tissue protector of the mineralocorticoid receptor. *Lancet* 1988; **ii**: 986–9.

8. Shimkets RA, Warnock DG, Bostitis CM, Nelson-Williams C, Hansson JH, Schambelan M, *et al*. Liddle's syndrome: heritable human hypertension caused by mutations in the β-subunit of the epithelial sodium channel. *Cell* 1994; **79**: 407–14.

9. Young M, Head G, Funder J. Determinants of cardiac fibrosis in experimental hyper-mineralocorticoid states. *Am J Physiol* 1995; **32**: E657–62.

10. Brilla CG, Matsubara LS, Weber KJ. Anti-aldosterone treatment and the prevention of myocardial fibrosis in primary and secondary hyperaldosteronism. *J Mol Cell Cardiol* 1993; **25**: 563–75.

11. Gomez-Sanchez EP. Intracerebroventricular infusion of aldosterone induces hypertension in rats. *Endocrinology* 1986; **118**: 819–23.

12. Liddle GW, Bledso T, Coppage WS. A familial renal disorder simulating primary aldosteronism but with negligible aldosterone secretion. *Trans Assoc Phys* 1983; **76**: 199–213.

13. Hansson JH, Nelson-Williams C, Suzuki H, Schild L, Shimkets R, Lu V, *et al*. Hypertension caused by a truncated epithelial sodium channel gamma subunit: genetic heterogeneity of Liddle syndrome. *Nat Genet* 1995; **11**: 76–82.

14. Connell JMC, Beastall GH, Davies DL, Buchanan K. Effect of low-dose dopamine infusion on insulin and glucagon-release in fasting normal man. *Horm Metab Res* 1986; **18**: 67–8.

15. Albiston AL, Obeyesekere VR, Smith RE, Krozowski ZS. Cloning and tissue distribution of the human 11β-hydroxysteroid dehydrogenase type 2 enzyme. *Mol Cell Endocrinol* 1994; **105**: R11–7.

16. Ulick S, Levine LS, Gunczler P, Zanconato G, Ramirez LC, Rauh W, et al. A syndrome of apparent mineralocorticoid excess associated with defects in the peripheral metabolism of cortisol. *J Clin Endocrinol Metab* 1979; **49**: 757–64.

17. Watson B, Bergman SM, Myracle A, Callen DF, Acton RT, Warnock DG. Genetic association of 11β-hydroxysteroid dehydrogenase type 2 (*HSD11B2*) flanking microsatellites with essential hypertension in blacks. *Hypertension* 1996; **28**: 478–82.

18. Farese RV, Biglieri EG, Shackleton CHL, Ironary I, Gomez-Fontez R. Licorice-induced hypermineralocorticoidism. *N Engl J Med* 1991; **325**: 1223–7.

19. DeSimone G, Tommaselli AO, Rossi R, Valentino R, Lauria R, Scopacasa F, et al. Partial deficiency of adrenal 11β-hydroxylase: a possible cause of primary hypertension. *Hypertension* 1985; **7**: 204–10.

20. Lifton RP, Dluhy RG, Powers M, Rich GM, Gutkin M, Fallo F, et al. Hereditary hypertension caused by chimaeric gene duplications and ectopic expression of aldosterone synthase. *Nat Genet* 1992; **2**: 66–74.

21. Conn JW. Primary aldosteronism, a new clinical entity. *J Lab Clin Med* 1955; **45**: 3–17.

22. Hiramatsu K, Yamada T, Yukimura Y, Komiya I, Ichikawa K, Ishihara M, et al. A screening test to identify aldosterone-producing adenoma by measuring plasma renin activity: results in hypertensive patients. *Arch Intern Med* 1981; **141**: 1589–93.

23. Gordon RD, Stowasser M, Klemm SA, Tunny TJ. High incidence of primary aldosteronism in 199 patients referred with hypertension. *Clin Exp Pharmacol Physiol* 1994; **21**: 315–8.

24. Lim PO, Rodgers P, Cardak K, Watson AS, MacDonald TM. Potentially high prevalence of primary aldosteronism in a primary care population. *Lancet* 1999; **353**: 40.

25. Abdelhamid S, Muller-Lobeck H, Pahl S, Remberger K, Bonhof J, Walb D, et al. Prevalence of adrenal and extra-adrenal Conn syndrome in hypertensive patients. *Arch Intern Med* 1996; **156**: 1190–5.

26. Rossi GR, Rossi E, Pavan E, Rosati N, Zecchel R, Semplicini A, et al. Screening for primary aldosteronism with a logistic multivariate discriminant analysis. *Clin Endocrinol* 1998; **49**: 713–23.

27. Fraser R, Murray GD, Connell JMC. Conn's syndrome: no longer a needle in a haystack? *Clin Endocrinol* 1998; **49**: 709–10.

28. Strowasser M, Gordon RD, Tunny TJ, Klemm SA, Finn WL, Krek AL. Familial hyperaldosteronism type II: five families with a new variety of primary aldosteronism. *Clin Exp Pharmacol Physiol* 1992; **19**: 319–22.

29. Idiopathic aldosteronism: a diagnostic artefact? *Lancet* 1979; **ii**: 1221–2.

30. Zarifs J, Lip GYH, Leatherdale B, Beevers G. Malignant hypertension in association with primary aldosteronism. *Blood Press* 1996; **5**: 250–4.

31. Rossi GP, Sacchetto A, Visentin P, Canali C, Graniero GR, Palatini P, et al. Changes in left ventricular anatomy and function in hypertension and primary aldosteronism. *Hypertension* 1996; **27**: 1039–45.

32. Gordon RD, Stowasser M, Klemm SA, Tunny TJ. Primary aldosteronism and other forms of mineralocorticoid hypertension. In: Swales JD (ed.): *Textbook of Hypertension.* Oxford: Blackwell Scientific, pp. 865–92.

33. Holland OB, Brown H, Kuhnert L, Fairchild C, Risk M, Gomez-Sanchez CE. Further evaluation of saline infusion for the diagnosis of primary aldosteronism. *Hypertension* 1984; **6**: 717–23.

34. Gordon RD, Jackson RV, Strakosch CR, Tunny TJ, Rutherford JC, McCosker J, *et al.* Aldosterone-producing adenoma: fludrocortisone suppression and left adrenal vein catheterization in definitive diagnosis and management. *Aust NZ J Med* 1979; **57**: 676–82.

35. Takeda M, Go H, Imai T, Nishiyama T, Morishita H. Laparoscopic adrenalectomy for primary aldosteronism: report of initial ten cases. *Surgery* 1994; **115**: 621–5.

10

Insulin resistance, hypertension and endothelial function

Introduction

The association between hypertension and hyperinsulinaemia is widely acknow-ledged, although the full clinical significance still requires detailed clarification. Nevertheless, in essential hypertension abnormalities of insulin-mediated glucose metabolism have been invoked to explain aspects of pathogenesis, complications and the responses to treatment. There remain controversies, however, with recent evidence both for and against 'the insulin hypothesis'. The following questions might be posed to explore the clinical relevance of insulin resistance, hyperinsulin-aemia and the interrelationships with hypertension, vascular endothelial function and responses to drug treatment:

1. Is insulin resistance associated with hypertension?
2. Do high insulin levels increase blood pressure?
3. (a) Does insulin have a vascular action?
   (b) Could blunting of insulin's vasodilator action cause hypertension?
4. (a) Could vascular endothelial dysfunction associated with hypertension cause insulin resistance?
   (b) Could primary insulin resistance result in endothelial dysfunction and pro-motion of hypertension?
5. Could an adverse lipid environment be the common antecedent linking insulin resistance and endothelial dysfunction/hypertension?
6. Could chronic inflammation play a role in the aetiology of insulin resistance and endothelial dysfunction/hypertension?
7. Do insulin-sensitizing drugs lower blood pressure?
8. What are the principal clinical issues?

Insulin resistance and hypertension

Studies using the hyperinsulinaemic euglycaemic clamp technique |1| have demon-strated that hyperinsulinaemia occurs in hypertension as a compensatory response to a reduction in insulin-mediated glucose uptake in skeletal muscle ('insulin resistance') |2, 3|. The known major determinants of insulin sensitivity are age, weight and body fat distribution; but it should be noted that there is a threefold variation in insulin sensitivity amongst subjects matched for these variables |4|. Insulin resistance is absent in secondary hypertension |5| but present in normotensive offspring of essential hypertensive patients |6, 7|, suggesting that it may be of pathophysiological relevance in this context.

Insulin resistance, hyperinsulinemia, and blood pressure: role of age and obesity.

E Ferrannini, A Natali, B Capaldo, M Lohtovirta, S Jacob, H Yki-Jarvinen.
Hypertension 1997; **30**: 1144–9.

BACKGROUND. In population surveys, blood pressure (BP) and plasma insulin concentration are related variables, but the association is confounded by age and obesity. Whether insulin resistance is independently associated with higher BP in normal subjects is debated. The authors analysed the database of the European Group for the Study of Insulin Resistance, made up of non-diabetic men and women from 20 centres, in whom insulin sensitivity was measured by the euglycaemic insulin clamp.

INTERPRETATION. In normotensive, non-diabetic Europeans, insulin sensitivity and age are significant, mutually independent correlates of BP, whereas body mass is not. The relation of BP to both insulin action and circulating insulin levels is compatible with distinct influences on BP by insulin resistance or compensatory hyperinsulinaemia.

It has been suggested that the relationship between insulin resistance and BP may be confounded by obesity, as Body Mass Index (BMI) has a strong negative correlation with insulin sensitivity |8|. However, in the above paper by Ferrannini and colleagues, it was shown, using pooled analysis of insulin sensitivity data from 333 subjects from various European centres, that both systolic and diastolic BP have a negative relationship with insulin sensitivity even after adjustment for age, gender, BMI and fasting serum insulin concentration, i.e. the association between BMI and BP may be mediated by insulin sensitivity. From this analysis, the authors estimated that in terms of cardiovascular risk a 30% reduction in insulin sensitivity was equivalent to a 1.4 mmHg rise in BP. Although this may not seem large at first glance, at a population level a rise of this order could result in a 17% relative increase in incidence of cerebrovascular disease and a 10% increase in incidence of ischaemic heart disease |9|.

Comment

Overall, it appears that insulin resistance is independently associated with BP levels.

Hyperinsulinaemia and blood pressure

An elevation in serum insulin concentrations in patients with essential hypertension was first noted over 30 years ago |**10**|, and a number of cross-sectional epidemiological studies have supported an association between insulin levels and BP |**11, 12**|. Whether hyperinsulinaemia is a cause, a consequence or an epiphenomenon in hypertension is hotly debated, but the relationship is certainly not direct and simple. For example, chronic artificial elevation of serum insulin concentrations increases BP in rats |**13**|, but has no effect in dogs |**14**|. Patients with insulinomas do not tend to have hypertension |**15**|. Nevertheless, prospective studies have shown that individuals with hyperinsulinaemia have a higher risk of going on to develop both hypertension |**16, 17**| and coronary events |**18**|.

Insulin resistance and the effect of insulin on blood pressure in essential hypertension.

T Heise, K Magnusson, L Heinemann, P T Sawicki. *Hypertension* 1998; **32**: 243–8.

BACKGROUND. The aim of this study was to investigate the effect of 2 weeks of insulin administration on BP and simultaneously to measure insulin sensitivity and insulin-induced vasodilation in obese hypertensive patients.

INTERPRETATION. Insulin infusion increased limb blood flow significantly in the healthy controls, but not in obese insulin-resistant hypertensive subjects. Obese hypertensive patients are resistant to the effects of insulin with regard to both glucose uptake and vasodilation. Administration of insulin exerts a small BP-lowering effect in these patients. These data strongly argue against the postulated pressor action of insulin in essential hypertension.

Comment

In the above well-designed study by Heise and colleagues, it was shown that administration of insulin to insulin-resistant non-diabetic obese hypertensives had, if anything, a BP-lowering effect, i.e. insulin has vasodilator properties. These data support the notion that the link between insulin action and BP is more closely related to insulin resistance (i.e. at a tissue or cellular level) than to high levels of circulating insulin.

Vascular effects of insulin

Does insulin have a vascular action?

It is now generally accepted that systemic hyperinsulinaemia results in significant limb vasodilation |**19–22**|, although the physiological relevance of insulin as a vasodilator has been questioned |**23**|. It has been suggested that changes in blood flow may be occurring via central mechanisms rather than as a result of direct stimulation of insulin in limb vascular beds, a concept that has been supported by studies demonstrating little or no vasodilation in response to intra-arterial insulin infusion |**24, 25**|.

 ## The vasodilating effect of insulin is dependent on local glucose uptake: a double-blind, placebo-controlled study.

S Ueda, J R Petrie, S J Cleland, H L Elliott, J M C Connell. *J Clin Endocrinol Metab* 1998; **83**: 2126–31.

BACKGROUND. During systematic hyperinsulinaemia in man, skeletal muscle vasodilation has consistently been demonstrated. However, most studies that have examined the vascular effect of local hyperinsulinaemia have reported either no effect or only weak vasodilation. The present studies were designed in a double-blind, placebo-controlled manner to evaluate the direct (local) vascular effect of insulin alone and in association with physiological concentrations of D-glucose.

INTERPRETATION. These data suggest that local uptake of D-glucose by insulin-sensitive tissues is an important determinant of insulin-mediated vasodilation.

The above study set out to test the hypothesis that insulin-mediated glucose uptake is a key step in the mechanism of insulin-mediated vasodilation. The authors concluded that local glucose uptake was an important determinant of insulin's vascular effect, a result that might explain conflicting results between local and systemic studies: when insulin is infused systemically, 20% glucose is co-infused to prevent hypoglycaemia, whereas this is unnecessary in intra-arterial studies. This result has led the authors |**26**| and others |**27**| to propose that the underlying mechanisms of insulin's metabolic and vascular actions are functionally coupled, which might help to explain some of the observed associations among defects in insulin action, endothelial dysfunction and hypertension.

Comment

What mechanisms underlie the relationship between insulin and BP? Firstly, as has been shown above, the hormone has depressor peripheral vasodilator actions mainly in skeletal muscle vascular beds. Secondly, it has pressor effects mainly via stimulation of the sympathetic nervous system |**19**| and enhancement of renal sodium absorption |**28, 29**|. The net physiological effect is a balance of pressor and depressor effects, and maintenance of BP. In pathophysiological states such as obesity, the balance may be disrupted by enhanced sympathetic activation in response to hyperinsulinaemia |**30**|, together with 'blunting' of insulin-mediated vasodilation (vascular insulin resistance) |**31**|.

Hypertension and impaired responsiveness to insulin

Insulin resistance in essential hypertension is characterized by impaired insulin stimulation of blood flow in skeletal muscle.

H Laine, M J Knuuti, U Ruotsalainen, M Raitakiari, H Iida, J Kapanen, *et al.*
Hypertension 1998; **16**: 211–9.

B ACKGROUND . **The objective of this study was to determine whether insulin-stimulated blood flow in patients with mild essential hypertension is altered.**

I NTERPRETATION . The ability of insulin to stimulate blood flow in patients with mild essential hypertension is impaired.

Comment

In the above study by Laine and colleagues, the technique of positron emission tomography was used to measure limb blood flow and muscle glucose uptake in lean patients with mild essential hypertension. They concluded that there was, indeed, evidence to suggest that insulin-stimulated muscle blood flow is impaired in hypertension. This result concurs with previous reports of a negative correlation between insulin-induced vasodilation and BP using less sensitive techniques for measurement of flow |**20, 32**|. In these studies supraphysiological doses of insulin were used to detect the relationship, and it has not so far been possible to confirm their findings using more physiological doses over shorter periods |**19, 33**|. Therefore, it remains unclear whether blunting of insulin-mediated vasodilation contributes to hypertension in insulin-resistant states via increased peripheral vascular resistance.

Summary

Taken together, the results of these two studies indicate that the metabolic and vascular effects of insulin are mechanistically related. However, it remains unclear which is the primary defect: thus does a blunted vasodilation response to insulin contribute to the development of hypertension or does increased peripheral vascular resistance create an insulin-resistant state?

Vascular endothelial dysfunction, hypertension and insulin resistance

Could vascular endothelial dysfunction associated with hypertension cause insulin resistance?

One common feature that has been proposed to account for the link between insulin resistance and BP is vascular endothelial dysfunction. Defects in basal and stimulated endothelial function have been demonstrated in some groups of patients with essential hypertension |**34–36**| and also in other insulin-resistant conditions such as obesity |37| and type II diabetes |38, 39|. In healthy volunteers, whole-body insulin sensitivity has been shown to correlate with basal endothelial nitric oxide production |40|. In addition, insulin appears to cause vasodilation, at least in part, by stimulation of endothelial nitric oxide production |41–43|, and insulin-mediated vasodilation has been shown to correlate positively with insulin-stimulated glucose uptake |26, 27, 44|. Decreased blood flow to nutritive capillary beds could conceivably result in insulin resistance via a reduction in substrate delivery to target tissues |20, 44|. Hence, primary endothelial dysfunction could contribute to high BP while at the same time causing blunting of insulin-mediated vasodilation and impaired insulin-mediated glucose uptake.

Vasodilation with sodium nitroprusside does not improve insulin action in essential hypertension.

A Natali, A Q Galvan, N Pecori, G Sanna, E Toschi, E Ferrannini.
Hypertension 1998; **31**: 632–6.

BACKGROUND. The vasodilation induced by systemic insulin infusion is mediated by nitric oxide and is impaired both in obese subjects and in patients with essential hypertension. Whether this vascular defect explains the metabolic resistance in insulin action is uncertain.

INTERPRETATION. The authors conclude that in overweight male patients with essential hypertension, increasing forearm perfusion with sodium nitroprusside does not attenuate the insulin resistance of forearm tissue.

Comment

If endothelial dysfunction blunts insulin-mediated vasodilation, one would predict that increasing blood flow to skeletal muscle vascular beds using vasodilators such as adenosine, bradykinin or sodium nitroprusside would result in an increase in glucose uptake. The above study by Natali and colleagues does not support this hypothesis. Despite local limb vasodilation with sodium nitroprusside, they were unable to demonstrate any improvements in insulin-mediated glucose uptake in a group of overweight male hypertensives. This negative finding is supported by two previous studies |45, 46|, and the conclusion must be that primary endothelial dysfunction with associated blunting of insulin-mediated vasodilation is unlikely to be a significant determinant of insulin resistance.

Could primary insulin resistance result in endothelial dysfunction and promotion of hypertension? Characterization of selective resistance to insulin signalling in the vasculature of obese Zucker (*fa/fa*) rats.

Z Y Jiang, Y-W Lin, A Clemont, E P Feener, K D Hein, M Igarashi, *et al.*
J Clin Invest 1999; **104**: 447–57.

BACKGROUND. Both insulin resistance and hyperinsulinaemia have been reported to be independent risk factors for cardiovascular disease. However, little is known regarding insulin signalling in the vascular tissue in insulin-resistant states. In this report, insulin signalling on the phosphatidylinositol 3-kinase (PI 3-kinase) and mitogen-activated protein (MAP) kinase pathways were compared in vascular tissues of lean and obese Zucker (fa/fa) rats in both ex vivo and in vivo studies.

INTERPRETATION. To our knowledge, these data provided the first direct measurements of insulin signalling in the vascular tissue, and documented a selective resistance to PI 3-kinase (but not to MAP kinase pathways) in the vascular tissue of obese Zucker rats.

A more compelling explanation for the relationship between insulin sensitivity, essential hypertension and endothelial function is suggested by experiments in cultured endothelial cells in which enzymes central to intracellular glucose metabolism were blocked, resulting in abolition of insulin-stimulated nitric oxide production |**47**|. Furthermore, it has been demonstrated recently that mice which are deficient in IRS-1, the major substrate of the insulin receptor and a functionally important step in the insulin-signalling pathway, also appear to have impaired endothelium-dependent vascular relaxation |**48**|. Thus primary insulin resistance in endothelial cells may contribute to vascular dysfunction, hypertension and its cardiovascular complications.

Comment

The above study by Jiang and colleagues provides the most convincing evidence to date that defects in the insulin-signalling pathway persist in vascular tissues of an insulin-resistant animal model. Thus primary 'vascular insulin resistance' may lead to relative endothelial dysfunction and promotion of hypertension. Results from vascular endothelial cell insulin receptor 'knock-out' studies are awaited with interest.

Insulin resistance, endothelial dysfunction, hypertension and the lipid environment

While it seems likely that defects in insulin action and endothelial dysfunction are causally associated, it is possible that both are influenced independently by a common antecedent. One of the strongest candidates for this 'third factor' is the 'atherogenic lipid profile', which has been shown to be associated with both insulin resistance and vascular endothelial dysfunction.

Elevated circulating free fatty acid levels impair endothelium-dependent vasodilation.

H O Steinberg, M Tarshoby, R Monestel. G Hook, J Cronin, A Johnson, *et al. J Clin Invest* 1997; **100**: 1230–9.

BACKGROUND. The authors have recently shown that insulin-resistant obese subjects exhibit impaired endothelial function. Here, they test the hypothesis that elevation of circulating free fatty acids (FFA) to levels seen in insulin-resistant subjects can impair endothelial function. They studied leg blood flow responses to graded intrafemoral artery infusions of the endothelial-dependent vasodilator methacholine chloride or the endothelium-independent vasodilator sodium nitroprusside during the infusion of saline and circulating FFA levels exogenously via a low- or high-dose infusion of Intralipid plus heparin or endogenously by an infusion of somatostatin (SRIF) to produce insulinopenia in groups of lean healthy humans.

INTERPRETATION. In conclusion, elevated circulating FFA levels cause endothelial dysfunction, and impaired endothelial function in insulin-resistant humans may be secondary to the elevated FFA concentrations observed in these parts.

Comment

In the above study, Steinberg and colleagues demonstrated that infusion of FFA caused acute endothelial dysfunction in insulin-resistant subjects. Interestingly, co-infusion of insulin restored endothelial function, suggesting a direct effect of insulin in promoting endothelial nitric oxide production.

The role of chronic inflammation in the aetiology of insulin resistance and endothelial dysfunction/ hypertension

Recently, it has been proposed that low-grade chronic inflammation may play a key role in the process of vascular endothelial dysfunction and atherosclerosis. In the following study on blood samples from over 100 healthy volunteers, C-reactive protein levels were significantly related not only to markers of endothelial activation, but also to surrogate measurements of insulin resistance and obesity. Furthermore, it was suggested that cytokines causing metabolic and vascular dysfunction could be released from centrally distributed adipose tissue, thus explaining the observed coexistence of insulin resistance, endothelial dysfunction and hypertension in centrally obese patients.

C-reactive protein in healthy subjects: association with obesity, insulin resistance, and endothelial dysfunction. A potential role for cytokines originating from adipose tissue.
J S Yudkin, C D A Stehouwer, J J Emeis, S W Coppack. *Arterioscler Thromb Vasc Biol* 1999; **19**: 972–8.

BACKGROUND. C-reactive protein, a hepatic acute phase protein largely regulated by circulating levels of interleukin-6, predicts coronary heart disease incidence in healthy subjects. The authors have shown that subcutaneous adipose tissue secretes interleukin-6 in vivo. This study sought associations of levels of C-reactive protein and interleukin-6 with measures of obesity and of chronic infection as their putative determinants. It also related levels of C-reactive protein and interleukin-6 to markers of the insulin resistance syndrome and of endothelial dysfunction.

INTERPRETATION. These data suggest that adipose tissue is an important determinant of a low-level, chronic inflammatory state as reflected by levels of interleukin-6, tumor necrosis factor-alpha and C-reactive protein, and that infection with *H. pylori*, *C. pneumoniae* and cytomegalovirus is not. Moreover, these data support the concept that such a low-level, chronic inflammatory state may induce insulin resistance and endothelial dysfunction, and thus link the latter phenomena with obesity and cardiovascular disease.

Comment

This is an interesting and plausible hypothesis. However, causal relationships cannot be proved from cross-sectional correlation studies, and further prospective research is required in this interesting area.

Effect of insulin-sensitizing drugs on blood pressure

Vasodilatory effects of troglitazone improve blood pressure at rest and during mental stress in type II diabetes mellitus.

B H Sung, H L Izzo Jr, P Dandona, M F Wilson. *Hypertension* 1999; **34**: 83–8.

BACKGROUND. The present study examined the haemodynamic mechanisms of BP lowering by troglitazone in patients with type II diabetes mellitus (DM) at rest and during a mental arithmetic test. Twenty-two patients with DM with normal to high-normal BP and 12 controls matched for age, gender, glucose tolerance and BP were studied.

INTERPRETATION. Improved insulin resistance rather than improved glycaemic control is associated with lower resting and stress BP values in patients with DM. A reduction in vascular resistance may be a primary haemodynamic mechanism of the manner in which troglitazone lowers BP. Insulin sensitizers may offer potential therapeutic advantage in subjects with DM with elevated BP.

Comment

Insulin-sensitizing agents, such as the thiazolidinedione derivatives ('glitazones') |49|, appear to exert their effects via peroxisome proliferator-activated receptor gamma on post-receptor binding steps in the transduction of the insulin response

|50|. Studies in man examining other primary endpoints have serendipitously reported significant reductions in BP |51, 52|. In the above study by Sung and colleagues, BP, both at rest and during a mental arithmetic test, was significantly reduced by troglitazone treatment, but not by glyburide, in a group of type II diabetic patients. This effect occurred in association with decreased peripheral resistance. Therefore, it appears that troglitazone influences metabolic and vascular pathways in parallel. Current research is attempting to elicit the intracellular mechanisms involved in these effects and, in doing so, may provide valuable insights into the physiological mechanisms responsible for the apparent coupling between insulin's metabolic and vascular actions and their relationship with vascular endothelial function.

Insulin resistance and cardiovascular disease: the clinical issues

Lifestyle issues and specific drug treatments

Having identified insulin resistance as a potential independent cardiovascular risk factor and having proposed lifestyle intervention and insulin-sensitizing drugs as potential risk-reduction strategies, it can be argued that the issue of insulin resistance still remains of academic interest rather than realistic clinical relevance. Although weight loss and aerobic exercise have been shown to improve insulin sensitivity, it is recognized that attempts in routine clinical practice to investigate major lifestyle changes are usually disappointing |53|. Additionally, the early promise of insulin-sensitizing drugs (glitazones) has been marred by the possibility of serious side-effects (and particularly the withdrawal of troglitazone), although this is currently under review.

Practical management issues

It is becoming clear that insulin-resistant subjects (i.e. these at high cardiovascular risk) benefit more from traditional cardiovascular risk-reduction management: therefore, it may be that the main clinical relevance of identifying insulin resistance is to target those individuals who warrant more aggressive cardiovascular risk reduction. For example, recent studies of type II diabetes subgroups in a number of BP-lowering trials have revealed a two- to three-fold increase in relative risk reduction for cardiovascular events |54–56| irrespective of the class of antihypertensive agent used. Furthermore, aiming for a target diastolic BP of < 80 mmHg compared with <90 mmHg resulted in a 50% further reduction in cardiovascular event rate in type II diabetic patients |55|, emphasizing the importance of aggressive risk reduction. In addition, it has long been known that diabetic patients benefit more than their non-diabetic counterparts from thrombolysis following myocardial infarction, as well as from cessation of smoking in terms of reduction of cardiovascular morbidity and mortality.

Antihypertensive drugs and insulin resistance

The reported deleterious metabolic effects of 'older' antihypertensive agents (β-blockers and diuretics) have been implicated by some in the shortfall in the reductions achieved (compared with those predicted) in mortality from coronary heart disease in treated hypertensive populations |57|.

Additionally, influential reports of improved insulin sensitivity during angiotensin converting enzyme (ACE) inhibitor drug treatment have led to the proposal of a variety of mechanisms by which the renin–angiotensin system might influence insulin responsiveness. However, many of these apparantly positive studies have used uncontrolled and/or flawed study designs, or indirect measures of insulin sensitivity, or have been conducted in subjects receiving potentially confounding medications |58|. One of the most widely cited and well-publicized studies in this area reported an improvement in insulin sensitivity in non-diabetic patients with hypertension randomized to captopril treatment versus hydrochlorothiazide |59|. The original oft-quoted study by Pollare et al. was designed as a cross-over study to compare captopril with hydrochlorothiazide, and did not include a direct comparison with placebo. However, data in the second treatment period were unsuitable for analysis, owing to a carry-over effect, and the results were presented separately for the two groups as comparisons with the baseline placebo period. The captopril group (n=23) at the start of treatment had similar measured insulin sensitivity to that of the diuretic-treated group (n=27) at the end of treatment. This suggests the possibility that the reported treatment effect may simply represent regression towards the mean. Despite these shortcomings, this trial has been extremely influential in support of the perception that ACE inhibitors improve insulin sensitivity.

The Landmark UK Prospective Diabetes Study has recently emphasized the benefits of antihypertensive treatment in type II diabetes, reporting similar efficacy of captopril and atenolol on diabetic complications in these patients. Furthermore, a recent study using the euglycaemic clamp technique has demonstrated that captopril does not effect insulin sensitivity in non-diabetic patients with essential hypertension |60|. Therefore, it can be concluded that there is, as yet, no compelling evidence for beneficial metabolic effects of ACE inhibitors over other classes of antihypertensive drugs. Instead, the clinical emphasis remains with 'tight' BP control with effective hypertensive drugs, alone and in combination.

Summary

Insulin resistance is associated with hypertension in man. In addition to its well-known metabolic actions, insulin causes vasodilation, which is dependent of both endothelial nitric oxide production and cellular glucose uptake. Insulin's metabolic and vascular actions appear to have a common physiological mechanism. Hence blunting of insulin-mediated vasodilation and subsequent increased peripheral vascular resistance could explain the observed association between insulin resistance and hypertension. There are three possible explanations for the observed association between insulin action and vascular endothelial function: (1) primary endothelial dysfunction may cause a reduction in blood flow to insulin-sensitive tissues, resulting in relative insulin resistance; (2) primary defects in the insulin-signalling pathway in vascular tissues may cause vascular dysfunction in parallel with metabolic insulin resistance; or (3) a 'third factor' may be influencing both insulin-mediated glucose uptake and endothelial function—potential candidates include lipid profile and cytokines. Treatment with thiazolidinediones in man enhances insulin sensitivity and lowers BP. Further elucidation of the intracellular mechanisms involved in the insulin-signalling pathway may reveal new therapeutic targets in cardiovascular and metabolic disorders.

References

1. DeFronzo RA, Tobin JD, Andres R. Glucose clamp technique: a method for quantifying insulin secretion and resistance. *Am J Physiol* 1979; **237**: E214–23.

2. Ferrannini E, Buzzigoli G, Bonadonna R, Giorico MA, Oleggini M, Graziadei L, *et al.* Insulin resistance in essential hypertension. *N Engl J Med* 1987; **317**: 350–7.

3. Lind L, Berne C, Lithell H. Prevalence of insulin resistance in essential hypertension. *J Hypertens* 1995; **13**: 1457–62.

4. Hollenbeck G, Reaven GM. Variations in insulin-stimulated glucose uptake in healthy individuals with normal glucose tolerance. *J Clin Endocrinol Metab* 1987; **64**: 1169–73.

5. Shamiss A, Carroll J, Rosenthal T. Insulin resistance in secondary hypertension. *Am J Hypertens* 1992; **5**: 26–8.

6. Beatty OL, Harper R, Sheridan B, Atkinson AB, Bell PM. Insulin resistance in offspring of hypertensive parents. *Br Med J* 1993; **307**: 92–6.

7. Endre T, Mattiasson I, Lennart Hulthen U, Lindgarde F, Berglund G. Insulin resistance is coupled to low physical fitness in normotensive men with a family history of hypertension. *J Hypertens* 1994; **12**: 81–8.

8. Jarrett RJ. In defence of insulin: a critique of syndrome X. *Lancet* 1992; **340**: 469–71.

9. Collins R, Peto R, MacMahon S, Hebert P, Fiebach N, Eberlein KA, *et al.* Blood pressure, stroke and coronary artery disease. Part 1: Prolonged differences in blood pressure: prospective observational studies corrected for the regression dilution bias. *Lancet* 1990; **335**: 765–74.

10. Welborn TA, Breckenridge A, Dollery CT, Rubenstein AH, Russell Fraser T. Serum insulin in essential hypertension and in peripheral vascular disease. *Lancet* 1966; **1**: 1336–7.

11. Modan M, Halkin H, Almog S, Lusky A, Eshkol A, Jhefi M, *et al.* Hyperinsulinaemia. A link between hypertension, obesity and glucose intolerance. *J Clin Invest* 1985; **75**: 809–17.

12. Feskens EJM, Tuomilehto J, Stengard JH, Pekkanen J, Nissinen A, Kromhout D. Hypertension and overweight associated with hyperinsulinaemia and glucose tolerance: a longitudinal study of the Finnish and Dutch cohorts of the Seven Countries Study. *Diabetologia* 1995; **38**: 839–47.

13. Brands MW, Mizelle HL, Gaillard DA, Hildebrandt DA, Hall JE. The haemodynamic response to chronic hyperinsulinaemia in conscious dogs. *Am J Hypertens* 1991; **4**: 164–8.

14. Brands MW, Hildebrandt DA, Mizelle HL, Hall JE. Sustained hyperinsulinaemia increases arterial pressure in conscious rats. *Am J Physiol* 1991; **260**: R764–8.

15. Fujita N, Baba T, Tomiyami T, Kodama T, Kako N. Hyperinsulinaemia and blood pressure in patients with insulinoma. *Br Med J* 1992; **304**: 1157.

16. Haffner SM, Valdez RA, Hazuda HP, Mitchell BD, Morales PA, Stern MP. Prospective analysis of the insulin-resistance syndrome (syndrome X). *Diabetes* 1992; **41**: 715–22.

17. Bao W, Srinivasan S, Berenson G. Persistent elevation of plasma insulin levels is associated with increased cardiovascular risk in children and young adults. *Circulation* 1996; **93**: 54–9.

18. Despres JP, Lamarche B, Mauriege P, Cantin B, Dagenais GR, Moorjani S, *et al.* Hyperinsulinaemia as an independent risk factor for ischaemic heart disease. *N Engl J Med* 1996; **334**: 952–7.

19. Anderson EA, Hoffman RP, Balon TW, Sinkey CA, Mark AL. Hyperinsulinemia produces both sympathetic neural activation and vasodilation in normal humans. *J Clin Invest* 1991; **87**: 2246–52.

20. Baron AD. Cardiovascular actions of insulin in humans. Implications for insulin sensitivity and vascular tone. *Bailliere's Clin Endocrinol Metab* 1993; **7**: 961–87.

21. Natali A, Taddei S, Galvan AQ, Camastra S, Baldi S, Frascerra S, *et al.* Insulin sensitivity, vascular reactivity and clamp-induced vasodilatation in essential hypertension. *Circulation* 1997; **96**: 849–55.

22. Utriainen T, Nuutila P, Takala T, Vicini P, Ruotsalainen U, Ronnemaa T, *et al.* Intact insulin stimulation of skeletal muscle blood flow, its heterogeneity and redistribution, but not of glucose uptake in non-insulin-dependent diabetes mellitus. *J Clin Invest* 1997; **100**: 777–85.

23. Yki-Jarvinen H, Utriainen T. Insulin-induced vasodilatation: physiology or pharmacology? *Diabetologia* 1998; **41**: 369–79.

24. Sakai K, Imaizumi T, Masaki H, Takeshita A. Intra-arterial infusion of insulin attenuates vasoreactivity in human forearm. *Hypertension* 1993; **22**: 67–73.

25. Natali A, Buzzigoli G, Taddi S, Sanatoro D, Cerri M, Pedrinelli R, *et al.* Effects of insulin on hemodynamics and metabolism in human forearm. *Diabetes* 1990; **39**: 490–500.

26. Cleland SJ, Petrie JR, Ueda S, Elliott HL, Connell JMC. Insulin-mediated vasodilation and glucose uptake are functionally linked in humans. *Hypertension* 1999; **33**(Suppl 2): 554–8.

27. Feldman RD, Hramiak IM, Finegood DT, Behme MT. Parallel regulation of the local vascular and systemic metabolic effects of insulin. *J Clin Endocrinol Metab* 1995; **80**: 1556–9.

28. DeFronzo RA, Cooke CR, Andres R, Faloona GR, David PJ. The effect of insulin on renal handling of sodium, potassium, calcium and phosphate in man. *J Clin Invest* 1975; **55**: 845–55.

29. Ferrannini E, Natali A. Insulin resistance and hypertension: connections with sodium metabolism. *Am J Kidney Dis* 1993; **21**(Suppl 2): 37–42.

30. Scherrer U, Randin D, Tappy L, Vollenweider P, Jequier E, Nicod P. Body fat and sympathetic nerve activity in healthy subjects. *Circulation* 1994; **89**: 2634–40.

31. Laakso M, Edelman SV, Brechtel G, Baron AD. Decreased effect of insulin to stimulate skeletal muscle blood flow in obese man: a novel mechanism for insulin resistance. *J Clin Invest* 1990; **85**: 1844–52.

32. Feldman RD, Bierbrier GS. Insulin-mediated vasodilation: impairment with increased blood pressure and body mass. *Lancet* 1993; **342**: 707–9.

33. Hunter SJ, Harper R, Ennis CN, Sheridan B, Atkinson AB, Bell PM. Skeletal muscle blood flow is not a determinant of insulin resistance in essential hypertension. *J Hypertens* 1997; **15**: 73–7.

34. Calver A, Collier J, Moncada S, Vallance P. Effect of local intra-arterial N(G)-monomethyl-L-arginine on patients with hypertension: the nitric oxide dilator mechanism appears abnormal. *J Hypertens* 1992; **10**: 1025–31.

35. Panza JA, Casino PR, Kilcoyne CM, Quyyumi AA. Role of endothelium-derived nitric oxide in the abnormal endothelium-dependent vascular relaxation of patients with essential hypertension. *Circulation* 1993; **87**: 1468–74.

36. Cockcroft JR, Chowienczyk PJ, Benjamin N, Ritter JM. Preserved endothelium-dependent vasodilatation in patients with essential hypertension. *N Eng J Med* 1994; **330**: 1036–40.

37. Steinberg HO, Chaker H, Leaming R, Johnson A, Brechtel G, Baron AD. Obesity/insulin resistance is associated with endothelial dysfunction. *J Clin Invest* 1996; **97**: 2601–10.

38. McVeigh E, Brennan GM, Johnston GD, McDermott BJ, McGrath LT, Henry WR, *et al.* Impaired endothelium-dependent and independent vasodilation in patients with type 2 (non-insulin-dependent) diabetes mellitus. *Diabetologia* 1992; **35**: 771–6.

39. Williams SB, Cusco JA, Roddy M, Johnstone MT, Creager MA. Impaired nitric oxide-mediated vasodilation in patients with non-insulin-dependent diabetes mellitus. *J Am Coll Cardiol* 1996; **27**: 567–74.

40. Petrie J, Ueda S, Webb DJ, Elliott HL, Connell JMC. Endothelial nitric oxide production and insulin sensitivity: a physiological link with implications for pathogenesis of cardiovascular disease. *Circulation* 1996; **93**: 1331–3.

41. Scherrer U, Randin D, Vollenweider P, Vollenweider L, Nicod P. Nitric oxide release accounts for insulin's vascular effects in humans. *J Clin Invest* 1994; **94**: 2511–15.

42. Steinberg HO, Brechtel G, Johnson A, Fineberg N, Baron AD. Insulin-mediated skeletal muscle vasodilation is nitric oxide dependent: a novel action of insulin to increase nitric oxide release. *J Clin Invest* 1994; **94**: 1172–9.

43. Cleland SJ, Petrie JR, Ueda S, Elliott HL, Connell JMC. Insulin vasodilatation is abolished by both L-NMMA and angiotensin II. *J Hypertens* 1997; **15**(Suppl 4): S71 (Abstract).

44. Baron AD, Steinberg HO, Chaker H, Leaming R, Johnson A, Brechtel G. Insulin-mediated skeletal muscle vasodilation contributes to both insulin sensitivity and responsiveness in lean humans. *J Clin Invest* 1995; **96**: 786–92.

45. Natali A, Bonadonna R, Santoro D, Galvan AQ, Baldi S, Frascerra S, *et al.* Insulin resistance and vasodilation in essential hypertension: studies with adenosine. *J Clin Invest* 1994; **94**: 1570–6.

46. Nuutila P, Raitakari M, Laine H, Kirvela O, Takala T, Utriainen T, *et al.* Role of blood flow in regulating insulin-stimulated glucose uptake in humans: studies using bradykinin, [^{15}O]water, and [^{18}F]fluoro-deoxy-glucose and positron emission tomography. *J Clin Invest* 1996; **97**: 1741–7.

47. Zeng G, Quon MJ. Insulin-stimulated production of nitric oxide is inhibited by wortmannin. *J Clin Invest* 1996; **98**: 894–8.

48. Abe H, Yamada N, Kamata K, Kuwaki T, Shimada M, Osuga J, *et al.* Hypertension, hypertriglyceridemia, and impaired endothelium-dependent vascular relaxation in mice lacking insulin receptor substrate-1. *J Clin Invest* 1998; **101**: 1784–8.

49. Petrie JR, Small M, Connell JMC. 'Glitazones', a prospect for non-insulin-dependent diabetes. *Lancet* 1997; **349**: 70–1.

50. Kotchen TA. Attenuation of hypertension by insulin-sensitizing agents. *Hypertension* 1996; **28**: 219–23.

51. Nolan JJ, Ludvik B, Beersden P, Joyce M, Olefsky J. Improvement in glucose tolerance and insulin resistance in obese subjects treated with troglitazone. *N Engl J Med* 1994; **331**: 1188–93.

52. Ogihara T, Rakugi H, Ikegami H, Mikami H, Masuo K. Enhancement of insulin sensitivity by troglitazone lowers blood pressure in diabetic hypertensives. *Am J Hypertens* 1995; **8**: 316–20.

53. NIH Technology Assessment Conference Panel. Methods for voluntary weight loss and control. *Ann Intern Med* 1993; **119**: 764–70.

54. Curb JD, Pressel SL, Cutler JA, Savage PJ, Applegate WB, Black H, *et al.* Effect of diuretic-based antihypertensive treatment on cardiovascular disease risk in older diabetic patients with isolated systolic hypertension. *JAMA* 1996; **276**: 1886–92.

55. Hansson L, Zanchetti I, Carruthers SG, Dahlof B, Elmfeldt D, Julius S, *et al.* Effects of intensive blood pressure lowering and low-dose aspirin in patients with hypertension. Principal results of the Hypertension Optimal Treatment (HOT) randomised trial. *Lancet* 1998; **35**: 1755–62.

56. UK Prospective Diabetes Study Group. Efficacy of atenolol and captopril in reducing risk of macrovascular and microvascular complications in type 2 diabetes. *Br Med J* 1998; **317**: 713–20.

57. Collins R, Peto R, MacMahon S, Herbert P, Fiebach NH, Eberlein KA, *et al.* Blood pressure, stroke and coronary heart disease. Part 2. Short-term reductions in blood pressure: overview of randomised drug trials in their epidemiological context. *Lancet* 1990; **335**: 827–38.

58. Donnelly R. Angiotensin-converting enzyme inhibitors and insulin sensitivity: metabolic effects in hypertension, diabetes and heart failure. *J Cardiovasc Pharmacol* 1992; **20**(Suppl 1): S38–S44.

59. Pollare TG, Lithell H, Berne C. A comparison of the effects of hydrochlorothiazide and captopril on glucose and lipid metabolism in patients with hypertension. *N Engl J Med* 1989; **321**: 672–86.

60. Wiggam MI, Hunter SJ, Atkinson AB, Ennis CN, Henry JS, Browne JN, *et al.* Captopril does not improve insulin action in essential hypertension: a double blind placebo-controlled study. *J Hypertens* 1998; **16**: 103–9.

Part IV

Current issues in practice

11

Angiotensin II receptor antagonists

Introduction

Angiotensin II receptor antagonist drugs are relatively new agents that have recently been licensed for the management of hypertension. They may also have a role in the management of heart failure, which is currently under investigation in a number of ongoing clinical trials, and their development has significantly advanced our understanding of the renin–angiotensin system

Angiotensin II receptor antagonists have been recognized as potential first-line antihypertensive drugs, and, with the current emphasis on 'tight' blood pressure control and its requirement for combination treatment regimens, there is a clear need for new and effective drug classes to expand the treatment options.

Background

Pharmacology

The principal actions of angiotensin II are vasoconstriction of the resistance vessels and stimulation of aldosterone production and release. Angiotensin II also has a facilitatory role within the sympathetic nervous system. Several different angiotensin II receptor subtypes have been identified, but the known cardiovascular functions are mediated via the AT_1 receptor (Fig. 11.1). An AT_2 receptor has also been clearly defined, but its physiological role remains obscure. It has been hypothesized, for example, that the regulatory role of angiotensin II in cell growth and proliferation reflects a dynamic equilibrium between its growth-promoting effects mediated via the AT_1 receptor and its antiproliferative effects mediated via the AT_2 receptor.

AT_1 receptor blockade versus ACE inhibition

There are several sites at which the renin–angiotensin II–aldosterone system (RAAS) might be inhibited or blocked, but in therapeutic terms, inhibition of angiotensin-converting enzyme (ACE) has to date proved to be the most successful (Fig. 11.2). However, ACE inhibition does not provide complete blockade of the RAAS because angiotensin II can be generated by non-ACE enzyme pathways, such as chymase, cathepsin, and CAGE (chymostatin-sensitive angiotensin-II-generating enzyme). Furthermore, ACE is also active in other metabolic pathways,

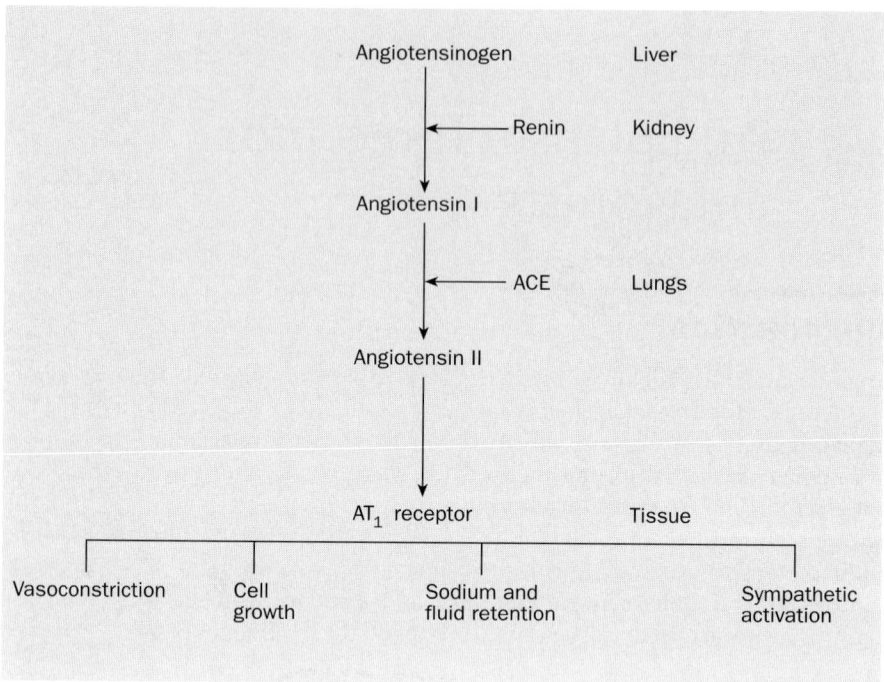

Fig. 11.1 Mediation of cardiovascular functions via the AT_1 receptor. ACE = angiotensin-converting enzyme.

and, most notably, in the guise of kininase II it is responsible for the breakdown of vasoactive kinins, principally bradykinin: during ACE inhibitor treatment, therefore, the breakdown of kinins is inhibited. The resultant accumulation of kinins has been implicated in the causation of ACE inhibitor cough. Since the angiotensin II receptor antagonists have no effect on kinin pathways, there is no problem with cough as an adverse effect. Furthermore, since the angiotensin II receptor antagonists act directly on the AT_1 receptor, complete blockade of the RAAS is produced irrespective of the enzyme pathway by which the angiotensin II has been generated.

Angiotensin II antagonist drugs

Since the development of the prototype agent, losartan, four further agents have become widely available—candesartan (cilexetil), irbesartan, telmisartan and valsartan. Although there are some differences in pharmacokinetics and specific pharmacological characteristics, all these agents (or their active metabolites) bind specifically to the AT_1 receptor. In general, the receptor-binding characteristics cannot be classified as 'competitive' according to classical pharmacological terminology, but instead the binding characteristics provide a longer-lasting antagonist effect, such

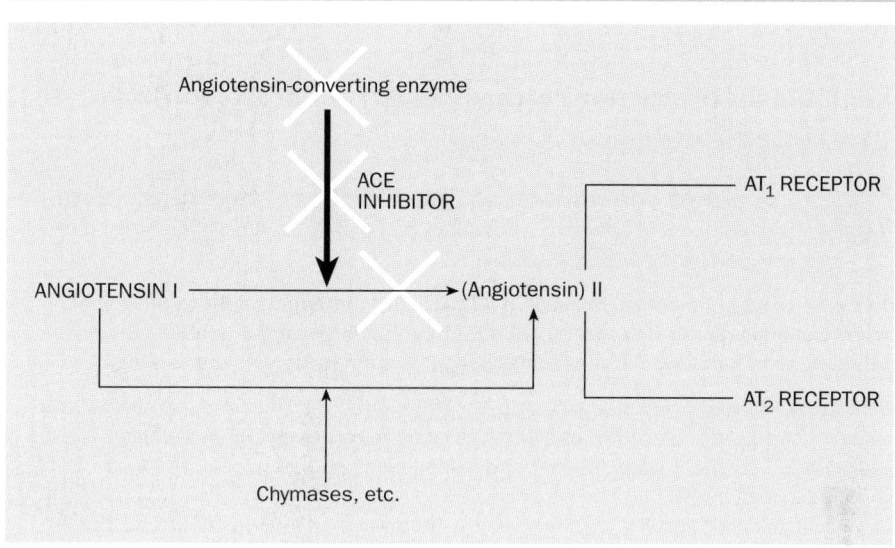

Fig. 11.2 Angiotensin II production effect of angiotensin-converting enzyme (ACE) inhibitor drugs.

that 'non-competitive' or 'insurmountable' or 'irreversible' are the terms that have become widely employed.

Clinical trials in hypertension and heart failure

To date, the clinical trials in hypertension have suggested that angiotensin II antagonists are well-tolerated agents with an antihypertensive efficacy that is comparable to other types of antihypertensive drug. However, there is not yet any evidence that angiotensin II antagonists are capable of reducing cardiovascular morbidity and mortality, although a number of long-term clinical trials is currently under way with several of these agents. In heart failure, a first published study suggested that losartan might be preferable to captopril, particularly because of a reduction in fatal myocardial infarction and sudden death. However, this possible benefit has not been substantiated in the follow-up study (Pitt *et al.* 1997; see ELITE, see p. 260), and the preliminary results of clinical trials with other angiotensin II antagonists have not yet provided evidence that angiotensin II receptor blockade is superior to ACE inhibition in the management of cardiac failure.

Clinical pharmacology

The selectivity of the action of angiotensin II receptor antagonists lends itself to clinical pharmacological studies in which the effectiveness of the receptor blockade can readily be quantified, typically by assessment of the responses to administered angiotensin II.

Angiotensin II receptor blockade in normotensive subjects

A direct comparison of three AT$_1$ receptor antagonists.
L Mazzolai, M Maillard, J Rossat, J Nussberger, H R Brunner, M Burnier.
Hypertension 1999; **33**: 850–5.

BACKGROUND. Use of angiotensin II AT$_1$ receptor antagonists for treatment of hypertension is rapidly increasing, yet direct comparisons of the relative efficacy of antagonists at blocking the renin–angiotensin system in humans are lacking.

INTERPRETATION. This study thus demonstrates that the first administration of the recommended starting dose of irbesartan induces a greater and longer-lasting angiotensin II receptor blockade than those induced by valsartan or losartan in normotensive subjects.

This clinical pharmacological study investigated the effectiveness of three different angiotensin II antagonists (losartan, valsartan and irbesartan) in a well-designed study in 12 normotensive subjects. In a double-blind, placebo-controlled, randomized, four-way cross-study each subject received single doses of each angiotensin II antagonist and placebo, and the effectiveness of the angiotensin II blockade was then assessed by three different methods: firstly, by the extent of the inhibition of the blood pressure response to the administration of exogenous angiotensin II; secondly, by an in vitro angiotensin II receptor binding assay; and, thirdly, by the reactive changes in plasma angiotensin II levels. Irbesartan appeared to produce the most marked blockade with the most effective and longest lasting inhibition of the BP response to administered angiotensin II (see Fig. 11.3).

Comment

This is a very well-designed and well-conducted clinical pharmacological study that describes three different but related methodologies and their usefulness in evaluating the effectiveness of angiotensin II receptor antagonist drugs. However, as a discriminating methodology for determining duration of action and overall effectiveness it is necessary to study comparable doses under steady-state conditions. Unfortunately for the clinician rather than the research worker, this single-dose evaluation, with dosages that may not be comparable, does not provide any useful evidence for discriminating among these three drugs in terms of their therapeutic benefits.

Conclusion

While there is a reasonably consistent body of evidence that losartan is not the most effective angiotensin receptor antagonist, there is a confusion of evidence surrounding the other drugs in this class. In fact, at present there is no sound evidence upon which the other agents might be separated. For the present, candesartan (cilexetil), irbesartan, telmisartan and valsartan can be considered to be equivalent.

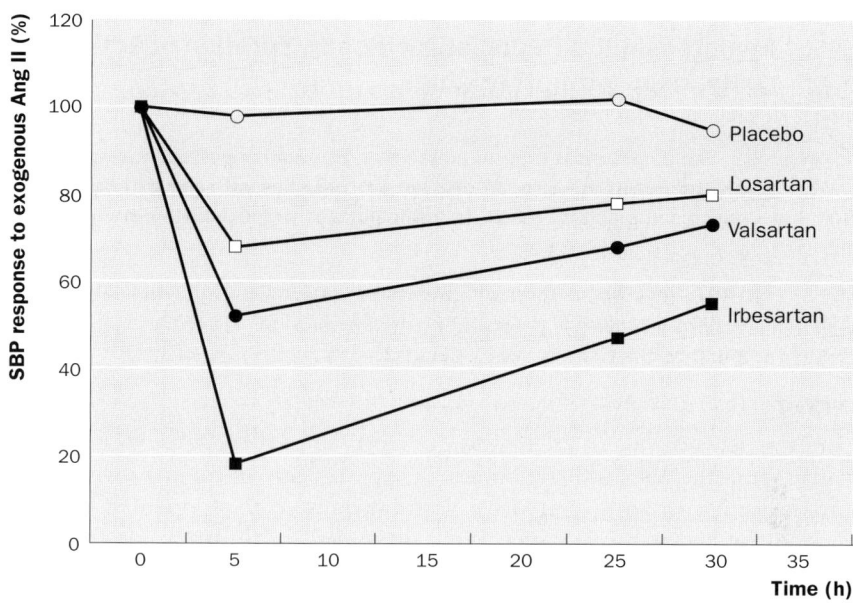

Fig. 11.3 Relative effectiveness of three angiotensin II (Ang II) antagonists in normotensive subjects. SBP = systolic blood pressure.

Clinical trials with angiotensin II antagonist drugs

There is no doubt that angiotensin II receptor (AT_1) antagonists constitute an exciting and important new class of antihypertensive drug. However, for any new agent, or any new class of drug, there remains a basic requirement that clinical usefulness be demonstrated at an early stage in terms of efficacy and tolerability. There is little doubt that the angiotensin II receptor antagonists, as a class, constitute a clear advance by virtue of their very good tolerability, both symptomatic and metabolic, and particularly their lack of any obvious class-specific adverse effect. However, it has not always proved possible to demonstrate clearly that their antihypertensive efficacy is comparable to that of established agents. In this respect, the prototype drug, losartan, for which there is the greatest volume of information, has failed to demonstrate that its BP-lowering effects are superior to those of established agents. Of greater concern is the evidence that suggests that losartan may, in fact, be less potent than comparator agents both within its own class and across the different antihypertensive drug classes.

Angiotensin II antagonists: efficacy, duration of action, comparison with other drugs.

H L Elliott. *J Hum Hypertens* 1998; **12**: 271–4.

BACKGROUND. The angiotensin II antagonists constitute an important new class of drug, with a low incidence of adverse effects; but early studies with the prototype, losartan, have raised some doubts about its antihypertensive 'potency' in the clinical setting.

INTERPRETATION. The preliminary results with newer angiotensin II antagonists suggest that they may have greater antihypertensive efficacy than losartan.

Comment

This short review was one of the first to question the antihypertensive efficacy of losartan as monotherapy for the treatment of hypertension. In comparative studies with drugs from other antihypertensive classes there were no reports that losartan had superior antihypertensive efficacy. While the majority of the comparative studies demonstrated, on statistical grounds, that losartan was equivalent to the comparator agent, the overall picture was that losartan tended to reduce BP by a few mmHg less than each of the comparator drugs. Furthermore, comparative studies between losartan and other angiotensin II receptor antagonists conveyed the same picture, whereby the competitor angiotensin II receptor antagonist was almost invariably superior to losartan in terms of BP reduction.

ABPM comparison of the antihypertensive profiles of the selective angiotensin II receptor antagonists telmisartan and losartan in patients with mild to moderate hypertension.

J M Mallion, J P Siche, Y Lacourcière, and the Telmisartan Blood Pressure Monitoring Group. *J Hum Hypertens* 1999; **13**: 657–64.

BACKGROUND. The antihypertensive efficacy and tolerability profiles of the selective AT_1 receptor antagonists telmisartan and losartan were compared with placebo in a 6-week multinational, multicentre, randomized, double-blind, double-dummy, parallel study of 233 patients with mild to moderate hypertension, defined as clinic diastolic blood pressure (DBP) $\geq$ 95 and $\leq$ 114 mmHg, clinic systolic blood pressure (SBP) $\geq$140 and $\leq$ 200 mmHg, and 24h ambulatory DBP $\geq$ 85 mmHg.

INTERPRETATION. Telmisartan 40 mg and 80 mg once daily were effective and well tolerated in the treatment of mild to moderate hypertension, producing sustained 24-hour BP control that compared favourably with losartan.

This was a multicentre, randomized, double-blind, double-dummy, parallel group study of 223 patients who received 6 weeks of treatment with placebo, or losartan 50 mg daily, or telmisartan 40 mg daily or telmisartan 80 mg daily. Overall, there were consistently greater BP reductions with the two different doses of telmisartan compared to losartan. In particular, telmisartan 80 mg daily was consistently significantly more effective than losartan 50 mg across the measured parameters (see Tables 11.1 and 11.2).

Table 11.1 Comparison of telmisartan and losartan—reductions in blood pressure (from baseline: placebo-corrected)–1

	Losartan (50 mg)	Telmisartan (40 mg)	Telmisartan (80 mg)
Daytime (06.00–22.00)	*6.6/4.4*	*9.4/6.4*	**11.2/7.4**
Night-time (22.00–0600)	*5.1/3.7*	**9.6/6.8**	**11.2/7.4**
'Trough' (00.00–0600)	3.7/2.4	**8.4/5.5**	**9.9/5.8**
Morning (06.00–12.00)	*5.3/2.8*	*8.1/5.3**	**10.3/6.2**

*P<0.05 versus placebo; **P<0.05 versus placebo and losartan. Adapted from Mallion *et al.* (1999).

Table 11.2 Comparison of telmisartan and losartan—reductions in blood pressure (from baseline: placebo-corrected)–2

	Losartan (50 mg)	Telmisartan (40 mg)	Telmisartan (80 mg)
Clinic BP	5.5/2.5	9.4/5.1	*11.1/6.2*
24-hour ABPM	6.2/4.1	*9.7/6.6*	*11.5/7.6*

*P ≤0.05 versus losartan. BP = blood pressure; ABPM = ambulatory blood pressure measurement. Adapted from Mallion *et al.* (1999).

Comment

This well-conducted study confirms the earlier concerns that losartan may not be the most effective agent within the class.

Efficacy and safety of telmisartan, a selective AT_1 receptor antagonist, compared with enalapril in elderly patients with primary hypertension.

B E Karlberg, L-E Lins, K Hermansson for the TEES Group. *J Hypertens* 1999; **17**: 293–302.

BACKGROUND. **To assess the antihypertensive efficacy and safety of the novel AT$_1$ receptor antagonist, telmisartan, compared with that of enalapril in elderly patients with mild to moderate hypertension.**

INTERPRETATION. These results demonstrate that telmisartan is well tolerated and is at least effective as enalapril in treating elderly patients with mild to moderate hypertension.

This was a 26-week, multicentre, double-blind, parallel group, dosage titration study involving 278 patients aged 65 years or more. Patients were randomly assigned to telmisartan across the dose range 20–40–80 mg or to enalapril from 5–10–20 mg according to the supine DBP response at trough. Both treatments lowered BP in a comparable and clinically meaningful manner, with mean changes from baseline of 22.1/12.9 mmHg for telmisartan and 20.1/11.4 mmHg for enalapril. Both regimens were well tolerated; however, 16% of patients receiving enalapril reported cough, compared with only 6.5% of those receiving telmisartan.

Comment

This conventional clinical trial illustrates again that comparable antihypertensive efficacy is more likely to be produced by one of the newer angiotensin II antagonists.

Comparison of the angiotensin II receptor antagonist irbesartan with atenolol for treatment of hypertension.

K O Stumpe, D Haworth, C Hoglund, L Kerwin, A Martin, T Simon, *et al.*
Blood Pressure 1998; **7**: 31–7.

BACKGROUND. **In this multicentre, double-blind study, the antihypertensive efficacy and safety of irbesartan were compared with those of atenolol in patients with mild to moderate hypertension.**

INTERPRETATION. In comparison to atenolol, irbesartan ≤ 150 mg provided at least equivalent BP control while demonstrating an excellent safety and tolerability profile.

This study in 231 patients with mild to moderate hypertension was a routine comparative clinical trial in patients with seated DBP in the range 95–110 mmHg. Treatments were initiated with irbesartan 75 mg or atenolol 50 mg daily and increased to respectively 150 mg and 50 mg according to the BP response, with the option to add hydrochlorothiazide and then nifedipine if seated DBP remained above 90 mmHg. Overall, there were no significant differences in the antihypertensive effect of the two drug treatment regimens, although the BP reduction (from baseline) was slightly greater with irbesartan: by 1.9 mmHg for SBP and by 0.6 mmHg for DBP. Adverse drug reports were similar, but serious adverse events and discontinuations because of adverse events were slightly greater in the atenolol group at 9.1% versus 4.5%. These authors concluded that irbesartan provided at least equivalent BP control in comparison to atenolol, while demonstrating an excellent safety and tolerability profile.

Comment

This routine clinical trial again illustrates the point that the newer angiotensin II antagonist appears better able to demonstrate antihypertensive comparability with representatives from other reference drug classes.

Angiotensin II type 1 (AT₁) receptor blockade in hypertensive women: benefits of candesartan cilexetil versus enalapril or hydrochlorothiazide.

K Malmqvist, T Kahan, M Dahl. *Am J Hypertens* 2000; **13**: 504–11.

BACKGROUND. Women have traditionally been treated with older types of antihypertensive drugs, mainly diuretics, often according to guidelines based on data from studies in men. Furthermore, women more frequently report side-effects from their medical treatment than do men, including dry cough found during ACE inhibitor treatment.

INTERPRETATION. Candesartan (cilexetil) 8–16 mm lowers SBP and DBP more effectively than enalapril, with less risk for dry cough. Candesartan (cilexetil) 8–16 mg lowers SBP and DBP more effectively than hydrochlorothiazide 12.5–25 mg, with less risk of hypokalaemia and hyperuricaemia. Quality of life was similar and well-maintained in all treatment groups. The favourable effect on SBP with candesartan (cilexetil) is of particular interest, since mean SBP is higher among post-menopausal women than in men of a similar age.

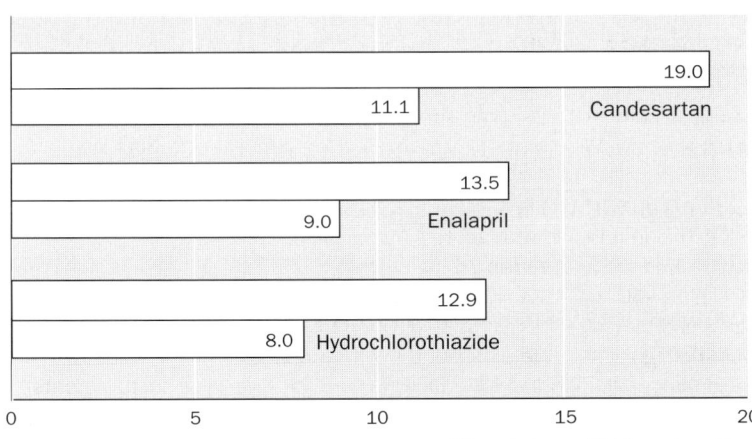

Fig. 11.4 Blood pressure reductions. Comparison of 12 weeks' treatment with candesartan, enalapril or hydrochlorothiazide.

This study in 429 women aged 40–69 years was a parallel group comparison of 12 weeks of treatment with candesartan (cilexetil) 8 or 16 mg, enalapril 10 or 20 mg or hydrochlorothiazide 12.5 or 25 mg. The BP reductions were significantly greater with candesartan compared to other treatments (Fig. 11.4). With candesartan BP was reduced by 19.0/11.1 compared to 13.5/9.0 with enalapril and 12.9/8.0 mmHg with hydrochlorothiazide.

Comment

The salient message is that candesartan is at least as effective as representative agents from alternative, established antihypertensive drugs.

Conclusion

These regulation clinical trials are important for generating a database, but seldom do they have real discriminatory power. However, the basic message remains unchanged: losartan appears to be the least effective, and the newer agents are more consistently able to demonstrate direct comparability with other reference drugs. But, which of the others—candesartan, irbesartan, telmisartan, valsartan—is the class leader?

Regression of left ventricular hypertrophy (LVH)

There is a considerable amount of background evidence implicating the renin–angiotensin–aldosterone system (RAAS) in the development of LVH and, consequently, there has been a considerable amount of interest in the effectiveness of ACE inhibitors in clinical studies. The same experimental rationale and the same experimental background has also been explored with angiotensin II receptor antagonists, with the same expectations that they might be particularly effective in promoting the regression of LVH. Additionally, since the angiotensin II receptor antagonists block non-ACE-dependent angiotensin II generation, such as occurs within the myocardium, there is the possibility that this class of drugs might be even more effective than the ACE inhibitor group.

 Increased left ventricular mass (LVM) after losartan treatment.
B Cheung. *Lancet* 1997; **349**: 1743–4.

BACKGROUND. Angiotensin II antagonists have the advantages over ACE inhibitors of specific blockade of the action of angiotensin II on the type 1 angiotensin receptor (AT$_1$) and a lower incidence of cough as a side-effect.

INTERPRETATION. This small study cannot exclude the possibility that long-term treatment with an angiotensin II antagonist may have a beneficial effect on LVH, but it would be difficult ethically to justify a placebo-controlled study of longer duration or the selection of patients with known LVH. Nevertheless, it would be disconcerting if losartan does have the unexpected effect of increasing LVM, [and] .... it may be prudent to have long-term data before it is used as a first-line agent in the treatment of hypertension.

Comment

As the author concedes, this study is substantially lacking in statistical power to draw definitive conclusions. Nevertheless, there was no regression of LVH and, overall, a disappointingly small reduction in BP after 12 weeks of treatment. In fact, the mean decrease in sitting DBP was 6.7 mmHg with losartan, and this conceals a range of blood pressure reduction values from 0.74 to 12.6 mmHg: these changes were not significantly different from the changes in BP induced by placebo.

Long-term effects of losartan on blood pressure and left ventricular structure in essential hypertension.

A Himmelmann, A Svensson, A Bergbrant, L Hansson. *J Hum Hypertens* 1996; **10**: 729–34.

BACKGROUND. In a 12-week, randomized, double-blind study, 24 patients with essential hypertension were given the angiotensin II antagonists losartan, or the beta-adrenoceptor-blocker atenolol.

INTERPRETATION. Losartan is effective in reducing BP during long-term treatment. No significant effect on LVM was observed, but there was an increase in LV wall thickness.

This was a small-scale study of 19 patients in whom LVM was reappraised after 26–32 months of treatment with losartan. Although BP on average was reduced from 156/103 to 131/83 mmHg, there was no significant change in LVM. There were, however, small but significant increases in septal and posterior wall thickness.

Comment

This was a small and non-definitive study with shortcomings in its design and methodology. The absence of any reduction in LVM despite a sizeable BP reduction is rather surprising, and raises questions about the effectiveness of losartan in the prevention and/or treatment of hypertensive LVH.

Pressure overload induces cardiac hypertrophy in angiotensin II type 1A receptor knock-out mice.

K Harada, I Komuro, I Shiojima, D Hayashi, S Kudoh, T Mizuno, *et al. Circulation* 1998; **97**: 1952–9.

BACKGROUND. Many studies have suggested that the renin–angiotensin system plays an important role in the development of pressure overload-induced cardiac hypertrophy. Moreover, it has been reported that pressure overload-induced cardiac hypertrophy is completely prevented by ACE inhibitors in vivo, and that the stored angiotensin II (Ang II) is released from cardiac myocytes in response to mechanical stretch and induces cardiomyocyte hypertrophy through the Ang II type 1 receptor (AT_1) in vitro.

INTERPRETATION. AT_1-mediated Ang II signalling is not essential for the development of pressure overload-induced cardiac hypertrophy.

Comment

This is a very interesting and thought-provoking study concerning the role of factors other than pressure overload in the development of hypertensive LVH. The AT_1 receptor is the 'effector' or 'signalling' locus within the RAAS and complete or marked reduction in cardiac hypertrophy would be predicted when functional responses mediated via the AT_1 receptor are eliminated. In this 'knock-out' animal model, elimination of the AT_1 receptor failed to prevent cardiac hypertrophy, thus raising considerable doubts about the proposed central role of angiotensin II and the RAAS in those non-haemodynamic processes that are anticipated in the development of LVH.

Influence of the angiotensin II antagonist valsartan on left ventricular hypertrophy in patients with essential hypertension.

P A Thürmann, P Kendi, A Schmidt, S Harder, N Rietbrock. *Circulation* 1998; **98**: 2037–42.

BACKGROUND. Left ventricular hypertrophy (LVH) represents an independent risk factor in patients with essential hypertension. Because reversal of LVH may be associated with an improvement of prognosis, the influence of new antihypertensive compounds, such as angiotensin II AT_1 receptor antagonists, on LVH should be determined.

INTERPRETATION. Antihypertensive treatment with the angiotensin II antagonist valsartan for 8 months produced a significant regression of LVH in predominantly previously untreated patients with essential hypertension. The drug may be safely administered in this subset of hypertensive patients; however, the long-term benefit in terms of risk reduction has still to be evaluated in further trials.

Comment

The evidence from this clinical study is consistent in showing that BP reduction leads to regression of LVH. However, there was no evidence of any additional benefit attributable to angiotensin II antagonist activity. In this illustrative study with valsartan, it is noteworthy that regression of LVH was actually achieved, whereas the earlier studies with losartan had failed to confirm even this basic requirement.

Effects of valsartan on left ventricular diastolic function in patients with mild or moderate essential hypertension: comparison with enalapril.

A Cuocolo, G Storto, R Izzo, G L Lovino, M Damiano, F Bertocchi, *et al.*
J Hypertens 1999; **17**: 1759–66.

BACKGROUND. This study compares the effects of an AT_1 angiotensin II receptor antagonist (valsartan) with those of an ACE inhibitor (enalapril) on left ventricular (LV) diastolic function in patients with mild or moderate essential hypertension and no evidence of LVH at echocardiography.

INTERPRETATION. Valsartan-induced renin–angiotensin system blockade is able to improve LV filling in patients with mild or moderate essential hypertension and impaired diastolic function. These findings support the hypothesis of a contribution of the renin–angiotensin system in the control of LV diastolic function in these patients.

This small-scale study of 24 patients used radionuclide ambulatory monitoring to investigate LV function at rest and during exercise testing. Patients received either valsartan (80–160 mg daily) or enalapril (20–40 mg daily) according to a double-blind cross-over randomization scheme. In brief summary, there were no significant differences between the two treatments in terms of their effects on LV diastolic function. A subgroup analysis was then used to suggest that valsartan had a greater beneficial effect on LV peak filling rate.

Comment

This small study is insufficiently powered to show anything other than the comparability of the two different treatments, which produced similar reductions in blood pressure. The small number of patients does not justify a *post hoc* subgroup analysis and it is not possible, in the light of a small but significant blood pressure reduction, to draw the conclusion that the renin–angiotensin system is implicated in the control of LV diastolic function in hypertensive patients. In fact, because of the reductions in BP with both active treatments it is not possible to draw any other conclusion than to suggest that BP reduction might be beneficial for LV diastolic function.

Conclusion

For the clinician, the practical message from all these studies is a reinforcement of the concept that the optimal means of preventing (or reversing) LVH is long-term BP control. While angiotensin II antagonists might usefully be incorporated into an effective antihypertensive combination regimen, there is no clinical evidence to favour their use on account of any additional 'tissue' effects.

Treatment of heart failure

The results of several major clinical outcome trials have clearly demonstrated the morbidity and mortality benefit associated with the use of ACE inhibitor drugs in patients with heart failure secondary to LV dysfunction.

Randomized trial of losartan versus captopril in patients over 65 with heart failure (Evaluation of Losartan in The Elderly Study, ELITE).

B Pitt, R Segal, F A Martinez, G Meurers, A J Cowley, I Thomas, *et al.*
Lancet 1997; **349**: 747–52.

BACKGROUND. **To determine whether specific angiotensin II receptor blockade with losartan offers safety and efficacy advantages in the treatment of heart failure over angiotensin-converting enzyme (ACE) inhibition with captopril, the ELITE study compared losartan with captopril in older heart failure patients.**

INTERPRETATION. In this study of elderly heart failure patients, treatment with losartan was associated with an unexpectedly lower mortality than that found with captopril. Although there was no difference in renal dysfunction, losartan was generally better tolerated than captopril and fewer patients discontinued losartan therapy. A further trial (ELITE II), evaluating the effects of losartan and captopril on mortality and morbidity in a larger number of patients with heart failure, is in progress.

The ELITE trial enrolled 722 patients aged 75 years or more with NYHA class II–IV heart failure and randomized them to receive either losartan or captopril for approximately 1 year of treatment. The primary endpoint was the tolerability assessment of renal function, for which there was no difference between the two treatments. However, there was the unexpected finding of a statistically significant reduction in all-cause mortality in the losartan group (17 deaths) compared to the captopril group (32 deaths).

Comment

This study produced an unexpected result in so far as all-cause mortality was significantly reduced by losartan relative to captopril. However, the sample size, study design and declared outcome measures were not sufficiently prospectively empowered to permit a definitive conclusion.

Comparison of candesartan, enalapril, and their combination in congestive heart failure. Randomized Evaluation of Strategies for Left Ventricular Dysfunction (RESOLVD) pilot study.

R S McKelvie, S Yusuf, D Pericak, A Avezum, R J Burns, J Probstfield, *et al.*
Circulation 1999; **100**: 1056–64.

B ACKGROUND . **The authors investigated the effects of candesartan (an angiotensin II antagonist) alone, enalapril alone, and their combination on exercise tolerance, ventricular function, quality of life, neurohormone levels and tolerability in congestive heart failure.**

I NTERPRETATION . Candesartan alone was as effective, safe, and tolerable as enalapril. The combination of candesartan and enalapril was more beneficial for preventing LV remodelling than either candesartan or enalapril alone.

Comment

This pilot study in 668 patients with NYHA-FC II to IV showed that candesartan monotherapy was similar but not superior to enalapril monotherapy in the management of patients with heart failure. The results of the main study have not yet been reported in full, but the preliminary announcements indicate that candesartan has no therapeutic advantages over enalapril.

Conclusion

There is now a considerable amount of evidence that ACE inhibitor drugs contribute positively to the management of patients with cardiac failure or LV dysfunction, or after myocardial infarction. Although, on a theoretical basis, angiotensin II antagonists might be expected to provide further benefits, there is no evidence so far that this is true.

Conclusions

There is no doubt that, as a class, angiotensin II receptor antagonists constitute a significant therapeutic advance. The good symptomatic tolerability profile and the lack of adverse metabolic effects are the principal advantages, but overall effectiveness remains to be clearly established, particularly for reducing cardiovascular morbidity and mortality. Unfortunately, although there is a considerable volume of clinical data on the prototype drug, losartan, these show that there are shortcomings in its effectiveness in terms of antihypertensive efficacy, regression of LVH and effectiveness in heart failure.

This review is not intended to be a comprehensive account of every study published in the past year or so; rather, it summarizes the current position of this class of drugs in the setting of practical clinical issues. There is no doubt that the newer agents have generated evidence of an antihypertensive efficacy that is more directly comparable to that of other antihypertensive drug classes, but, as yet, there are no outcome studies to confirm their effectiveness. Furthermore, although there is accumulating evidence to suggest that losartan is the least effective agent, there are as yet no definitive discriminatory studies to determine which of the alternative agents is 'best'. In summary, selective angiotensin II receptor antagonist drugs constitute a major therapeutic advance: but how much of an advance remains to be quantified, and which agent(s) are the 'best buys' has still to be clarified.

12

24-hour blood pressure measurement: current issues

Introduction

The recent guidelines from national and international authorities are consistent in their recommendations for 'tighter' blood pressure (BP) control, particularly in patients at high risk of cardiovascular disease. However, despite the volume of evidence that adverse cardiovascular outcomes are correlated more closely with the values derived from 24-hour BP assessments, rather than those derived from conventional clinic measurements, several practical considerations prevent the widespread applicability of 24-hour ambulatory blood pressure monitoring (ABPM). The following are the major areas of debate:

- Guidelines for the use of the 24-hour ABPM
- 24-hour BP values and cardiovascular morbidity and mortality
- 24-hour BP control: practical examples

Ambulatory blood pressure monitoring

The following extracts are taken from the recent guidelines to illustrate the current consensus view:

The sixth report of the Joint National Committee on Prevention, Detection, Evaluation, and Treatment of High Blood Pressure.
Joint National Committee on Prevention, Detection, Evaluation, and Treatment of High Blood Pressure and the National High Blood Pressure Education Program Coordinating Committee. *Arch Intern Med* 1997; **157**: 2413–46.

EXTRACT. Normal BP values taken by ambulatory measurement (1) are lower than clinic readings while patients are awake (< 135/85 mmHg); (2) are even lower while patients are asleep (< 120/75 mmHg); and (3) provide measures of systolic and diastolic BP load (throughout 24 hours) |**1, 2**|. In the majority of individuals, BP falls by

10–20% during the night; this change is more closely related to patterns of sleep and wakefulness than to time of day (as illustrated by the fact that the BP rhythm follows the inverted cycle of activity in nightshift workers) |3|.

Prospective data relating ambulatory BP to prognosis are limited to two published studies, which suggest that, in patients in whom an elevated clinic pressure is the only abnormality, ABP may identify a group at relatively low risk of morbidity |4–6|.

ABPM is most clinically helpful and most commonly used in patients with suspected white-coat hypertension; but it is also helpful in patients with apparent drug resistance, hypotensive symptoms with antihypertensive medications, episodic hypertension and autonomic dysfunction |2|. However, this procedure should not be employed indiscriminately, as in the routine evaluation of patients with suspected hypertension.

1999 World Health Organization–International Society of Hypertension Guidelines for the Management of Hypertension.

Guidelines subcommittee. *J Hypertens* 1999; **17**: 151–83.

EXTRACT. Non-invasive semi-automatic and automatic devices are now available for BP measurement at home and for ABPM over periods of 24 hours or more. Both of these approaches provide useful additional clinical information and have a place in the management of the hypertensive patient, but in both cases there are three important limitations:

- First, there are limited data available on the prognostic value of both home and ambulatory BP measurements |7, 8|. Further prospective studies are required to determine whether such measurements offer material advantages over conventional BP measurements for the prediction of morbidity and mortality. Therefore information obtained via these methods must be regarded as supplementary to conventional measurements, not as a substitute for them.
- Second, studies conducted in the general population and in hypertensive individuals have demonstrated that BP values obtained by home measurement or by ambulatory monitoring are several mmHg lower than those obtained by office measurements, with 24-hour average or home BP values of around 125/80 mmHg corresponding to clinic pressures of 140/90 mmHg |9|.
- Third, the devices used should be checked for accuracy and performance over time against other well-validated BP measurement devices, using standardized protocols.

ABPM also offers the advantages of providing a more realistic setting for BP measurements, and of improving patient perceptions and adherence to treatment. More important, however, is the large body of evidence indicating that the target organ damage (TOD) associated with hypertension is more closely related to 24-hour or daytime average BP than to clinic BP |8, 10|, particularly if few office values are obtained |11|. There is also evidence that pretreatment ambulatory BP has a prognostic value |12, 13|, and recent prospective studies suggest that regression of TOD such as LVH is more closely related to changes in 24-hour average than to changes in office BP values |**14**|. While ABP monitoring is not a substitute for office measurement, it provides an important research tool for investigations of normal and deranged mechanisms of cardiovascular regulation, of the clinical relevance of phenomena such as BP variability and nocturnal hypotension, and of the time course and homogeneity of the antihypertensive effect of newer drugs or drug combinations |**8, 15**|.

Guidelines for management of hypertension: report of the third working party of the British Hypertension Society.

L E Ramsay, B Williams, G D Johnston, G A MacGregor, L Poston, J F Potter, *et al. J Hum Hypertens* 1999; **13**: 569–92.

E x t r a c t . All outcome trials on hypertension have been based on surgery or clinic BP, not on ABPM, and it is therefore difficult to provide firm guidance based on evidence for use of this technique. Nevertheless, ABPM is widely used and may be valuable in special circumstances. ABPM provides numerous measurements over a short time, and so reduces variability when compared to the average of a limited number of surgery or clinic readings |**11, 16**|. BP by ABPM correlates more closely with TOD, presumably in part because of reduced variability and measurement error |**4, 6**|.

ABPM may be indicated in the following circumstances:

- When BP shows unusual variability;
- In hypertension resistant to drug therapy, defined as BP >150/90 mmHg on a regimen of three or more antihypertensive drugs;
- When symptoms suggest the possibility of hypotension; and
- To diagnose 'white-coat hypertension'.

The term 'white-coat hypertension' is widely used to describe consistent hypertension in the clinic coexisting with consistent normotension by ABPM. There is a systematic clinic–ABPM difference in the population that is related to the level of clinic BP, and white-coat hypertension is considered to be present only when the clinic–ABPM difference exceeds the population average difference |**17**|.

It is not necessary or feasible to perform ABPM to exclude white-coat hypertension in *all* hypertension patients. It is *not* indicated in patients who are at high coronary heart disease (CHD)/cardiovascular disease (CVD) risk. This includes patients who already have TOD or cardiovascular complications and those who have an estimated 10-year CHD risk of 15% or higher. In these patients treatment decisions should be based on surgery or clinic pressures rather than ABPM, as was the case in outcome trials of hypertension treatment. ABPM is also unnecessary in patients with mild hypertension (140–159/90–99 mmHg) with no TOD, no cardiovascular complications and an estimated 10-year CHD risk <15%. These patients may be left untreated without using ABPM, but must be followed up.

ABPM may alter management when the average clinic BP is greater than 160/100 mmHg, there is no TOD or cardiovascular complications, *and* the estimated 10-year CHD risk is <15%. Here elevated BP is the only indication of high CHD/CVD risk, and for antihypertensive treatment, normal BP values by ABPM may alter the treatment decision.

Some important points to bear in mind when interpreting ABPM records need emphasis. The average daytime BP should be used for treatment decisions, not the average 24-hour BP. BP measured by ABPM is systematically lower than surgery or clinic measurements in hypertensive and normotensive people |**17, 18**|. Because of this, treatment thresholds and targets must be adjusted downwards when making decisions based on ABPM data. Precise adjustment is complex, but the average difference between clinic and daytime mean pressures determined by ABPM is approximately 12/7 mmHg |**17, 18**|. Thus an ABPM average daytime BP of 148/83 mmHg is approximately equivalent to a surgery BP of 160/90 mmHg, and this may require treatment in some patients. Recommended targets for ABPM measurement and for conventional clinic BP measurements are given in Table 12.1.

Table 12.1 Treatment targets

	Clinic BP (mmHg)		Mean daytime ABPM (mmHg)	
	No diabetes	**Diabetes**	**No diabetes**	**Diabetes**
Optimal BP	< 140/85	< 140/80	< 130/80	< 130/75
Audit standard	< 150/90	< 140/85	< 140/85	< 140/80

BP = blood pressure; ABPM = ambulatory blood pressure monitoring.

Comment

These extracts from the recent guidelines summarize the current recommendations concerning the use of ABPM in clinical practice. While there are some differences in points of detail, the principal practical messages are consistent:

1. Prospective (outcome) data for ABPM itself are very limited and there are no outcome studies in which treatment has been directed in accordance with the ABPM values.

2. ABPM is not (yet) recommended as part of the routine work-up of every hypertensive patient, but instead should be reserved for those in whom there are specific management issues.

3. ABPM values are invariably lower than clinical BP readings: relative to the clinic BP, the ABPM daytime average value (which is generally preferred to the full 24-hour average) will typically be lower by 10–15 mmHg systolic and 5–10 mmHg diastolic BP.

Conclusion

The overwhelming conclusion is that ABPM is important and valuable but not recommended for indiscriminate or routine use in every hypertensive patient. Instead,
where major management decisions might be implicated—to withhold antihypertensive treatment in an otherwise low-risk patient, for example, or to intensify treatment in a high-risk patient with apparently 'resistant' hypertension—then
the information derived from ABPM is likely to constitute an important and deci-
sive factor.

24-hour BP and cardiovascular morbidity and mortality

The long-term consequences of uncontrolled hypertension manifest through the
development of cardiovascular TOD. However, the predictive power of the conventional clinic BP measurement is relatively weak, whereas a number of studies
have described closer relationships with the BP values derived from 24-hour BP
measurements [19, 20]. Thus, the concept has arisen that TOD is more likely to
occur when the BP remains elevated throughout the whole 24-hour period. This
concept of a BP 'load' throughout 24 hours has typically been seen in studies assessing LVM; and, generally, there are much closer relationships between measures of
LVM and the values derived from 24-hour BP assessments than with those derived
from conventional clinic BP measurements [21]. For example, the correlations illus-

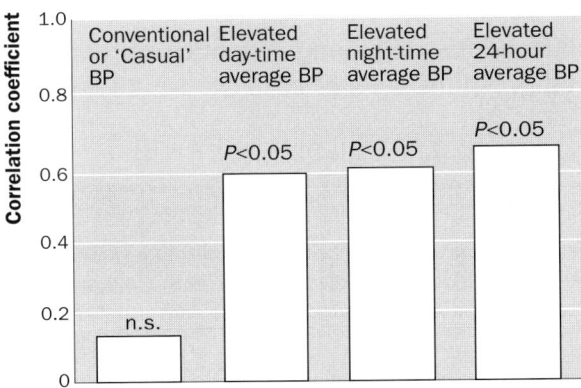

Fig. 12.1 Correlations between left ventricular mass measurements and derived
ambulatory blood pressure (BP) monitoring values; n.s. = not significant (adapted from
White *et al.* [21]).

trated in Fig. 12.1 show that values derived from 24-hour BP assessment correlate much more closely with LVM than those obtained with a conventional clinic BP measurement. Furthermore, it can be seen that persistence of an elevated overnight BP contributes significantly to the increase in LVM and the development of LVH.

Table 12.2 24-h average blood pressure correlates with different types of target organ damage

- Overall target organ damage score
- Left ventricular mass
- Impaired left ventricular function
- (Micro)albuminuria
- Brain damage (cerebral lacunae)
- Retinopathy
- Intima-media thickness (carotid)

Although many studies have focused on measurement of LVM as an index of TOD, similar relationships have been identified between 24-hour BP measurements and other types of TOD (Table 12.2). Thus, it is reasonable to assume that the level of BP throughout 24 hours is the principal determinant of TOD, and this concept is entirely consistent with the results of the classical longitudinal study by Perloff *et al.* |4|, which showed that ambulatory values provided prognostic power additional to that obtained by conventional BP measurements. This seminal observation has since been confirmed by the results of several other studies; but further evidence of the predictive power of derived 24-hour BP values is seen in the following studies.

Predicting cardiovascular risk using conventional versus ambulatory blood pressure in older patients with systolic hypertension.

J A Staessen, L Thijs, R Fagard, E T O'Brien, D Clement, P W de Leeuw, *et al.*, for the Systolic Hypertension in Europe Trial Investigators. *JAMA* 1999; **282**: 539–46.

BACKGROUND. The clinical use of ambulatory blood pressure monitoring (ABPM) requires further validation in prospective outcome studies. The aim is to compare the prognostic significance of conventional and ABPM in older patients with isolated systolic hypertension.

INTERPRETATION. In untreated older patients with isolated systolic hypertension, ambulatory systolic BP was a significant predictor of cardiovascular risk over and above conventional BP.

A total of 808 untreated hypertensive patients aged >60 years participated in this substudy, which was part of the Systolic Hypertension in Europe trial (SYST-EUR). The conventional BP measurement was taken as the mean of six pre-treatment readings (two measurements in the sitting position at three visits, each 1 month apart) and the baseline ambulatory BP assessment was also obtained prior to drug treatment.

In the placebo group, an increment of 10 mmHg in 24-hour systolic BP average was associated with an increased relative risk rate for most outcome measurements: for example, total mortality was increased by 23% and cardiovascular mortality by 34%. Of particular interest was the finding that, statistically, the night-time systolic BP more accurately predicted endpoints than the daytime level. In other words, the persistence of a (relatively) high BP overnight was an adverse prognostic feature.

Comment

This study confirms the expectation that the values derived from 24-hour BP assessments, prior to treatment, are more powerful predictors of cardiovascular risk. It is noteworthy that this predictive power was apparent particularly in the placebo group, but was less apparent in the active treatment group. This apparent anomaly presumably arises because the prognosis is altered by antihypertensive treatment and BP reduction, so that the achieved BP during antihypertensive drug treatment becomes a more important predictor than the pre-treatment value.

Reference values for 24-hour ambulatory blood pressure monitoring based on a prognostic criterion. The Ohasama Study.

T Ohkubo, Y Imai, I Tsuji, K Nagai, S Ito, H Satoh, *et al. Hypertension* 1998; **32**: 255–9.

BACKGROUND. Although reference values for ambulatory blood pressure monitoring (ABPM) have been investigated in several population studies, these values were derived from cross-sectional observations and were based merely on the statistical distribution of BP values. Therefore, we conducted a prospective cohort study to identify reference values for 24-hour BP in relation to prognosis.

INTERPRETATION. This is the first report to propose reference values for 24-hour ambulatory BP (ABP) based on a prognostic criterion.

This is an interesting study because it was a prospective examination attempting to identify reference values for 24-hour ABP in relation to prognosis. Data were obtained from 1542 subjects (565 men) aged 40 years and over, and during the follow-up period, 6.2 years on average, there were 117 deaths. The salient findings were that 24-hour average BP values >134/79 mmHg were associated with increased cardiovascular risk, whereas BP in the range 120–133 mmHg for systolic and 65–78 mmHg for diastolic BP predicted the best prognosis. Interestingly, BP values below 119/64 mmHg were related to increased risks for non-cardiovascular mortality.

Comment

As the authors declare, this is the first report to relate 24-hour ABP values to outcome information (i.e. here, death) rather than to an intermediate or surrogate endpoint such as LVM.

Prognostic value of ambulatory blood pressure monitoring in refractory hypertension. A prospective study.

J Redon, C Campos, M L Narciso, J L Rodicio, J M Pasual, L M Ruilope.
Hypertension 1998; **31**: 712–8.

BACKGROUND. The objective of this study was to establish whether ABP offers a better estimate of cardiovascular risk than does its clinical BP counterpart in refractory hypertension.

INTERPRETATION. Higher values of ABP result in a worse prognosis in patients with refractory hypertension, supporting the recommendation that ABPM is useful in stratifying the cardiovascular risk in patients with refractory hypertension.
    This was a prospective study in 86 patients with essential hypertension and diastolic BP > 95 mmHg despite treatment with three or more antihypertensive drugs, including a thiazide diuretic. Patients were divided into tertiles of average diastolic blood pressure according to the ABPM: the average diastolic BP was < 88 mmHg (n=29) in the lowest tertile; 88–97 mmHg (n=29) in the middle tertile; and > 97 mmHg (n=28) in the highest tertile. Interestingly, while there were significant differences in systolic and diastolic BP according to the ABPM, there were no differences between the groups for office BP, either at the beginning or at the end of the period of observation. The incidence of cardiovascular events was significantly lower, at 2.2 per 100 patient-years in the lowest tertile, compared to 9.5 per 100 patient-years in the middle tertile and 13.6 per 100 patient-years in the upper tertile of ABP. The probability of event-free survival was also significantly different when comparing the lowest tertile with the other two groups. Thus, ABP in the highest tertile was an independent risk factor for the incidence of cardiovascular events, with a relative risk of 6.2.

Comment

In one sense, this is not a novel or surprising result. However, it confirms the prognostic superiority of derived ABPM in a particular subgroup of patients, namely those resistant to multiple antihypertensive drug treatments. Of particular interest, however, was the observation that those patients at greatest risk could not be clearly identified via the conventional clinic BP measurements. It was only in relation to their derived ambulatory BP values that the adverse prognostic significance was identified.

Conclusion

This important finding is consistent with the guidelines from the international authorities whereby ABPM is advised only in those patients where it might affect the management decision and lead to a change in drug treatment. Following the example of this study, even greater efforts with multiple drug combination treatments might be attempted in those patients identified as being at the highest risk. This might even be supported by advice to the patient that adverse effects should be considered acceptable (if they are relatively minor) if intensified drug treatment then leads to a significant improvement in BP control and prognosis.

24-hour BP control: practical examples

Recent studies from the UK and the USA have clearly identified the shortcomings of current antihypertensive treatment strategies in so far as < 50% of hypertensive patients are identified and satisfactorily treated to achieve the recommended treatment targets for clinic BP |22, 23|. This was confirmed in a recent Italian study which was of additional and particular interest because the study design incorporated home and 24-hour ambulatory measurements in addition to conventional clinic BP measurements.

Poor BP control

Blood pressure control in the hypertensive population.
G Mancia, R Sega, C Milesi, G Cesana, A Zanchetti. *Lancet* 1997; **349**: 454–7.

BACKGROUND. In large-scale surveys of individuals with hypertension, those whose clinic BP is reduced to 140/90 mmHg or less have been found to represent only a small fraction of the hypertensive population. We assessed whether these results arise because of a white-coat effect elevating clinic BP.

INTERPRETATION. In the hypertensive population the number of patients with inadequate BP control is high not only when assessed in the clinic, but also when assessed by ABPM or at home. The high BP values commonly found in treated hypertensive individuals cannot be accounted for by a white-coat effect, but by a true lack of daily life BP control.

Clinic, home and ABP measurements were obtained in 651 randomly selected patients. Patients were classified as treated hypertensive (n=207: i.e. those receiving antihypertensive drug treatments); or, according to their clinic BP measurements, as either normotensive individuals (n=1042), or untreated hypertensive patients with clinic BP > 140 mmHg systolic and/or > 90 mmHg diastolic (n=402). The salient finding was that there was no significant difference between untreated and treated hypertensive patients with average clinic BP values of respectively 148/93.3 versus 147/90.2 mmHg. In those classified as normotensive, the average clinic BP was 120/78.1 mmHg. The number of treated hypertensive patients found to have BP within the normal limits was small not only on the basis of clinic BP values, but also on the basis of home and ABP values. In other words, the average home and 24-hour BP showed lower values than clinic BPs in all patient groups as expected, but remained similarly higher in both untreated and treated hypertensive individuals when compared with normotensive individuals.

Comment

This report from Italy confirms the reports from other countries that the identification and treatment of hypertensive patients is inadequate. However, of particular interest in this study was the additional finding that, for the groups as a whole, where clinic BP control was poor, the corresponding home and ambulatory BP measurement also indicated poor BP control.

Conclusion

This study again indicates the potential applicability of 24-hour BP monitoring for the refining of management decisions. There is confirmation that poor BP control in the clinic setting translates to poor BP control generally. This does not overlook the fact that there may be individual exceptions with a pronounced 'white-coat' effect, but as a generalization, where clinical BP control is poor, daily life BP control is poor. Of additional interest in the above study were the BP profiles throughout 24 hours in the different patient groups (Fig. 12.2). While there is modest separation of the diastolic BP profiles during the daytime period in the treated and untreated hypertensive patients, there is no clear separation during the early morning period, i.e. the final hours of the 24-hour monitoring period. This suggests that the drug treatments taken by these patients tended to have an inadequate duration of action, such that 24-hour BP control was not being provided.

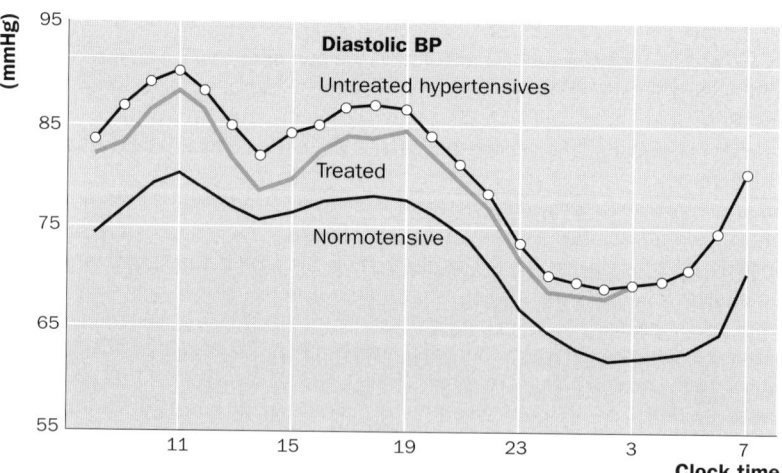

Fig. 12.2 Diastolic blood pressure (BP) profiles throughout 24 hours in normotensive, untreated hypertensive and treated hypertensive individuals (adapted from Mancia *et al.*, 1997).

Optimal BP control throughout 24 hours

Although the above study identified a lack of full 24-hour BP control, there is not yet any definitive evidence that BP control throughout 24 hours is superior to 'intermittent' or 'incomplete' control. However, a considerable volume of indirect evidence suggests that this is likely.

 Ambulatory blood pressure is superior to clinic blood pressure in predicting treatment-induced regression of left ventricular hypertrophy.

G Mancia, A Zanchetti, E Agebiti-Rosei, G Benemio, R De Cesaris, R Fogari, *et al.* for the SAMPLE study group. *Circulation* 1997; **95**: 1464–70.

BACKGROUND. In cross-sectional studies, ambulatory blood pressure (ABP) correlates more closely than clinic BP with the organ damage of hypertension. Whether ABP predicts development or regression of organ damage over time better than clinic BP, however, is unknown.

INTERPRETATION. In hypertensive subjects with left ventricular hypertrophy (LVH), regression of LVH was predicted much more closely by treatment-induced changes in ABP than in clinic BP. This provides the first longitudinally controlled evidence that ABP may be clinically superior to traditional BP measurements.

In this detailed study of 206 essential hypertensive patients with LVH, several different BP measurements were obtained before and after 1 year of treatment. BP values were obtained by 24-hour home BP monitoring and by conventional clinic measurements. It was noted that the pretreatment LV mass measurement correlated significantly with the 24-hour value, but not with either the clinic or home BP values. While this is confirmatory, there were additional and novel findings that the improvement in BP related to a reduction in LVM index was not the reduction in clinic or home BP, but was the reduction in the 24-hour average BP.

Comment

This important study illustrates the concept that 24-hour control of BP is an important requirement. Although the endpoint of LVH, and its regression, is a surrogate measure for cardiovascular outcome, the findings that pretreatment LVM was related to 24-hour BP and that the regression during treatment was correlated with the reduction in 24-hour BP are consistent with the idea that 24-hour BP control constitutes optimal BP control.

There are additional considerations that relate to an antihypertensive effect that is consistently maintained throughout 24 hours. The following might be considered features of an optimal antihypertensive treatment:

- Effective BP control throughout 24 hours and an overall decrease in BP load;
- 'Smooth' and consistent antihypertensive activity with no increase in BP variability;

- Attenuation of the early morning BP surge; and
- Once-daily dosing (in the interests of compliance).

Conclusion

There is no doubt that 24-hour BP monitoring and the blood pressure values derived from this technique have provided additional and important insights into the relationships between hypertension and cardiovascular morbidity and mortality. Of particular practical importance is the evidence that patients at high risk, or alternatively patients at low cardiovascular risk, can be clearly identified by 24-hour BP measurement, but not by conventional clinic BP measurement. This observation has practical importance with respect to the need for intensified treatment in a high-risk patient and the avoidance of unnecessary treatment in a low-risk patient. This is the strategy endorsed by the guidelines from the national and international authorities, which, at present, do not recommend 24-hour ABPM as part of the routine assessment of each individual hypertensive patient. Thus 24-hour ABPM is recommended only for selected patients. The fundamental reason for this recommendation resides in the fact that the benefits of antihypertensive drug treatment have been established through clinical trials that have used conventional clinic BP measurements and targets. As yet, there is no definitive prospective clinical outcome trial that has relied upon 24-hour BP values and targets. There are also the practical considerations of the expense of time and resources that would be incurred if 24-hour BP measurements had to be obtained in every hypertensive patient and repeated on each occasion that a treatment change was implemented.

Accumulated evidence clearly indicates that 24-hour control of BP is a desirable therapeutic goal. In turn, with the preference for once-daily antihypertensive treatment, there follows the clear inference that drugs with a protracted duration of action are to be preferred. Thus in line with the current emphasis on 'tight' BP control, there is therefore an additional practical recommendation to prescribe appropriately long-acting agents either as monotherapy or in combination therapy.

References

1. Appel G, Stason WB. Ambulatory blood pressure monitoring and blood pressure self measurement in the diagnosis and management of hypertension. *Ann Intern Med* 1993; **118**: 867–82.
2. Pickering T, for an American Society of Hypertension *ad hoc* panel. Recommendations

for the use of home (self) and ambulatory blood pressure monitoring. *Am J Hypertens* 1995; **9**: 1–11.

3. Sternberg H, Rosenthal T, Shamiss A, Green M. Altered circadian rhythm of blood pressure in shift workers. *J Hum Hypertens* 1995; **9**: 349–53.

4. Perloff D, Sokolow M, Cowan R. The prognostic value of ambulatory blood pressures. *JAMA* 1983; **249**: 2792–8.

5. Perloff D, Sokolow M, Cowan R, Juster RP. Prognostic value of ambulatory blood pressure measurements: further analysis. *J Hypertens* 1989; 7 (Suppl 3): S3–S10.

6. Verdecchia P, Porcellati C, Schillaci G, Borgioni C, Ciucci A, Battistelli M, *et al.* Ambulatory blood pressure: an independent predictor of prognosis in essential hypertension. *Hypertension* 1994; **24**: 793–801.

7. Ohkubo T, Imai Y, Tsuji I, Nagai K, Kato J, Kikuchi N, *et al.* Home blood pressure measurement has a stronger predictive power for mortality than dose screening blood pressure measurement: a population-based observation in Ohasama, Japan. *J Hypertens* 1998; **16**: 971–5.

8. Mancia G, Di Rienzo M, Parati G. Ambulatory blood pressure monitoring use in hypertension research and clinical practice. *Hypertension* 1993; **21**: 510–24.

9. Mancia G, Sega R, Bravi D, De Vito G, Valagussa F, Cesana G, *et al.* Ambulatory blood pressure normality: results from the PAMELA study. *J Hypertens* 1995; **13**: 1377–90.

10. Zanchetti A, Bond MG, Henning M, Neiss A, Mancia G, Dal Palu XC, *et al.* On behalf of the ELSA Investigators. Risk factors associated with alterations in carotid intima-media thickness in hypertension: baseline data from the European lacidipine Study on Atherosclerosis. *J Hypertens* 1998; **16**: 946–61.

11. Fagard RH, Staessen JA, Thijs L. Prediction of cardiac structure and function by repeated clinic and ambulatory blood pressure. *Hypertension* 1997; **29**: 22–9.

12. Redon J, Campos C, Narciso ML, Rodicio JL, Pasquale JM, Ruilope LM. Prognostic value of ambulatory blood pressure monitoring in refractory hypertension; a prospective study. *Hypertension* 1998; **31**: 712–8.

13. Ohkubo T, Imai Y, Tsuji I, Nagai K, Ito S, Satoh H, *et al.* Reference values for 24-hour ambulatory blood pressure monitoring based on a prognostic criterion: Ohasama study. *Hypertension* 1998; **32**: 255–9.

14. Mancia G, Zanchetti A, Agabiti-Rosei E, Benemio G, De Cesaris R, Fogari R, *et al.*, for the SAMPLE Study group. Ambulatory blood pressure is superior to clinic blood pressure in predicting treatment-induced regression of left ventricular hypertrophy. *Circulation* 1997; **95**: 1464–70.

15. Mancia G, Omboni S, Parati G. Assessment of antihypertensive treatment by ambulatory blood pressure. *J Hypertens* 1997; **15** (Suppl 2): S43–S50.

16. Fagard R, Staessen J, Thijs L, Amery A. Multiple standardised clinic blood pressure may predict left ventricular mass as well as ambulatory monitoring. A meta-analysis of comparative studies. *Am J Hypertens* 1995; **8**: 533–40.

17. Parati G, Omboni S, Staessen J, Thijs L, Fagard R, Ulian L, *et al.* Limitations of the difference between clinic and daytime blood pressure as a surrogate measurement of the 'white-coat hypertension' effect. *J Hypertens* 1998; **16**: 23–9.

18. Staessen JA, O'Brien ET, Atkins N, Amery AK. Ambulatory blood pressure in normotensive compared with hypertensive subjects. *J Hypertens* 1993; **11**: 1289–97.

19. Mancia G. Ambulatory blood pressure monitoring: research and clinical applications. *J Hypertens* 1991; **8** (Suppl 7): S1–S13.

20. Devereux RB, Pickering TG. Relationship between the level, pattern and variability of ambulatory blood pressure and target organ damage in hypertension. *J Hypertens* 1991; **9** (Suppl 8): S34–8.

21. White WB, Dey HM, Schulman P. Assessment of the daily blood pressure load as a determinant of cardiac function in patients with mild–moderate hypertension. *Am Heart J* 1989; **118**: 782–95.

22. Burt VL, Whelton P, Roccella EJ, Brown C, Cutler JA, Higgins M, *et al.* Prevalence of hypertension in the US adult population: results from the third National Health and Nutrition Examination Survey, 1988–1991. *Hypertension* 1995; **25**: 305–13.

23. Colhoun HM, Dong W, Poulter N. Blood pressure control, screening and management and control in England, results from the Health Survey for England 1994. *J Hypertens* 1998; **16**: 747–53.

13

Surrogate measures in cardiovascular disease

Introduction

In terms of the sheer volume of evidence, the risks of uncontrolled hypertension and the benefits of antihypertensive drug treatment are indisputable. However, the association between hypertension and cardiovascular events, fatal and non-fatal, is indirect in so far as intermediate pathological processes are also implicated. Furthermore, despite the fact that blood pressure (BP) may be 'normalized', cardiovascular disease continues to account for most morbidity and mortality among treated hypertensive patients.

Amongst the most important 'intermediate' or 'surrogate' measures of hypertensive cardiovascular disease are:

1. The development of left ventricular hypertrophy;
2. The progressive changes that lead to the development of atheromatous disease of the arterial system; and
3. The appearance of microalbuminuria as a marker for renal dysfunction/damage.

Left ventricular hypertrophy

Left ventricular hypertrophy (LVH) constitutes a major independent cardiovascular risk factor such that the cardiovascular risk of the hypertensive patient is increased beyond that associated with the level of hypertension itself. For example, in the Framingham study, the presence of the 'voltage and strain' electrocardiographic pattern was associated with a doubling of the risk of cardiovascular disease relative to hypertension alone. Thus the presence of LVH is a risk factor for all the major manifestations of cardiovascular disease: for example, LVH is associated with a two- to threefold increase in non-fatal myocardial infarction and a fivefold increase in sudden cardiac death.

The electrocardiogram (ECG) diagnosis of LVH has limitations, particularly in relation to its sensitivity, and it has now largely been superseded by echocardiographic assessments, which provide a more sensitive and specific method of assessing

LVH. It is now well established that echocardiographic LVH is an important adverse prognostic factor. Overall, therefore, LVH can be regarded as a surrogate marker for the adverse cardiovascular consequence of uncontrolled hypertension.

Echocardiographic measurement

The Sixth Report of the Joint National Committee on prevention, detection, evaluation and treatment of high BP recommended that an extensive (optimal) preliminary investigation for risk stratification in the hypertensive patient should include assessment of the lipid profile, the status for diabetes and renal function/disease, and limited echocardiography. However, a fully quantitative echocardiographic examination is not universally recommended as part of the initial investigations for evaluation and management of arterial hypertension, and this primarily reflects concerns about the ability of the technique to monitor adequately changes in left ventricular geometry in individual patients. These concerns arise because of the variability of the methodology. This issue of the reproducibility and the clinical usefulness of repeated measurements of left ventricular mass (LVM) in the hypertensive patient was specifically explored in the following study.

Reliability and limitations of echocardiographic measurements of left ventricular mass for risk stratification and follow-up in single patients: the RES trial.

G de Simone, M L Muiesan, A Ganau, C Longhini, P Verdecchia, V Palmieri, *et al.*, on behalf of the Working Group on Heart and Hypertension of the Italian Society of Hypertension. *J Hypertens* 1999; **17**: 1955–63.

BACKGROUND. The objective of this study was to investigate the clinical reliability of repeated measurement of LVM in a single patient.

INTERPRETATION. Measurement of LVM in single patients allows reliable risk stratification on the basis of the presence of LVH. The probability of a true change in LVM over time is maximized for a single-reader difference greater that 9% of the initial value, although differences of 10–13% might also have clinical relevance.

In this study, M-mode echocardiography was undertaken in 261 participants and repeated, on average, 5 days later. There were 131 hypertensive and 130 normotensive patients, mean age 45 years, mean Body Mass Index 24.7 kg/m, with an equal sex distribution amongst the patients, who were recruited in 16 centres in Italy. In terms of the quality of the M-mode tracings, it was adjudged that 29% were optimal and 50% were sufficient. The salient result was that the categorical consistency was 87% for the identification of hypertensive patients with LVH. However, a significant but small degree of intra- and inter-observer variability was noted, and there was also negligible regression toward the mean.

Comment

The small but significant amount of technical variability in the M-mode measurements in this study suggests that it is not appropriate to use repeated measurement of LVM in the 'routine' or indiscriminate assessment and follow-up of patients attending a hypertension clinic. Of specific technical interest was the fact that posterior wall thickness was identified as the least reliable variable in the overall calculations used to compute LVM. However, where the measurements can be obtained systematically and according to a standardized protocol, the derived information can usefully be applied to guide the management strategy in an individual hypertensive patient. The obvious implication is that the identification of LVH should lead to intensive antihypertensive treatment, and the effectiveness of that treatment can be confirmed by the evidence of regression of LVH at a subsequent echocardiographic examination.

Regression of LVH

LVH can be regarded as an adaptive or compensatory response to increased BP and, although the focus of antihypertensive treatment should be upon BP reduction, there also should be an awareness of the potential benefits of promoting the regression of hypertension-induced structural changes. Despite the volume of evidence relating LVH to adverse cardiovascular outcomes, and despite the evidence that antihypertensive treatment may lead to the regression of LVH, the prognostic significance of the improvement in this surrogate parameter is still to be determined by an appropriate prospective study. The following study is therefore an important indicator of the potential benefits of the regression of LVH through effective antihypertensive treatment.

Prognostic significance of serial changes in left ventricular mass in essential hypertension.

P Verdecchia, G Schillaci, C Borgioni, A Ciucci, R Gattobigio, I Zampi, *et al.*
Circulation 1998; **97**: 48–54.

BACKGROUND. Increased left ventricular mass (LVM) predicts an adverse outcome in patients with essential hypertension. The purpose of this study was to determine the relation between changes in LVM during antihypertensive treatment and subsequent prognosis.

INTERPRETATION. In essential hypertension, a reduction in LVM during treatment is a favourable prognostic marker that predicts a lesser risk for subsequent cardiovascular morbid events. Such an association is independent of baseline LVM, baseline clinical and ambulatory BP, and degree of BP reduction.

This study of 430 patients with essential hypertension involved 24-hour ambulatory BP measurements in addition to echocardiography before and after antihypertensive drug treatment. During the follow-up, 31 patients suffered a first morbid cardiovascular event, but with an event rate of 1.78 per 100 person-years in the group with a decrease in LVM and a significantly greater event rate of 3.03 per 100 person-years in the group with an increase in LVM (P=0.029). Further statistical analysis in the group at lesser cardiovascular risk (i.e. with a decrease in LVM during treatment) identified that the benefit was independent of age and baseline LVH on the ECG. This finding was confirmed in the subset with increased LVM at baseline: thus, those who achieved regression of LVH had a lower event rate of 1.08 per 100 person-years compared to those patients who did not achieve regression of LVH, who had an event rate of 6.27 per 100 person-years.

Comment

The most important result of this study is that the reduction of LVM in response to treatment in otherwise uncomplicated essential hypertension had a favourable impact on prognosis because it was predictive of a lesser risk for the development of subsequent cardiovascular disease. This benefit was independent of baseline LVM, baseline clinic and ambulatory BPs and the BP responses to antihypertensive drug treatment. It must be recognized, however, that this is a relatively small study in relatively young hypertensive patients with a relatively short duration of follow-up. Nevertheless, the results of other ongoing clinical trials should confirm whether or not the results of this observational study are valid. Despite these reservations, however, this is an important study because it also suggests that M-mode echocardiography is a clinically valuable and cost-effective investigation because it permits the risk stratification of patients with essential hypertension. Thus those who fail to achieve a reduction in LVM or regression of LVH should be considered at increased risk for subsequent cardiovascular disease and, accordingly, targeted for a more aggressive therapeutic approach.

LVH: causative factors

Mechanical effects of hypertension

Hypertension leads to an increase in wall stress, and this is the fundamental stimulus for the development of LVH. However, a number of other factors contributes to the increased risk of adverse cardiovascular outcomes, and these include myocardial ischaemia, coexisting coronary artery disease, left ventricular dysfunction, structural myocardial changes and ventricular arrhythmias. Initially, however, hypertrophy of the left ventricular myocardium is a compensatory response attempting to restore wall stress to a normal level and thereby preserving left ventricular systolic function and reducing the possibility of myocardial perfusion abnormalities. However, this adaptive response is not limitless, and eventually there is a deterioration in both cardiac function and myocardial perfusion if the BP remains elevated.

Neuroendocrine factors

In addition to the mechanical effects, 'stretching' of the myocardium promotes protein synthesis and activation of a number of important cellular signals, which also contribute to the development of cardiac hypertrophy. The adrenergic and renin–angiotensin–aldosterone systems have also been implicated in the pathogenesis of LVH, and there is a wealth of experimental evidence implicating, in particular, angiotensin II and aldosterone. For example, angiotensin II has direct cardiac actions that stimulate cardiac contractility, increase protein synthesis, etc., and it also has indirect actions via the effects of aldosterone, which is implicated in myocyte hypertrophy and myocardial fibrosis. While the experimental evidence is voluminous in implicating angiotensin II as a necessary mechanistic factor, there are some inconsistencies.

Pressure overload induces cardiac hypertrophy in angiotensin II type 1A receptor knock-out mice.

K Harada, I Komuro, I Shiojima, D Hayashi, S Kudoh, T Mizuno, *et al.* *Circulation* 1998; **97**: 1952–9.

BACKGROUND. **Many studies have suggested that the renin–angiotensin system plays an important role in the development of pressure overload-induced cardiac hypertrophy. Moreover, it has been reported that pressure overload-induced cardiac hypertrophy is completely prevented by angiotensin-converting enzyme (ACE) inhibitors in vivo and that the stored angiotensin II (Ang II) is released from cardiac myocytes in response to mechanical stretch and induces cardiomyocyte hypertrophy through the Ang II type I receptor (AT_1) in vitro.**

INTERPRETATION. AT_1-mediated Ang II signalling is not essential for the development of pressure overload-induced cardiac hypertrophy.

Comment

This is an interesting experiment in which a 'knock-out' mouse model still developed LVH despite being totally deficient in angiotensin II (AT_1) receptors. This finding clearly raises doubts about the proposed central and causative role of the renin–angiotensin–aldosterone system in the development of LVH in man. At a more philosophical level, the finding also sounds a cautionary note about the risk of directly and simplistically extrapolating from experimental to clinical evidence!

Regression of LVH by antihypertensive drug treatment

A question which is frequently asked is, 'Which antihypertensive drug is most effective in promoting the regression of LVH?' Unfortunately, there is no individual study in which an adequate number of patients has been appropriately randomized in a double-blind manner to one or two (or more) treatments and assessed after not less than 6 months of treatment with a validated measure of LVM. Accordingly, much reliance has been placed on meta-analytical techniques, despite the well-recognized shortcomings of this approach. In some of these meta-analyses, and in line with the experimental evidence, ACE inhibitor drugs appear to be the most effective, agents for promoting regression of LVH. Correspondingly, there is an overall impression that beta-blockers are not particularly effective and there is the suggestion for thiazide diuretics that part of their measured effect is attributable to their volume-depleting action, leading to shrinkage of the left ventricular cavity, which is then interpreted as an overall reduction in LVM.

The shortcomings of meta-analytical techniques are considerable because they depend on the 'quality' of the studies that are included (or not included). For example, in one meta-analysis in which basic criteria of inclusion were pre-defined, such as the incorporation of only randomized studies comparing two or more treatments and with a blinded measurement technique, only 39 of 471 published studies fulfilled the relevant criteria |**1**|. In this particular analysis, ACE inhibitor drugs appeared to be associated with the greatest reduction in LVM by 13.3%, followed by calcium channel blockers at 9.3%, diuretics at 6.8% and beta-blockers at 5.5%. While this result appears to support the widely held view that ACE inhibitor drugs are the most effective agents for promoting the regression of LV hypertrophy, different meta-analyses using different criteria give different results.

Reversibility of left ventricular hypertrophy and malfunction by antihypertensive treatment.

G L Jennings, J Wong. In: L Hansson, W H Birkenhäger (eds). *Handbook of Hypertension. Volume 18: Assessment of Hypertensive Organ Damage.* Amsterdam: Elsevier Science 1997, p. 6.

BACKGROUND. **Cardiac hypertrophy is a feature of many of the common cardiovascular diseases including ischaemic heart disease, cardiomyopathies, valvular disease and hypertension. For the most part, treatment has been directed towards alleviating factors contributing to cardiac load, implying that hypertrophy is generally secondary to mechanical stretch. In hypertension, however, there has been considerable discussion on the strategies for optimal regression of cardiac hypertension as a goal of treatment of changes in BP.**

INTERPRETATION. The reasons for the recent emphasis on regression of cardiac hypertrophy in hypertension are multiple. They include the recognition from epidemiological data that left ventricular hypertrophy (LVH) is a potent marker of outcome, and is particularly associated with risk of sudden death. Basic studies have shown that factors other than mechanical load can influence the development of LVH and its regression. These considerations lead to the following important questions that are the subject of this chapter: does regression of LVH occur in human hypertension, is regression beneficial, when it does occur, and do different antihypertensive therapies exert selective effects on cardiac hypertrophy independent of their effects on blood pressure?

Comment

This comprehensive review and meta-analysis calculates a closer comparability in the effectiveness of the different classes of antihypertensive drug (see Fig. 13.1). Earlier indications that beta-blockers might be the least effective class in promoting regression of LVH appear to be confirmed, but there is no confirmation of any clear benefits attributable to ACE inhibitor drugs, since the ACE inhibitor group and the calcium channel blocker group appear to be similar. Furthermore, despite insinuations about changes in internal diameter being misinterpreted as changes in LVM, the overall effectiveness of thiazide diuretics appears to be consistent with the effects of other drugs. In summary, effective BP control with treatment based upon an ACE inhibitor or a calcium channel blocker or a thiazide diuretic leads to similar reductions in LVM.

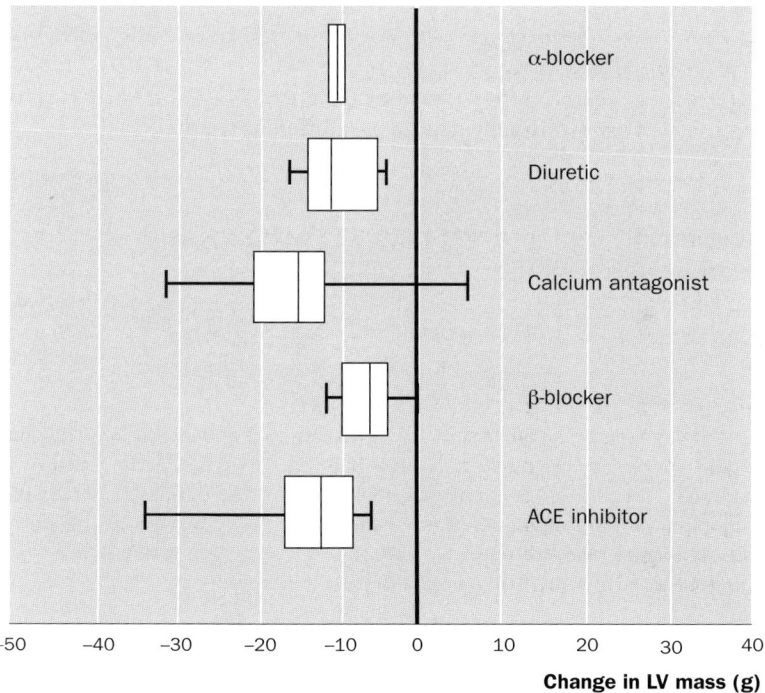

Fig. 13.1 Effectiveness of different classes of hypertensive drug in promoting regression of left ventricular (LV) hypertrophy (adapted from Jennings and Wong 1997). ACE = angiotensin-converting enzyme.

Confirmation of the effectiveness of thiazide diuretics in promoting the regression of LVH is provided in the following paper.

Effect of treatment of isolated systolic hypertension on left ventricular mass.

E O Ofili, J D Cohen, J A St Vrain, A Pearson, T J Martin, N D Uy, *et al.*
JAMA 1998; **279**: 778–80.

BACKGROUND. **Left ventricular hypertrophy (LVH) is a common problem among elderly patients with isolated systolic hypertension (ISH), but the effect of treatment of ISH on left ventricular mass (LVM) is not known.**

INTERPRETATION. Treatment of ISH with a diuretic-based regimen reduced LVM. This was a subgroup study of 104 patients who participated in the Systolic Hypertension in the Elderly Programme (SHEP), in which it was shown conclusively that antihypertensive treatment (based upon the diuretic, chlorthalidone) was associated with significant cardiovascular benefits, particularly through a 36% reduction in stroke events. In this substudy with a minimum follow-up of 3 years, 80% of subjects continued to receive

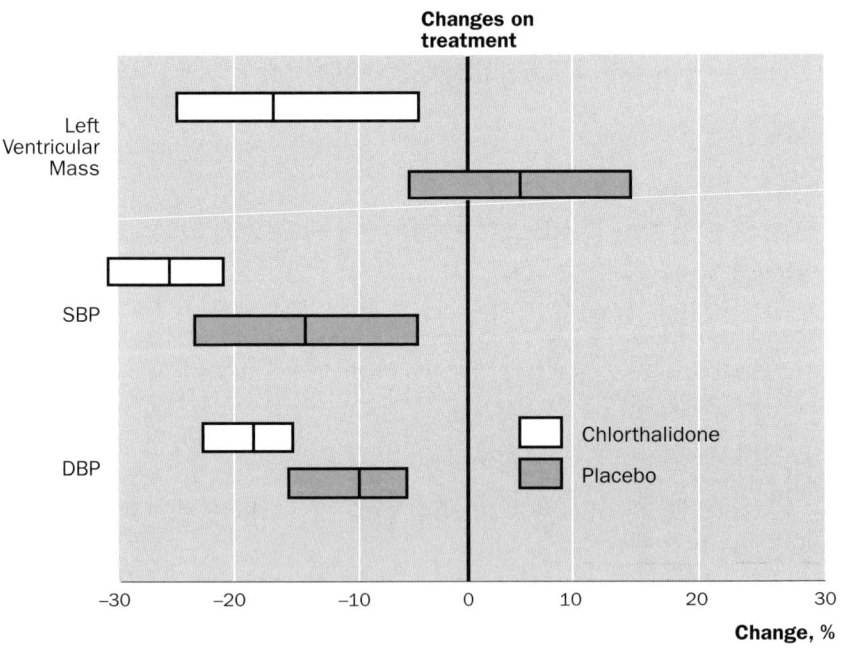

Fig. 13.2 Effect of antihypertensive treatment with chlorthalidone diuretic on left ventricular mass (adapted from Ofili *et al.*, 1998). SBP = systolic blood pressure; DBP = diastolic blood pressure.

treatment with chlorthalidone alone by the end of year 3. The LVM index declined by an average of 13% in the active group compared to a 6% increase in the placebo group (see Fig. 13.2). According to a multivariate analysis, the change in LVM was significantly correlated with the change in BP, particularly the reduction in SBP (r=0.40; P<0.003). The reduction in LVM in the active treatment group reflected an actual decrease in wall thickness, since there were insignificant effects on LV end diastolic dimension (5% reduction with chlorthalidone compared to a 2% reduction in the placebo group).

Summary

Overall, no class of drug can be clearly and consistently shown to be superior for the treatment of LVH, although at least there now appears to be overall agreement that beta-blockers are the least effective group. Other antihypertensive drug classes generally have comparable effects with, on average, 12–13% reductions in LVM. Whilst there may be differential drug effects, as identified in the experimental setting, it has not proved possible to confirm these effects in clinical studies.

Similarly, it has not proved possible to demonstrate clearly that factors other than blood pressure reduction are important in promoting reductions in LVM in hypertensive patients. It is obviously possible that subtle mechanistic changes are simply overwhelmed by the beneficial effects of good BP control. Thus, on the basis of the available clinical evidence, it appears that the reduction in LVM is primarily influenced by the magnitude of the BP reduction and the duration of effective anti-hypertensive drug treatment, rather than by the class of drug itself.

Atheromatous vascular disease

Hypertension, along with cigarette smoking, hypercholesterolaemia and diabetes, is associated with 'premature vascular ageing' and the development of atheromatous vascular disease. These two recent review commentaries have illustrated the current areas of research interest and highlighted the potential role of vascular measurements as surrogate markers for the cardiovascular risk of hypertension.

Arterial mechanics predict cardiovascular risk in hypertension.
M E Safar, J-P Siche, J-M Mallion, G M London. *J Hypertens* 1997; **15**: 1605–11.

BACKGROUND. **Systolic and diastolic BP are the exclusive mechanical factors considered as predictors of cardiovascular risk for members of populations of normotensive and hypertensive subjects. However, if hypertension is considered as a mechanical factor acting on the arterial wall with deleterious consequences, the totality of the BP curve should be considered in order to investigate the risk.**

INTERPRETATION. The purpose of this review is to show that in addition to systolic and diastolic BPs, other haemodynamic indexes with particular relevance for cardiac complications and that originate from pulsatile pressure should be taken into account, namely brachial pulse pressure, pulse pressure amplification, early wave reflections and pulse wave velocity.

Vessel wall properties and cardiovascular risk.
R Cockcroft, I B Wilkinson. *J Hum Hypertens* 1998; **12**: 343–4.

BACKGROUND. **Stiffening of the arteries, resulting in decreased compliance, is a consequence of the normal ageing process. It is accompanied by an increase in systolic and pulse pressure, and an increased risk of cardiovascular morbidity or mortality. Risk factors for the development of atherosclerosis, such as hypertension, diabetes, hypercholesterolaemia, smoking and obesity are associated with 'premature vascular ageing' and increased arterial stiffness.**

INTERPRETATION. To date, both primary and secondary prevention of coronary heart disease has focused almost exclusively on modification of conventional risk factors. However, accumulating evidence suggests that increased vascular stiffness is not just a marker for atheromatous disease, but may also be an important additional risk factor, promoting atherogenesis and acting as a link between existing risk factors and cardiovascular disease.

Comment
These reviews summarize the current thinking relating to pulse pressure, arterial stiffness or compliance, intima–media thickness and endothelial function. The following studies illustrate some of the clinical applications.

Carotid-artery intima and media thickness as a risk factor for myocardial infarction and stroke in older adults.
D H O'Leary, J F Polak, R A Kronmal, T A Manolio, G L Burke, S K Wolfson, for the Cardiovascular Health Study Collaborative Research Group. *N Engl J Med* 1999; **340**: 14–22.

BACKGROUND. **The combined thickness of the intima and media of the carotid artery is associated with the prevalence of cardiovascular disease. The authors studied the associations between the thickness of the carotid artery intima and media and the incidence of new myocardial infarction or stroke in persons without clinical cardiovascular disease.**

INTERPRETATION. Increases in the thickness of the intima and media of the carotid artery, as measured non-invasively by ultrasonography, are directly associated with an increased risk of myocardial infarction and stroke in older adults without a history of cardiovascular disease.

This was a large study of 5858 subjects aged 65 years or more in whom non-invasive measurements of the intima and media of the common and internal carotid arteries were made with high-resolution ultrasonography. Correlations were then sought with a range of outcome variables over a median follow-up period of 6.2 years. The incidence of cardiovascular events correlated with measurements of carotid artery intima–media (IM) thickness. A relative risk of 3.87 for myocardial infarction or stroke (adjusted for age and sex) was calculated for the quintile with the highest IM thickness as compared with the quintile with the lowest IM thickness. The association between cardiovascular events and IM thickness remained significant after adjustment for traditional risk factors. The results of the separate analysis for myocardial infarction and stroke paralleled those for their combined endpoint.

Comment

In this analysis of elderly subjects there were clear correlations between the development of atherosclerotic vascular disease, as assessed by IM thickness, and adverse cardiovascular outcomes, particularly myocardial infarction and stroke.

Although the volume of information is significantly less for IM thickness, there are clear parallels with LVH in their respective roles as surrogate markers for cardiovascular disease. For example, as for echocardiographic assessment of LVM, methodological concerns remain about the reproducibility of the measurements such that specific methodological validation analyses have been undertaken.

Baseline reproducibility of B-mode ultrasonic measurement of carotid artery intima–media thickness: the European Lacidipine Study on Atherosclerosis (ELSA).

R Tang, M Hennig, B Thomasson, R Scherz, R Ravinetto, R Catalini, *et al.* for the ELSA Investigators. *J Hypertens* 2000; **18**: 197–201.

BACKGROUND. The European Lacidipine Study on Atherosclerosis (ELSA) is a prospective, randomized, double-blind, multinational interventional trial to determine the effect of 4-year treatment using the calcium antagonist lacidipine versus the beta-blocker atenolol on the progression of carotid atherosclerosis in 2259 asymptomatic hypertensive patients.

INTERPRETATION. The results demonstrate that by implementing standardized protocols and strict quality control procedures, highly reliable ultrasonic measurements of carotid artery IM thickness can be achieved in large multinational trials.

IM thickness was measured by B-mode ultrasound in this evaluation, which sought to establish the acceptability and reproducibility of this technique. Each patient was scanned twice at baseline and scanned again at four annual visits, with 80% of the replicate scans being performed by the same observer; 50% of the replicate scans were read by the same reader. The overall coefficient of the reliability was 0.859 for the maximum IM thickness of the carotid bifurcation (CBM_{max}), 0.872 for the mean maximum IM thickness of 12 standard sites on the common carotid artery (M_{max}) and 0.794 for the overall maximum IM thickness (T_{max}). The reliability for CBM_{max} was stable during the baseline period ($r=0.848$ to 0.953) and was uniform among the 23 field centres ($r=0.798$ to 0.926) with intra- and inter-reader reliabilities of 0.915 and 0.872, respectively.

Comment

The ELSA study is one of many that have used intima–media (IM) thickness of the carotid artery wall as a surrogate marker for cardiovascular morbidity and mortality. However, because of methodological shortcomings in previous studies, particular care was taken to standardize the procedures of measurement and to demonstrate the reproducibility (and, thereby, the clinical usefulness) of the techniques.

Summary

The first study confirms that IM thickness is an appropriate surrogate marker for adverse cardiovascular outcomes. The second study, the ELSA study, illustrates the methodological requirements for standardizing the procedures to make the technique sufficiently reproducible for the clinical purpose of prospective long-term evaluations. Unfortunately, earlier attempts to apply these techniques in clinical studies have typically been confounded by a lack of reproducibility in the measurement techniques. It is hoped that the results of the ELSA study can clarify whether or not baseline measurements of IM thickness and the changes induced by treatment are predictive of morbid and mortal cardiovascular events.

IM thickness obviously reflects structural changes in the vessel wall, but there is considerable research interest in the associated functional changes that accompany and, presumably, precede the processes involved in the structural alterations. Endothelial function/dysfunction is thought to be one of the most important early indicators of vascular disease. Whether endothelial dysfunction is a risk factor or only a risk marker, however, remains a subject of debate.

Endothelial dysfunction in cardiovascular disease: risk factor, risk marker, or surrogate endpoint?
H L Elliott. *J Cardiovasc Pharmacol* 1998; **32** (Suppl 3): S67–S73.

BACKGROUND. Endothelial dysfunction is a feature of the early stages of atherosclerotic cardiovascular disease. It also is almost invariably associated with the recognized cardiovascular risk factors, including those that are irreversible (such as age and family history) and those that are reversible (such as hypertension and hypercholesterolaemia). It remains a subject of debate whether endothelial dysfunction can be considered to be an independent risk factor or, perhaps more plausibly, an intermediate or surrogate endpoint.

INTERPRETATION. While the relevance to research into cardiovascular pathophysio-logy is not in dispute, there remains uncertainty about its relevance as a therapeutic target. Overall, the available evidence suggests that targeting of the conventional, major risk factors remains the primary strategy, but an ancillary effect on intermediate endpoints, such as an improvement in or reversal of endothelial dysfunction, constitutes an additional potential benefit.

Comment

This short review focuses attention upon the clinical issues surrounding endothelial dysfunction. It is not yet possible to answer definitively the question that was posed; but there is no doubt that endothelial dysfunction is the earliest manifestation of vascular disease, albeit as a non-specific response to a range of insults including hypertension, dyslipidaemia, diabetes mellitus and cigarette smoking. There is not yet sufficient outcome evidence to confirm whether or not endothelial function can be considered to be a surrogate endpoint (in the same way as LVH or carotid IM thickness, for example), but there are clinical studies investigating whether or not treatment can induce beneficial changes and whether or not these changes can lead to outcome benefits beyond the obvious factors such as BP control or lipid-lowering treatment.

Nifedipine improves endothelial function in hypercholesterolaemia, independently of an effect on blood pressure or plasma lipids.

M C Verhaar, M L H Honing, T van Dam, M Zwart, H A Koomans, J J P Kastelein, *et al. Cardiovasc Res* 1999; **42**: 752–60.

BACKGROUND. **Dihydropyridine calcium antagonists have been shown to retard atherogenesis in animal models and to prevent the development of early angiographic lesions in human coronary arteries. Endothelial dysfunction is an early event in the pathogenesis of cardiovascular disease. The authors investigated whether nifedipine could improve endothelial function in hypercholesterolaemia, independently of changes in BP or plasma lipids.**

INTERPRETATION. These data show that nifedipine improves endothelial function in hypercholesterolaemia. It is suggested from the in vitro experiments that this effect is due to reduced nitric oxide (NO) degradation.

This study employed forearm venous occlusion plethysmography to assess the vasodilator responses to endothelium-dependent and endothelium-independent vasodilators in 11 patients with familial hypercholesterolaemia before and after 6 weeks' treatment with nifedipine Gastrointestinal Therapeutic System (GITS) and in 12 matched controls. In a subgroup of six control subjects forearm vascular function was also assessed before and after 6 weeks of nifedipine GITS treatment. The salient results were that endothelium-dependent vasodilatation was impaired in hypercholesterolaemic subjects, with only a 47% increase in forearm blood flow compared to a 99% increase in the control subjects. Treatment with nifedipine completely restored endothelium-dependent vasodilation, whereas it had no influence on basal forearm blood flow or endothelium-independent vasodilation. Nifedipine did not alter forearm vascular responses in the control subjects and did not significantly alter BP or plasma lipids. These in vivo investigations were supported by in-vitro investigations in which NO production was unaltered by nifedipine but production of the NO antagonist, superoxide, was impaired. For this reason, the authors concluded that nifedipine improves endothelial function by a mechanism that reflects reduced NO degradation.

Effects of calcium antagonism and HMG-coenzyme reductase inhibition on endothelial function and atherosclerosis: rationale and outline of the ENCORE trials.

G Sütsch, M Büchi, A M Zeither, T Meinertz, P G Hugenholtz, R Jenni, *et al.* on behalf of the ENCORE Trial Investigators. *Eur Heart J* 1999; **1** (Suppl M): M27–M32.

BACKGROUND. **For ENCORE I, four groups of 100 patients each with coronary artery disease (CAD) undergoing percutaneous transluminal coronary angioplasty (PTCA) will be recruited. After PTCA, endothelial function is assessed by intracoronary methods, i.e. infusion of increasing dosages of acetylcholine in a non-obstructed coronary segment. Coronary responses to acetylcholine will be measured by quantitative coronary angiography (QCA) and Doppler flow velocity measurements. Endothelial-independent responses are tested by i.c. adenosine and nitroglycerine, respectively. Patients will then be randomly assigned in a double-blind fashion to four treatment groups: placebo, nifedipine (30–60 mg/day) or their combination. Studies will be repeated at 6 months. This trial will determine whether or not in patients with CAD calcium antagonists and/or a statin alone or in combination improve endothelial function within 6 months.**

INTERPRETATION. The ENCORE II trial will last 2 years, and aims at correlating endothelial function (as assessed by QCA and intravascular ultrasound, IVUS) and structural atherosclerosis in patients treated with cerivastatin, 200 receiving 200 μg/day and 200 receiving 800 μg/day, compared with 200 patients having a combination treatment with cerivastatin (800 μg/day) and nifedipine (30–60 mg). Endothelial-dependent responses of epicardial coronary arteries to acetylcholine at baseline as well as structural vascular changes as assessed by IVUS will be correlated and followed over 2 years. At the end of the 2 years another acetylcholine test, QCA and IVUS will be performed.

The principal aim of these complementary studies is an assessment of endothelium-dependent responses in patients with known CAD. Treatment will be with a calcium channel blocker and a statin, alone or in combination, and the follow-up assessments will determine whether endothelial dysfunction and/or its improvement is associated with progression or regression of atherosclerotic CAD and possibly with clinical events.

Summary

The first study illustrates the clinical research approach to assessing endothelial function in human subjects. The study is well-designed and carefully conducted but, as the authors concede, it was not a randomized, placebo-controlled assessment. Nevertheless, the conclusion that treatment with the calcium channel blocker, nifedipine, improves endothelial function in hypercholesterolaemia suggests that there may be benefit from this pharmacological intervention beyond any simple change in BP or serum cholesterol. The larger ENCORE trials seek to extend this concept of an additional and potentially protective vascular effect by investigating patients with known vascular disease. There is, however, an immediate difference in so far as these patients will already have structural vascular changes, whereas these would be absent or at a much less advanced stage in the subjects studied by Verhaar and colleagues. While the results of the ENCORE trials, and particularly the results in terms of clinical events, are awaited with interest, it may be that the pre-existing structural changes will compromise the identification of any functional improvement attributable to the drug treatments beyond their lipid- and BP-lowering effects.

Microalbuminuria

Microalbuminuria is defined as a urinary albumin concentration of 30–200 mg/l and is thought to reflect the glomerular manifestation of a systemic capillary leak |2|. Microalbuminuria is used clinically to monitor incipient diabetic nephropathy, but it is also known to be a useful predictor of outcome, including mortality, in a number of clinical situations, including hypertension |3|.

Microalbuminuria predicts cardiovascular events and renal insufficiency in patients with essential hypertension.

R Bigazzi, S Bianchi, D Baldari, V M Campese. *J Hypertens* 1998; **16**: 1325–33.

BACKGROUND. Some patients with essential hypertension manifest greater than normal urinary albumin excretion (UAE). Authors of a few retrospective studies have suggested that there is an association between microalbuminuria and cardiovascular risk.

INTERPRETATION. This study suggests that hypertensive individuals with microalbuminuria manifest a greater incidence of cardiovascular events and a greater decline in renal function than do patients with normal UAE.

This was a retrospective cohort analysis of 141 hypertensive patients who were followed up for approximately 7 years. In this study, microalbuminuria was defined as an average UAE in the range 30–300 mg/24 hours in three urine collections obtained at baseline. At baseline, 54 of these patients had microalbuminuria and 87 patients had a normal urinary albumin excretion rate (AER). The two groups were similar in age, weight, BP and creatinine clearance rates, although the serum levels of cholesterol and uric acid were higher in those with microalbuminuria, whereas high-density lipoprotein cholesterol was lower in those with microalbuminuria. During follow-up, 12 cardiovascular events occurred in the patients with microalbuminuria (an event rate of 21.3%), whereas only two such events occurred in the 87 patients with a normal urinary AER ($P<0.0002$). Additionally, the creatinine clearance rates decreased more rapidly in the patients with microalbuminuria at outset, with a rate of decline of 12.1 ml/min versus 7.1 ml/min. A stepwise logistic regression analysis showed that UAE, cholesterol concentration and diastolic BP were independent predictors of adverse cardiovascular outcomes.

Treatment of diabetic nephropathy

It is a widely held view that ACE inhibitor drugs might have effects beyond BP reduction and an added ability to provide renal protection. While there is no doubt that an ACE inhibitor is the cornerstone of treatment for diabetic nephropathy, there remains some doubt as to whether or not there are benefits beyond BP reduction.

Randomized placebo-controlled trial of lisinopril in normotensive patients with insulin-dependent diabetes and normoalbuminuria or microalbuminuria.
The EUCLID Study Group. *Lancet* 1997; **349**: 1787–92.

BACKGROUND. Renal disease in people with insulin-dependent diabetes (IDDM) continues to pose a major health threat. Inhibitors of angiotensin-converting enzyme (ACE) slow the decline of renal function in advanced renal disease, but their effects at earlier stages are unclear, and the degree of albuminuria at which treatment should start is not yet known.

INTERPRETATION. Lisinopril slows the progression of renal disease in normotensive IDDM patients with little or no albuminuria, although the greatest effect was in those with microalbuminuria (AER ≥ 20 µg/min). Our results show lisinopril does not increase the risk of hypoglycaemic events in IDDM.

This was a randomized, double-blind, placebo-controlled trial of the ACE inhibitor lisinopril in 530 men and women with type 1 diabetes mellitus and with normoalbuminuria or microalbuminuria. All patients were considered to be normotensive, with BP not more than 155/90 mmHg. On entry, the mean BP was 121/80 in the placebo group and 122/79 mmHg in the lisinopril group. The great majority of patients had normal albuminuria, with only 14% in the placebo group and 19% in the lisinopril group having micro- or macroalbuminuria. For patients who completed 24 months in the trial there was a significant difference in albuminuria, with a reduction by 38.5 µg/min in those with microalbuminuria at baseline (P=0.001) and by 0.23 µg/min in those with normal albuminuria at baseline (P=0.6). The principal conclusion from this study was that lisinopril was of clinical benefit in patients with type 1 diabetes mellitus who have early signs of renal disease without hypertension. The authors additionally recommended that the treatment of early-stage renal disease, even in normotensive patients, should include an ACE inhibitor drug.

Comment

This is another paper that demonstrates the ability of ACE inhibitor drug treatment to improve the clinical profile of diabetic patients with a significant reduction in albumin excretion rate. This adds to the volume of information that ACE inhibition is an important initial treatment in such patients. However, it should be noted that there was a small but significant difference in BP in the two groups, whereby DBP was 77 mmHg in the placebo group and 74 mmHg in the lisinopril group (P=0.0001). This BP difference was maintained throughout the rest of the trial. Once again this raises the issue as to whether or not the improvements in UAE were attributable to ACE inhibition or, simply, to BP reduction.

Effects of intensified antihypertensive treatment in diabetic nephropathy: mortality and morbidity results of a prospective controlled 10-year study.
A K Trocha, C Schmidtke, U Didjurgeit, I Mühlhauser, R Bender, M Berger, et al. *J Hypertens* 1999; **17**: 1497–503.

BACKGROUND. The aim of this study was to describe the effect of intensified antihypertensive therapy based on a structured teaching and treatment programme on the prognosis of hypertension type 1 (insulin-dependent) diabetic patients with kidney disease.

INTERPRETATION. Intensified antihypertensive treatment, based on a hypertension teaching and treatment programme, reduces long-term morbidity and mortality in patients with diabetic nephropathy.

This was a controlled, prospective, parallel group study, albeit in a relatively small number of 91 hypertensive patients with type 1 diabetes mellitus. Patients were assigned to intensified antihypertensive treatment, with specialist follow-up, or to routine antihypertensive treatment as provided by family physicians, local hospitals and consultants. During the follow-up period of 10 years, there were 7 deaths in the intensive treatment group and 22 deaths in the routine treatment group (P=0.0008), and a cardiovascular cause was identified in 3 and 17 of these patients, respectively. For one of the main secondary endpoints, namely renal replacement treatment, 11 patients in the intensified group reached regular dialysis treatment compared to 18 patients in the routine treatment group. Of particular interest was the antihypertensive drug treatment

Table 13.1 Antihypertensive treatment in diabetic nephropathy: blood pressure (BP) control

	Intensified group	Routine group	Significance
Baseline	$^{154}/_{92}$	$^{143}/_{87}$	*P<0.05 for both systolic and diastolic BP
Year 5	$^{148}/_{85}$	$^{156}/_{88}$	*P<0.005 for the systolic BP difference
Year 10	$^{151}/_{87}$	$^{150}/_{89}$	

Adapted from Trocha *et al.* (1999).

Table 13.2 Antihypertensive treatment in diabetic nephropathy: choice of drug

	Intensified group		Routine group	
	5Y	**10Y**	**5Y**	**10Y**
ACE inhibitors	12	41	43	41
Beta-blockers	69	60	27	33
Calcium channel blockers	41	46	39	41
Diuretics	67	76	52	63

Adapted from Trocha *et al.* (1999).

regimen in the two groups. After 10 years of treatment, 41% of patients in both groups were receiving an ACE inhibitor (Table 13.1). Thus in terms of 'exposure' to ACE inhibition there was no difference between the two groups to explain the differences in outcome. However, there were significant differences in the blood pressure values and in the number of antihypertensive drugs, which averaged 2.2 after 5 years and 2.7 after 10 years in the intensified treatment group, compared to corresponding numbers of 1.6 and 2.1 in the routine treatment group (Table 13.2).

Comment

This is an interesting study from which the principal message appears to be that intensified antihypertensive drug treatment and improved BP control is more important than the pharmacological characteristics of any given antihypertensive drug class. It is also important to note that multiple drug treatments were inevitably required to achieve this control, and these findings are entirely consistent with the outcome benefits produced by 'tight' BP control with combinations of antihypertensive drugs [4].

Conclusion

Although BP is the most extensively studied of the cardiovascular risk factors, it must be recognized that its measurement is both indirect and relatively crude, and that an elevation of BP predisposes to intermediate cardiovascular changes prior to the development of morbid and mortal events. In our attempts to refine our approaches to patient management, and also to define which patients are at greatest risk, attention has recently been focused on a number of intermediate or surrogate endpoints.

As has been described for the cases of LVH, vascular changes and micro-albuminuria, there are clear and important correlations between the surrogate endpoints and adverse cardiovascular outcomes, and there is also evidence that therapeutic intervention can exert a beneficial influence. However, the method-ologies are not simple and not readily applicable in routine practice. There is only limited evidence that improvement in the surrogate measure leads to outcome benefit, i.e. a reduction in cardiovascular events, and there is not yet clear evidence that ancillary properties add significantly to the benefits of BP reduction. Thus although it is important to continue to study these intermediate factors and to try to modify them, at the present time the balance of evidence suggests that 'tight' BP control is the primary requirement. The practical message therefore remains that BP control is more important than pharmacological characteristics.

References

1. Schmieder RE, Martus P, Klingbeil A. Reversal of left ventricular hypertrophy in essen-tial hypertension: a meta-analysis of randomised double-blind studies. *JAMA* 1996; **275**: 1507–13.

2. Jensen JS, Borch-Johnsen K, Jensen G, Feldt-Rasmussen B. Microalbuminuria reflects a generalised transvascular albumin leakiness in clinical healthy subjects. *Clin Sci* 1995; **88**: 629–33.

3. Damsgaard EM, Froland A, Jorgensen OD, Mogensen CE. Microalbuminuria as predic-tor of increased mortality in elderly people. *BMJ* 1990; **300**: 297–300.

4. United Kingdom Prospective Diabetes Study Group. Tight blood pressure control and risk of macrovascular and microvascular complications in type II diabetes: UKPDS 38. *BMJ* 1998; **317**: 703–13.

14

Cost-effectiveness in cardiovascular therapeutics

Introduction

The cost implications of providing optimal treatment for cardiovascular disorders are the subject of considerable debate at the present time. In the UK, for example, where cardiovascular disease constitutes the single most common cause of death, the focus continues to be on prevention and treatment of coronary heart disease (CHD) and its complications, using strategies for which there is clear evidence from clinical trials. However, there would be substantial cost implications if the primary and secondary prevention of CHD were to be undertaken with the drug treatments, entry criteria and treatment targets defined in these clinical trials. Thus to control these costs, and to maximize the absolute benefits in terms of preventing the greatest number of cardiovascular events, there are strong recommendations for identifying and treating patients at the highest risk of developing a major cardiovascular event within the next 5–10 years. Among the most important practical issues for the general practitioner, therefore, are effective hypertension management and cost-effective strategies for reducing cholesterol, particularly in patients at high cardiovascular risk.

Unfortunately, in the UK and in many countries throughout the world, concerns about costs continue to hamper efforts to implement the strategies that are known to be effective for the primary and secondary prevention of cardiovascular disease. This applies particularly to the drug treatment of hypertension and hypercholesterolaemia—for which the clinical trial evidence of benefit is strongest—and the problems are especially well illustrated in the recommendations for the use of lipid-lowering drug treatments (statins). For example, in the UK it is recommended that statin treatment should be targeted to those patients with a 3% (or greater) annual risk of a major CHD event. However, drug treatment for hypertension is recommended for those with an annual CHD risk above 1.5%. Thus there is a paradox, whereby the patient whose 'risk' is attributable to hypertension warrants treatment, but the patient with an identical 'risk' due to hypercholesterolaemia does not warrant treatment; this creates considerable confusion. Furthermore, there is no evidence base for this arbitrary distinction because there is already clinical trial evidence (in the AFCAPS/TexCAPS study [1]) that there are outcome benefits if lipid-lowering drug treatment is administered to patients with an annual CHD risk as low as 0.6%. However, the additional patient load and the necessary lipid-lowering drug costs are deemed to be 'unaffordable' at the present time. As a consequence of such cost concerns and financial constraints, there is currently an undue emphasis on drug acquisition costs and a tendency to use the least expensive drug, on the assumption that this will automatically be the most cost-effective treatment.

Cost-effective antihypertensive drug treatment

With respect to a single drug class, it is fortunate in hypertension that the greatest volume of evidence has been derived from studies using the least expensive antihypertensive drug as the baseline treatment, i.e. thiazide diuretics. Furthermore, with the shift in emphasis towards the treatment of patients at high risk of cardiovascular disease, and with the increasing number of elderly hypertensives in Westernized societies, there is an increasing demand that resources be directed towards the treatment of elderly patients. In short, targeting treatment to elderly hypertensive patients is effective and evidence-based and it is also justifiable on the basis that it is extremely cost-effective. However, the question arises: are there hidden costs with thiazide diuretics because of their well-recognized adverse metabolic effects: glucose intolerance, adverse lipid effects, hypocalaemia, etc.?

Influence of long-term, low-dose, diuretic-based, antihypertensive therapy on glucose, lipid, uric acid, and potassium levels in older men and women with isolated systolic hypertension.

P J Savage, S L Pressel, D Curb, E B Schrom, W B Applegate, H R Black, *et al.*, for the SHEP Cooperative Research Group. *Arch Intern Med* 1998; **158**: 741–51.

BACKGROUND. **Earlier studies, often of short duration, have raised concerns that antihypertensive therapy with diuretics and beta-blockers adversely alters levels of other cardiovascular disease risk factors.**

INTERPRETATION. Antihypertensive therapy with low-dose chlorthalidone (supplemented if necessary) for isolated systolic hypertension lowers blood pressure and its cardiovascular disease complications and has relatively mild effects on other cardiovascular disease risk factor levels.

This is a further and retrospective analysis of the Systolic Hypertension in the Elderly Programme which involved 4736 participants. Treatment was based upon chlorthalidone, 12.5 or 25 mg, supplemented by the addition of atenolol 25 or 50 mg as required, or reserpine. After 3 years of treatment, there was a blood pressure reduction of 13/4 mmHg attributable to the diuretic-based antihypertensive treatment and significant outcome benefits with, for example, a 36% reduction in stroke events. With respect to adverse metabolic effects, new cases of diabetes were reported in 8.6% of the participants in the active treatment group and in 7.5% of the placebo group; this was a non-significant difference. For the measured metabolic parameters, the predicted adverse effects of active treatment were apparent (Table 14.1), but the effects were generally small.

Table 14.1 Metabolic parameters in SHEP: differences due to active treatment

	Change	Significance
Glucose	+0.2 mmol/l	(P<0.01)
Total cholesterol	+0.09 mmol/l	(P<0.01)
HDL cholesterol	−0.02 mmol/l	(P<0.01)
Total triglycerides	+0.9 mmol/l	(P<0.001)
Creatinine	+2.8 µmol/l	(P<0.001)
Potassium	−0.3 mmol/l	(P<0.001)

Adapted from Savage et al. (1998). SHEP = Systolic Hypertension in the Elderly Programme; HDL = high-density lipoprotein.

Comment

Thiazide diuretics remain the cornerstone of antihypertensive drug treatment in elderly hypertensive patients, and their cost-effectiveness cannot be questioned in terms of the evidence of reduced cardiovascular morbidity and mortality. In these elderly patients, however, changes in a range of metabolic parameters were identified, and, although these changes were generally small, there was an overall adverse effect on the metabolic profile. However, there is no clear evidence (to date) that any alternative type of antihypertensive drug treatment is able to provide a better outcome, even though the metabolic effects may be neutral (or even beneficial).

Conclusion

Thiazide diuretics are clearly the most cost-effective antihypertensive drugs. Their place as a first-line antihypertensive drug treatment, particularly for the elderly hypertensive patient, cannot be challenged, although some concerns remain. For example, these metabolic effects (after 3 years of treatment) may not be relevant for elderly hypertensive patients because the more immediate benefits of blood pressure reduction may simply overwhelm the potentially negative consequences of the long-term adverse metabolic effects. In contrast, however, there is already evidence that long-term treatment (for over 10 years) leads to quantitatively similar adverse metabolic effects, and, in younger patients, concerns remain that the benefits of blood pressure reduction might be compromised.

A further issue is that combination drug treatment will be required to obtain the tighter blood pressure targets that are now widely recommended and, obviously, there will also be patients who are unable to tolerate a thiazide diuretic and who therefore require an alternative treatment. In short, in terms of the evidence base, it is impossible to resolve the cost-effectiveness argument for the alternative types of antihypertensive drug treatment. The more immediate question, however, is, 'Which is the most cost-effective agent within each antihypertensive drug class?'

CHD prevention with statins

The evidence base for the effectiveness of statins in reducing morbidity and mortality, particularly in high-risk patients, is well established but the cost implications are considerable if all 'at risk' patients are to receive drug treatment. The cost of a non-discriminatory primary prevention strategy was explored via the results of the West of Scotland Coronary Prevention Study (WOSCOPS): the results are illustrative.

The West of Scotland Coronary Prevention Study: economic benefit analysis of primary prevention with pravastatin.
J Caro, W Klittich, A McGuire, I Ford, J Norrie, D Pettitt, *et al.*, for the West of Scotland Coronary Prevention Study Group. *BMJ* 1997; **315**: 1577–82.

BACKGROUND. **The objective of this study was to estimate the economic efficiency of using pravastatin to prevent the transition from health to cardiovascular disease in men with hypercholesterolaemia.**

INTERPRETATION. In subjects without evidence of prior myocardial infarction but who have hypercholesterolaemia, the use of pravastatin yields substantial health benefits at a cost that is not prohibitive overall and can be quite efficient in selected high-risk subgroups.

This economic benefit analysis was derived from the WOSCOPS study, which investigated the use of pravastatin in 6595 men aged 45–64 years with a mean cholesterol concentration of 7 mmol/l and no evidence of previous myocardial infarction. The summarizing calculation was that if 10 000 men in this age group received treatment with a lipid-lowering drug (pravastatin), the development of serious cardiovascular disease during the next 5 years would be prevented in 318 men at a total treatment cost of £20 million. These authors calculated that 31.4 men would have to be treated to prevent one major CHD event, and that this would cost £20 375 per life-year if no allowance was made for the cost savings due to the potential health benefits. However, if the treatment availability was restricted to the 40% of men at highest risk, then 22.5 men would require treatment to prevent one CHD event, and this would require £13 995 per life year gained (again discounting the potential health benefits).

Comment

In addition to their cost calculations these authors remind us that, for the individual patient, the transition from health to cardiovascular disease (i.e. primary prevention) represents a much larger 'loss' than that experienced in moving from one degree of illness to another (i.e. secondary prevention). In other words, a decision to focus only on secondary prevention would force a healthy person to experience and survive a cardiovascular event in order to become eligible for treatment. It can be argued that, since such experience of serious illness involves more than just hospital costs and life-years gained, the overall benefits achieved with primary prevention are actually greater than those of secondary prevention. However, this 'holistic' argument has been submerged by concerns about the costs of drug treatment, and the authors of this analysis effectively reverse their initial recommendation for primary prevention as a global strategy. Instead, the authors adopt the 'compromise' position whereby the identification and treatment of patients at highest absolute risk constitutes the most cost-effective approach to lipid-lowering treatment.

Conclusion

This analysis illustrates the problem and the beginnings of the confusion that surrounds the findamental issue of cost-effective treatment: i.e. which patient 'deserves' drug treatment? However, the real practical difficulty then becomes the identification of the most cost-effective treatment strategy, i.e. not only which patient, but which drug? However, since a complex methodology is required to take account of all cost issues, the principal, if not the sole, consideration has degenerated towards an obsession with the drug acquisition cost. The shortcomings of this oversimplistic approach are illustrated in a short report from physicians in New Zealand.

Increased thrombotic vascular events after change of statin.

M Thomas, J Mann. *Lancet* 1998; **352**: 1830–1.

BACKGROUND. These authors have described an increase in serum lipids after the introduction of a referencing pricing for HMG-CoA (3-hydroxy-3-methyl-glutaryl coenzyme A) reductase inhibitors in New Zealand. When patients receiving simvastatin were charged more for prescriptions, there was a general switch to fluvastatin, the only fully subsidized statin to be made available. As a result of this policy, patients received insufficient doses of a less potent drug, which predictably altered their lipid control.

INTERPRETATION. Switching patients to less potent statins and/or consequent increase in lipid may act to unleash otherwise quiescent atheroma, with plaque instability, leading to an increase in vascular events. In addition, these findings caution against sudden increases in cholesterol that may be associated with a change in or cessation of therapy.

Comment

This report illustrates the potential problems when cost alone (i.e. drug acquisition cost) is the sole criterion. In terms of the outcome data there are shortcomings because of the 'before-and-after' design of the study, and there also are limitations relating to drug and dose comparability. Nevertheless, the message is compelling in so far as the cheaper drug was significantly less effective for reducing cholesterol. More important, and of greater concern, was the poorer patient outcome because of the significantly greater number of arterial thrombotic events.

Conclusion

The current emphasis on cost-effective treatments is being misinterpreted and undermined by the fixation on drug acquisition costs. The cost of the drug can only be considered to be the deciding factor when two (or more) drugs have been clearly shown to be equivalent in their principal pharmacological effect, which in this case is cholesterol reduction. Even this fundamental requirement appears to have been overlooked in this case, as is evidenced by the significant increases in cholesterol levels following the substitution of fluvastatin for simvastatin. Additionally (and probably even more important), the drugs should also be known to be approximately equivalent in their abilities to reduce CHD events. Although the data on the CHD event rate are not sufficiently robust in scientific terms (primarily because of the 'before-and-after' design) in this study, one drug (simvastatin) has an extensive and sound evidence base, while the other (fluvastatin) has a very limited evidence base. Thus if the drugs (in their usual doses) are not equivalent in their lipid-lowering effectiveness, and this, in turn, results in more patients suffering events and requiring other interventional costs, then the drug acquisition cost becomes essentially irrelevant, and it is certainly not cost-effective to recommend a cheaper, but inferior, medication.

The wider and more relevant issues of cost-effectiveness have been specifically explored in a further analysis of the 4S trial which illustrates the types of calculations necessary if account is to be taken of the whole picture of costs and benefits.

Effect of simvastatin treatment on cardiovascular resource utilization in impaired fasting glucose and diabetes.

W H Herman, C M Alexander, J R Cook, S J Boccuzzi, T A Musliner, T R Pedersen, *et al.*, for the Scandinavian Simvastatin Survival Study Group. *Diabetes Care* 1999; **22**: 1771–8.

BACKGROUND. The Scandinavian Simvastatin Survival Study (4S) showed that simvastatin treatment reduced cardiovascular events in hypercholesterolaemic subjects with CHD. The clinical benefits of therapy were similar in all three subgroups: normal fasting glucose (NFG, n=3237), impaired fasting glucose (IFG, n=678), and diabetes (n=483). This analysis compared the cost of simvastatin treatment with the cost of cardiovascular disease-related hospitalization in the three subgroups.

INTERPRETATION. Simvastatin significantly reduced cardiovascular disease-related hospitalization and total hospital days for all three groups and significantly reduced length of stay for the diabetic group in addition to providing significant clinical benefits. The benefits were greatest in the diabetic group, with estimated cost savings within trial from simvastatin treatment.

In this analysis of 4398 patients (out of 4444) who participated in the Scandinavian Simvastatin Survival Study, it was calculated that simvastatin treatment cost about US $6000 per patient. The patients were further subdivided into three subgroups, with 678 patients identified as having IFG and 483 patients with type II diabetes mellitus. The remainder had NFG values. Not unexpectedly, treatment was most cost-effective in those patients at highest risk, i.e. those with diabetes mellitus. Cardiovascular disease-related hospitalizations were reduced by 40% in diabetic patients (P=0.007) and the average length of hospital stay was reduced by 2.4 days (P=0.021). Taking these benefits into account in the cost calculation showed that there was a net saving of $1801 per diabetic subject within the trial. The benefits were of lesser absolute magnitude in the other patient groups, but nevertheless it was calculated that the cost savings through reduced hospitalizations 'repaid' 60% of the drug acquisition cost in the main group of patients and 74% of the drug cost in the group with IFG. Additionally, fewer patients suffered events!

Comment

This analysis obviously looks beyond the drug acquisition costs to explore the wider issues of cost-effectiveness, and clearly illustrates that cost savings can be derived from an effective treatment because events can be prevented and hospitalization costs reduced. Thus there can actually be financial savings from an investment in relatively expensive drug treatments, particularly for high-risk patients, because serious cardiovascular events and their resultant treatment costs can be reduced. There are also savings in terms of human costs, since fewer events will presumably create less anxiety and distress for the patient and his/her family.

Conclusion

This study clearly illustrates the need to take account of the wider issues involved in calculating the costs of a drug treatment, and the acquisition costs of a specific agent, relative to the potential outcome benefits.

Cost-effectiveness comparisons with statins

In both hypertension and hypercholesterolaemia, the clinical trial evidence has progressively led to more rigorous treatment target levels for blood pressure and cholesterol, respectively. It is inevitable, therefore, that attainment of lower targets will require higher doses and/or more potent drugs and/or combinations of drugs. Again, there are obvious cost implications, and again questions are raised, first about the comparative efficacy of specific drugs, and secondly about the cost-effectiveness of individual agents.

Cost of treating to a modified European Atherosclerosis Society LDL-C target. Comparison of atorvastatin with fluvastatin, pravastatin and simvastatin.

D G Smith, S J Leslie, T D Szucs, S McBride, L M Campbell, C Calvo, *et al.*
Clin Drug Invest 1999; **7**: 185–93.

B A C K G R O U N D . **The objective of this study was to compare the cost of treating hypercholesterolaemic patients to the modified European Atherosclerosis Society low-density lipoprotein cholesterol (LDL-C) target using atorvastatin, fluvastatin, pravastatin and simvastatin.**

I N T E R P R E T A T I O N . In patients with CHD and/or peripheral vascular disease, the LDL-C target is achieved faster using fewer resources and at a significant cost saving with the use of atorvastatin rather than fluvastatin, pravastatin or simvastatin.

In this study of 330 patients with hyperlipidaemia and also with CHD or peripheral vascular disease a comparative assessment was made with atorvastatin, fluvastatin, pravastatin and simvastatin. The study was based upon the concept of attaining an LDL cholesterol target of < 2.6 mm/l and the effectiveness and cost-effectiveness of the different statins was assessed with titration steps at 12-week intervals. A significantly greater number of patients achieved the LDL target with atorvastatin (89% of patients) as against both fluvastatin and pravastatin, at 61% and 50%, respectively. There was no significant difference in attainment rate between atorvastatin (89%) and simvastatin (80%). Overall, patients achieved the LDL target significantly faster with lower doses of atorvastatin and required significantly fewer clinic visits. The cost calculations indicated that the LDL target was attained more effectively with atorvastatin than with other statins. The study calculated that the cost in 1997 sterling values of attaining the target was £501 for atorvastatin versus £1130 for fluvastatin, £906 for pravastatin and £612 for simvastatin.

Comment

This study also illustrates the relevance of looking beyond the drug acquisition costs to try to calculate costs related to drug effectiveness in terms of achieving the primary therapeutic target, i.e. the attainment of a rigorous cholesterol target.

The issues of comparative efficacy and cost-effectiveness are further explored in terms of prescribing costs via the following two studies.

Efficacy and safety of cerivastatin, 0.2 mg and 0.4 mg, in patients with primary hypercholesterolaemia: a multinational, randomized, double-blind study.

L Ose, O Luurila, J Eriksson, A Olsson, H Lithell, B Widgren, on behalf of the Cerivastatin Study Group. *Curr Med Res Opin* 1999; **15**: 228–40.

B A C K G R O U N D . **Elevated serum cholesterol level is a key risk factor for cardiovascular morbidity and mortality.**

INTERPRETATION. Cerivastatin 0.2 mg/day and 0.4 mg/day was found to lower LDL cholesterol and total cholesterol levels in a dose-dependent manner, with both doses exhibiting a good safety profile.

Following a 6-week placebo run-in, this parallel group study compared the efficacy of cerivastatin 0.2 mg daily and 0.4 mg daily during a 24-week treatment period in a total of 494 patients. There was a significantly greater reduction in LDL cholesterol ($P<0.0001$) by 38.4% from baseline in the 0.4 mg group (n=332 patients) than the decrease of 31.5% in the 0.2 mg group (n=162 patients).

Comment

The overall conclusion of this study was that cerivastatin reduced LDL cholesterol in a dose-dependent manner. It was additionally commented that there appeared to be a significant gender difference, with a reduction by 44.4% in women as against 37% in men. This apparent gender difference achieved a borderline statistical significance ($P<0.046$), but the subgroup comparison was not a primary consideration and involved relatively small numbers of patients, with no information provided about the pretreatment LDL levels in the two sexes.

Comparative dose efficacy study of atorvastatin, lovastatin, and fluvastatin in patients with hypercholesterolaemia (the CURVES study).

P Jones, S Kafonek, I Laurora, D Hunninghake. *Am J Cardiol* 1998; **81**: 582–7.

BACKGROUND. The objective of this multicentre, randomized, open-label, parallel group, 8-week study was to evaluate the comparative dose efficacy of the 3-hydroxy-3-methyl-glutaryl coenzyme A (HMG-CoA) reductase inhibitor atorvastatin 10, 20, 40 and 80 mg compared with simvastatin 10, 20 and 40 mg, pravastatin 10, 20 and 40 mg, lovastatin 20, 40 and 80 mg, and fluvastatin 20 and 40 mg.

INTERPRETATION. Atorvastatin 10, 20 and 40 mg produced greater ($P\leq0.01$) reductions in LDL cholesterol (–38%, –46% and –51%, respectively) than the milligram equivalent doses of simvastatin, pravastatin, lovastatin and fluvastatin. Atorvastatin 10 mg produced LDL cholesterol reductions comparable to or greater than simvastatin 10, 20 and 40 mg ($P<0.02$), pravastatin 10, 20 and 40 mg, lovastatin 20 and 40 mg and fluvastatin 20 and 40 mg. Atorvastatin 10, 20 and 40 mg produced greater reductions in total cholesterol ($P<0.01$) than the milligram equivalent doses of simvastatin, pravastatin, lovastatin and fluvastatin. All reductase inhibitors studied had similar tolerability. There was no incidence of persistent elevations in serum transaminases or myositis.

Comment

This study evaluated the responses to five different agents in a total of 534 hypercholesterolaemic patients. The greatest differences were seen with fluvastatin, which consistently produced the smallest reductions in LDL cholesterol, and atorvastatin, which consistently produced the greatest reductions in LDL cholesterol.

Conclusions

Data from these two studies have been linked to the drug acquisition costs to derive another parameter upon which the prescribing clinician might judge the cost-effectiveness of different statins. For example, based on current UK pricing (£), the percentage reduction in LDL cholesterol can be expressed in terms of a monetary cost per unit of LDL cholesterol reduction (see Table 14.2). From this type of analysis, it appears that cerivastatin and atorvastatin are the most cost-effective agents, whereas simvastatin and pravastatin are the least cost-effective.

The principles underlying this approach are basically sound and, particularly where there are financial restrictions, the concept is valid and the cost comparisons might be very useful. However, the precision of such a cost-effectiveness analysis depends directly upon the quality of the data from which it is derived. For example, the CURVES study is one of the few studies directly comparing several different agents in a homogeneous patient population, and the conclusions derived from it might therefore be considered to be reasonably robust. However, concerns might then be expressed as to whether or not the study population was sufficiently large to draw definitive statistical conclusions and whether or not the study was sufficiently representative and reproducible for the results to be generally applicable. Correspondingly, to incorporate data on an additional agent it was necessary to add the data from a second report (with cerivastatin), but the second study contains no direct cross-comparative data with other statins. The question then arises as to whether or not the results from the two studies are compatible, because it cannot be automatically assumed that the magnitude of the responses to any statin would necessarily be comparable in two different study populations.

At a more fundamental level, however, there arises the question of the measure of 'effectiveness'. While reduction of LDL cholesterol is the principal and shared pharmacological effect of all statins (and this analysis suggests that atorvastatin and cerivastatin are the most cost-effective), the evidence of benefit in terms of reduced

Table 14.2 Cost-effectiveness of different statins targeted to the dose producing a reduction of greater than 30% in low-density lipoprotein (LDL) cholesterol (cost expressed as UK £ per month per 1% reduction in LDL cholesterol)

	Dose	Reduction in LDL-C (%)	Cost (£)
Atorvastatin	10 mg	38	0.50
Cerivastatin	200 mg	31	0.56
	400 mg	38	0.46
Fluvastatin	Insufficient data		?
Pravastatin	40 mg	34	0.87
Simvastatin	20 mg	35	0.85
	40 mg	41	0.72

cardiovascular morbidity and mortality is overwhelmingly superior with prava-statin and simvastatin (and lovastatin).

Cost-effectiveness in high-risk patients

Type II diabetic patients

Patients with type II diabetes mellitus and with hypertension and/or microalbu-minuria are at increased cardiovascular risk, and intensive treatment is warranted. There remains an important emphasis on blood pressure reduction, but it is well recognized that blood pressure control is often difficult, so that combinations of antihypertensive drugs are usually required in these patients. Is the attainment of 'tight' blood pressure control and the expense of multiple antihypertensive drug treatments warranted?

Cost-effectiveness analysis of improved blood pressure control in hypertensive patients with type II diabetes mellitus: UKPDS 40.

United Kingdom Prospective Diabetes Study Group. *BMJ* 1998; **317**: 720–6.

BACKGROUND. **The objective of this study was to estimate the economic efficiency of tight blood pressure control, with angiotensin-converting enzyme inhibitors or beta-blockers, compared with less tight control in hypertensive patients with type II diabetes.**

INTERPRETATION. Tight control of blood pressure in hypertensive patients with type II diabetes substantially reduced the cost of complications, increased the interval without complications and survival, and had a cost-effectiveness ratio that compares favourably with many accepted health care programmes.

Comment

The mean costs for treatment and complications per patient over the duration of the study are shown in Table 14.3, and it can be seen that, while tight blood pressure control increased the antihypertensive drug costs by an average of £613, there were no significant differences in relation to antidiabetic therapies, other drug treat-ments or clinic visits. Overall, therefore, the drug acquisition costs and the costs for the clinic visits were £740 higher in the tight control group relative to the less tight control group. In turn, hospitalization was the most important cost in terms of complications, with those assigned to tight blood pressure control reducing this cost by about £674. Putting all the different components together, however, the higher acquisition costs of antihypertensive therapy in the tight blood pressure control group were offset by lower complication costs, so that the total costs per

Table 14.3 'Tight, versus 'less tight' blood pressure control costs per patient (1997 sterling values)

	Less tight	Tight
Antihypertensive drugs	608	1221
Antidiabetic drugs	1189	1312
Other drugs	43	41
Clinical visits	1664	1671
Subtotal (1)	**3504**	**4631**
Hospital costs	3603	2930
Outpatient costs	1304	1301
Specific treatment (eyes, kidneys)	672	400
Subtotal (2)	**5579**	**4630**
Total costs	**9083**	**8876**

patient were almost equal for the two groups at £9083 in the less tight control group and £8876 in the tight control group.

Conclusion

This study again illustrates the wider issues that require to be taken into account when costs are calculated in relation to drug treatment and potential outcome benefits. The main message was that intensive treatment of high-risk patients is both justifiable and cost-effective, because the cost savings derived from events prevented outweighed the extra drug acquisition costs.

In this important clinical setting, there are two major practical issues: (1) is blood pressure reduction the principal requirement? and (2) are ACE inhibitor drugs mandatory because they have benefits beyond blood pressure reduction? In short, should an ACE inhibitor drug automatically be introduced to diabetic patients at an early (prophylactic) stage?

Routine treatment of insulin-dependent diabetic patients with ACE inhibitors to prevent renal failure: an economic evaluation.

B A Kiberd, K K Jindal. *Am J Kidney Dis* 1998; **31**: 49–54.

BACKGROUND. The objective of this study was to determine how effective angiotensin-converting enzyme (ACE) inhibitors must be in preventing diabetic nephropathy to warrant routine administration to insulin-dependent diabetic patients. Three treatment strategies were compared.

INTERPRETATION. Routine ACE inhibitor therapy could prove to be cost-effective, especially if high-risk individuals could be identified. A prospective trial examining this goal should be considered.

In this study, three treatment strategies were compared: (1) screening for microalbuminuria and treatment of incipient nephropathy; (2) routine administration of an ACE inhibitor 5 years after diagnosis of diabetes; and (3) identification of patients at high risk for nephropathy, who were routinely treated, whereas low-risk patients were treated with an ACE inhibitor only if they developed hypertension and/or macroproteinuria. These authors calculated that strategy 2 would produce as many quality-adjusted life-years as strategy 1 at nearly the same cost if routine drug therapy reduced the rate of development of microalbuminuria by 26% in all patients.

Comment

This is not a definitive study, but it is an interesting approach to a complex problem. It is an illustrative example of the type of study that is required to address the whole issue of drug costs and cost-effectiveness appropriately. In pragmatic terms, however, the principal shortcoming of this study is that the reduction of proteinuria is, of itself, virtually irrelevant, because it has no proven outcome cost or implications. The important endpoints, and the important cost issues, are preservation of renal function (and the avoidance of dialysis treatment, for example) and, ultimately, prevention of cardiovascular events.

Patients with stroke

Treatment and secondary prevention of stroke: evidence, costs, and effects on individuals and populations.

G J Hankey, C P Warlow. *Lancet* 1999; **354**: 1457–63.

BACKGROUND. This review of the effectiveness of treatment for acute stroke and methods of secondary prevention shows that the highest priority for providers of a stroke service must be to establish a stroke unit and a multidisciplinary team that delivers organized stroke care.

INTERPRETATION. Acute ischaemic stroke patients should be immediately started on aspirin 300 mg daily, and, if possible, many of them should be entered into further trials of thrombolysis and other promising treatments. After the acute phase, aspirin should be continued in a lower dose, 75 mg daily; smoking should be discouraged; high blood pressure should be treated, initially with a diuretic; and fibrillating ischaemic stroke/transient ischaemic attack survivors should be anticoagulated long-term with warfarin or given aspirin if anticoagulation is not sensible. Statins are probably indicated in patients who already have symptomatic CHD. Adding dipyridamole to aspirin, substituting clopidogrel for aspirin, and carotid endarterectomy are all expensive interventions to prevent stroke, but if ways could be found to focus them on those patients at especially high risk, they would become more affordable.

Comment

The abstract from this review succinctly summarizes the practical advice relevant to secondary prevention of stroke. Two eminent authorities in stroke medicine address all the issues relating to acute stroke interventions and the benefits of specialized stroke units. While immediate management issues obviously fall within the remit of the specialist centre, the secondary prevention issues are of much more concern to the non-specialist physician, the generalist and the GP. These latter issues are discussed in detail.

Conclusion

It is perhaps not surprising that the most effective interventions focus upon the conventional risk factors and the importance of smoking cessation, antihypertensive drug treatment and cholesterol-lowering drugs. In turn, these are associated with relative risk reductions of respectively 33%, 28% and 24%. According to the cost calculations, the most cost-effective treatment is, not surprisingly, voluntary smoking cessation, which costs nothing. However, if medical pharmacological treatment such as nicotine patches is involved, then the cost rises to approximately £9000 per stroke avoided. In turn, the costs of antihypertensive treatment will obviously vary according to the choice of drug, and the examples quoted show that diuretic treatment could prevent one stroke per annum at a cost of approximately £600, whereas ACE inhibitor treatment would cost approximately £8000. Correspondingly, treatment to prevent one stroke with a cholesterol-lowering drug (statin) would cost approximately £19 000. In short, cessation of smoking (by voluntary efforts) and blood pressure reduction (especially by thiazide diuretic treatment) are the most cost-effective strategies.

Conclusions

The optimal treatment of patients at increased cardiovascular risk involves drugs and combinations of drugs that are designed to improve the overall cardiovascular risk profile, particularly though reduction in blood pressure and improvements in the lipid profile. With the setting of increasingly aggressive blood pressure and cholesterol targets and with the emphasis on aggressive treatment for high-risk patients, there is an inevitable requirement for increased drug usage and, therefore, expenditure. As was illustrated by the direct comparisons of the 'statins', however, there are pitfalls to be avoided and hidden costs to be incorporated, and among these factors the most important consideration is the cost saving that accrues when major cardiovascular events are prevented and when hospital admissions are either avoided or reduced in length. Because of financial constraints, however, a disproportionate emphasis is currently being placed on drug acquisition costs in the search for the most cost-effective treatment. Inevitably, this creates an unfortunate emphasis on the cheapest available agent. While this applies as much to antihypertensive drugs as it does to lipid-lowering drugs, the greater homogeneity within the lipid-lowering group permits more direct comparisons. Although there is a corresponding cost-effectiveness debate within the antihypertensive drug groups, the more diverse nature of the antihypertensive drug classes and their profiles for adverse effects, both short-term and long-term, make cost-effectiveness comparisons particularly difficult.

It is obviously simplistic to focus only on the drug acquisition costs, but this, unfortunately, is often seen as the most obvious and the easiest course of action. The reality is that the cheapest agent in terms of the drug acquisition cost (with the possible exception of thiazide diuretics in hypertension) is almost certainly not the most cost-effective.

Reference

1. Downs JR, Clearfield M, Weis S, Whitney E, Shapiro DR, Beere FA, *et al.* Primary prevention of acute coronary events with lovastatin in men and women with average cholesterol levels. *JAMA* 1998; **279**: 1615–22.

Index of Papers Reviewed

Part III Hypertension: emerging concepts

Davies E, Holloway CD, Ingram MC, Inglis GC, Friel EC, Morrison C, *et al.* Aldosterone excretion rate and blood pressure in essential hypertension are related to polymorphic differences in the aldosterone synthase gene (*CYP11B2*). *Hypertension* 1999; 33: 703–7. **157, 203**

Devlin AM, Brosnan MJ, Graham D, Morton JJ, McPhasen AR, McIntyre M, *et al.* Vascular smooth muscle cell polyploidy and cardiomyocyte hypertrophy due to chronic NOS inhibition in vivo. *Am J Physiol Heart Circ Physiol* 1998; 43: H52–9. **186**

Ferrannini E, Natali A, Capaldo B, Lohtovirta M, Jacob S, Yki-Jarvinen H. Insulin resistance, hyperinsulinemia, and blood pressure: role of age and obesity. *Hypertension* 1997; 30: 1144–9. **230**

Forte P, Copland M, Smith LM, Milne E, Sutherland J, Benjamin N. Basal nitric oxide synthesis in essential hypertension. *Lancet* 1997; 349: 837–42. **178**

Goonasekera CDA, Shah V, Rees DD, Dillon MJ. Nitric oxide activity in childhood hypertension. *Arch Dis Child* 1997; 77: 11–6. **179**

Heise T, Magnusson K, Heinemann L, Sawicki PT. Insulin resistance and the effect of insulin on blood pressure in essential hypertension. *Hypertension* 1998; 32: 243–8. **231**

Inoue N, Kawashima S, Kanazawa K, Yamada S, Akita H, Yokoyama M. Polymorphism of the NADH/NAD(P)H oxidase *p22 phox* gene in patients with coronary artery disease. *Circulation* 1998; 97: 135–7. **194**

Jiang ZY, Lin Y-W, Clemont A, Feener EP, Hein KD, Igarashi M, *et al.* Could primary insulin resistance result in endothelial dysfunction and promotion of hypertension? Characterization of selective resistance to insulin signalling in the vasculature of obese zucker (*fa/fa*) rats. *J Clin Invest* 1999; 104: 447–57. **234**

Kamitani A, Wong ZYH, Fraser R, Davies DL, Connor JM, Foy CJW, *et al.* Human α-adducin gene, blood pressure, and sodium metabolism. *Hypertension* 1998; 32: 138–43. **160**

Kato N, Sugiyama T, Morita H, Nabika T, Kurihara H, Yamori Y, *et al.* Lack of evidence for association between the endothelial nitric oxide synthase gene and hypertension. *Hypertension* 1999; 33: 933–6. **168, 183**

Kato N, Sugiyama T, Nabika T, Morita H, Kurihara H, Yazaki Y, *et al.* Lack of association between the α-adducin locus and essential hypertension in the Japanese population. *Hypertension* 1998; 31: 730–3. **161**

Kerr S, Brosnan MJ, McIntyre M, Reid JL, Dominiczak AF, Hamilton CA. Superoxide anion production is increased in a model of genetic hypertension: role of the endothelium. *Hypertension* 1999; 33: 1353–8. **191**

Kupari M, Hautanen A, Lankinenn L, Koskinen P, Virolainen J, Nikkila H, *et al.* Association between human aldosterone synthase (*CYP11B2*) gene polymorphisms and left ventricular size, mass, and function. *Circulation* 1998; 97: 569–75. **158**

Lacolley P, Gautier S, Poirier O, Pannier B, Cambien F, Benetos A. Nitric oxide synthase gene polymorphisms, blood pressure and aortic stiffness in normotensive and hypertensive subjects. *J Hypertens* 1998; 18: 31–6. **181**

Laine H, Knuuti MJ, Ruotsalainen U, Raitakiari M, Iida H, Kapanen J, *et al.* Insulin resistance in essential hypertension is characterized by impaired insulin stimulation of blood flow in skeletal muscle. *Hypertension* 1998; 16: 211–9. **233**

Litchfield WR, Anderson BF, Weiss RJ, Lifton RP, Dluhy RG. Intracranial aneurysm and hemorrhagic stroke in glucocorticoid remediable aldosterone. *Hypertension* 1998; 31: 445–50. **212**

Joint National Committee on Prevention, Detection, Evaluation, and Treatment of High Blood Pressure and the National High Blood Pressure Education Program Coordinating Committee. The sixth report of the Joint National Committee on Prevention, Detection, Evaluation, and Treatment of High Blood Pressure. *Arch Intern Med* 1997; 24: 2413–46. **263 (27)**

Jones P, Kafonek S, Laurora I, Hunninghake D. Comparative dose efficacy study of atorvastatin, lovastatin, and fluvastatin in patients with hypercholesterolaemia (the CURVES study). *Am J Cardiol* 1998; 81: 582–7. **305 (130)**

Karlberg BE, Lins L-E, Hermansson K, for the TEES Group. Efficacy and safety of telmisartan, a selective AT_1 receptor antagonist, compared with enalapril in elderly patients with primary hypertension. *J Hypertens* 1999; 17: 293–302. **253**

Kiberd BA, Jindal KK. Routine treatment of insulin-dependent diabetic patients with ACE inhibitors to prevent renal failure: an economic evaluation. *Am J Kidney Dis* 1998; 31: 49–54. **308**

Mallion JM, Siche JP, Lacourcière Y, and the Telmisartan Blood Pressure Monitoring Group. ABPM comparison of the antihypertensive profiles of the selective angiotensin II receptor antagonists telmisartan and losartan in patients with mild to moderate hypertension. *J Hum Hypertens* 1999; 13: 657–64. **252**

Malmqvist K, Kahan T, Dahl M. Angiotensin II type 1 (AT_1) receptor blockade in hypertensive women: benefits of candesartan cilexetil versus enalapril or hydrochlorothiazide. *Am J Hypertens* 2000; 13: 504–11. **255**

Mancia G, Sega R, Milesi C, Cesana G, Zanchetti A. Blood pressure control in the hypertensive population. *Lancet* 1997; 349: 454–7. **271**

Mancia G, Zanchetti A, Agebiti-Rosei E, Benemio G, De Cesaris R, Fogari R, et al.

for the SAMPLE Study Group. Ambulatory blood pressure is superior to clinic blood pressure in predicting treatment-induced regression of left ventricular hypertrophy. *Circulation* 1997; 95: 1464–70. **273**

Mazzolai L, Maillard M, Rossat J, Nussberger J, Brunner HR, Burnier M. A direct comparison of three AT_1 receptor antagonists. *Hypertension* 1999; 33: 850–5. **250**

McKelvie RS, Yusuf S, Pericak D, Avezum A, Burns RJ, Probstfield J, et al. Comparison of candesartan, enalapril, and their combination in congestive heart failure. Randomized Evaluation of Strategies for Left Ventricular Dysfunction (RESOLVD) pilot study. *Circulation* 1999; 100: 1056–64. **260**

O'Leary DH, Polak JF, Kronmal RA, Manolio TA, Burke GL, Wolfson SK, for the Cardiovascular Health Study Collaborative Research Group. Carotid-artery intima and media thickness as a risk factor for myocardial infarction and stroke in older adults. *N Engl J Med* 1999; 340: 14–22. **286**

Ofili EO, Cohen JD, St Vrain JA, Pearson A, Martin TJ, Uy ND, et al. Effect of treatment of isolated systolic hypertension on left ventricular mass. *JAMA* 1998; 279: 778–80. **284**

Ohkubo T, Imai Y, Tsuji I, Nagai K, Ito S, Satoh H, et al. Reference values for 24-hour ambulatory blood pressure monitoring based on a prognostic criterion. The Ohasama Study. *Hypertension* 1998; 32: 255–9. **269**

Ose L, Luurila O, Eriksson J, Olsson A, Lithell H, Widgren B, on behalf of the Cerivastatin Study Group. Efficacy and safety of cerivastatin, 0.2 mg and 0.4 mg, in patients with primary hypercholesterolaemia: a multinational, randomized, double-blind study. *Curr Med Res Opin* 1999; 15: 228–40. **304**

Pitt B, Segal R, Martinez FA, Meurers G, Cowley AJ, Thomas I, et al. Randomized

General Index

A

ABCD (Appropriate Blood Pressure Control in Diabetes) 117
ACE inhibitors 5, 8, 35, 73, 247–8, 249
  ALLHAT 74, 75
  ASCOT 77
  BHS guidelines 54
  CAPPP 11–14, 106–7
  diabetes mellitus 36, 116–18, 118–19, 292–3, 294, 308, 308–9
  HYVET 89
  insulin sensitivity effect 118–19, 239
  JNC VI guidelines 35
  left ventricular hypertrophy regression 282, 283
  STOP-Hypertension–2 15, 16
  Treatment Trialists' Collaboration 93
  UKPDS 102, 105
acetylsalicylic acid, see aspirin
adducin, genetic studies 160–2
adipose tissue cytokines 236–7
adrenal adenoma, see Conn's adenoma
adrenal gland imaging 223
adrenal hyperplasia, bilateral 205, 217, 223, 224
AFCAPS/TexCAPS (Airforce/Texas Coronary Atherosclerosis Prevention Study) 121–2, 123, 297
aldosterone, renal vascular injury in stroke-prone hypertensive rats (SHRSP) 218–20
aldosterone synthase 204, 205
  CYP11B2 gene polymorphism 157–60, 201, 202–5
aldosteronism, primary 204–5, 212–23
  adrenal pathology 217
  cardiovascular effects 218
  mechanisms of hypertension 218
  renal damage 218
  screening 215–16, 220–1
ALLHAT (Antihypertensive therapy and Lipid-Lowering Heart Attack prevention Trial) 74–7
alpha-adducin genetic polymorphism 160–2
alpha-blockers, ALLHAT 74, 75, 76
ambulatory blood pressure measurement (ABPM) 27, 28, 29, 30, 263–74
  angiotensin II receptor antagonists 252–3

cardiovascular morbidity/mortality 267–71
cardiovascular risk 268–9
  refractory hypertension 270
guidelines 263–7
  BHS 46–7, 265–6
  JNC VI 263–4
  WHO-ISH 264–5
hormone replacement therapy 139–40
inadequately treated hypertension 271–2
left ventricular hypertrophy 273–4, 279–80
reference values (Ohasama study) 269–70
amiloride 15, 207, 224
  see also co-amilozide
amlodipine 35
  ALLHAT 74, 75
  ASCOT 78
  FACET 116, 117
  VALUE 84, 87
angiotensin II receptor antagonists 247–61
  antihypertensive efficacy 252–3
  clinical trials 249, 251–6
  left ventricular hypertrophy studies 256–9
  pharmacology 247, 249–51
  relative effectiveness 250, 251
angiotensin AT_1 receptor 247, 248
  cardiac hypertrophy in knock-out mice 257–8, 281
angiotensin AT_2 receptor 247
angiotensin receptor blocker (ARB) 35, 36, 54, 82–7
angiotensin-converting enzyme (ACE) gene polymorphism 155–6
angiotensinogen gene
  essential hypertension association 154–5, 201
  M235T polymorphism 152–4, 155
anti-platelet therapy 10–11
antihypertensive agents
  ALLHAT 74–7
  angiotensinogen M235T polymorphism 153–4
  ASCOT 77–9
  concordance (adherence) strategies 33, 35
  coronary heart disease secondary prevention 59
  cost-effectiveness 298–300
  diabetes mellitus 101–11, 116–18
    ABCD 117

The Year in Hypertension

FUTURE VOLUMES

The Year in Hypertension will be appearing
on a regular basis

To receive more information about the next issue, or to
reserve a copy on publication, please contact
the address below

Clinical Publishing Services
Oxford Centre for Innovation
Mill Street
Oxford OX2 0JX UK

T: +44 1865 811116
F: + 44 1865 251550
E: gresford@compuserve.com
W: www.clinicalpublishing.co.uk